Clinical Guide to Primary Angioplasty

T0174673

Clinical Guide to Primary Angioplasty

Edited by

Stephen Brecker
St. Georges Hospital
London, U.K.

Martin Rothman
London Chest Hospital
London, U.K.

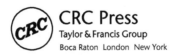

CRC Press
Taylor & Francis Group
Boca Raton London New York

CRC Press is an imprint of the
Taylor & Francis Group, an **informa** business

CRC Press
Taylor & Francis Group
6000 Broken Sound Parkway NW, Suite 300
Boca Raton, FL 33487-2742

First issued in paperback 2019

ISBN-13: 978-1-84184-673-6 (hbk)
ISBN-13: 978-0-367-38400-5 (pbk)

A CIP record for this book is available from the British Library.

Library of Congress Cataloging-in-Publication Data

To Lucy, Joshua and Liorah

Foreword

The highest level of achievement in evidence-based medicine is to conclusively demonstrate a mortality benefit of an evolving new therapy compared with the previously accepted standard of care. There is now overwhelming evidence that primary angioplasty results in an approximately 2% reduction in mortality when compared with thrombolytic therapy, and primary angioplasty has been accepted worldwide as a Class I (level of evidence A) indication for the treatment of ST-segment elevation myocardial infarction (STEMI). However, the gap between evidence-based medicine and clinical execution can sometimes be cavernous, requiring special efforts to bring a preferred procedure-based therapy to widespread use in the community. *Clinical Guide to Primary Angioplasty* represents one of those important "special efforts" which provides the educational underpinnings to aid the clinical practitioner in establishing a state-of-the-art acute MI treatment center.

Clinical Guide to Primary Angioplasty is a comprehensive academic primer, a technical "how to" manual, and a logistic roadmap to overcome environmental speed bumps. The editors have chosen wisely a collection of international experts constituting consensus and varying opinions on therapy nuances and strategies. This easy-to-use and digest volume deals with every clinical situation associated with primary angioplasty therapy, including many of the more recent controversial technical topics, such as optimal adjunctive pharmacology and changing angioplasty technique considerations (e.g., use of drug-eluting stents and the need for aspiration thrombectomy). Moreover, given the regional nature of health care delivery, it is refreshing to see different perspectives on the same topic from a broad spectrum of global thought leaders.

Clinical Guide to Primary Angioplasty should be viewed as required reading for any health care professional involved with acute MI treatment. At a time when angioplasty has been under siege by critics claiming nondefinitive treatment advantages relative to medical therapy or surgery for many coronary syndromes, the aggressive promulgation of primary angioplasty to all practitioners should be viewed as a shining example of the striking clinical value of lesser-invasive catheter-based interventions. *Clinical Guide to Primary Angioplasty* is an outstanding educational tool and in a concise yet thorough volume surpasses the myriad of other less focused and less practical texts. The editors and authors should be congratulated on creating one of those special "gap-bridging" efforts to make optimal application of primary angioplasty, the uniform treatment strategy for patients with STEMI.

Martin B. Leon, MD
Professor, Columbia University Medical Center
Chairman Emeritus, Cardiovascular Research Foundation
New York, New York, U.S.A.

Preface

Primary angioplasty for myocardial infarction has evolved over the years, first being undertaken over 20 years ago but only now gaining worldwide acceptance. The protracted roll out of primary angioplasty has been due to the real logistic difficulties in delivering a door-to-balloon time of under 90 minutes, 24 hours a day, seven days a week, both in cities and in rural areas. It is only now that more than 50% of eligible patients are being treated this way in developed health care delivery systems. We think therefore, it is timely to produce a text covering all the major issues surrounding primary angioplasty.

We hope that readers find *Clinical Guide to Primary Angioplasty* to be a comprehensive guide to the basis, technique, and evidence for primary angioplasty as a reperfusion strategy in acute ST segment elevation myocardial infarction. Our aim was to be very clinically oriented and relevant to everyday clinical practice and we hope we have succeeded. For cardiologists, nurses, and physiologists/technicians actively involved in a primary angioplasty program, we hope this volume will be a useful resource providing a solid grounding in the how, what, and why of primary angioplasty. We believe providers of health care services planning a primary angioplasty service will find useful information on the logistics of how to deliver a fast, efficient, and safe treatment for the millions of individuals worldwide who suffer from acute ST segment elevation myocardial infarction every year.

Stephen Brecker
Martin Rothman

Contents

Contributors

Yasir Abu-Omar Department of Cardiothoracic Surgery, Papworth Hospital, Cambridge, U.K.

Joseph S. Alpert University of Arizona College of Medicine, Tucson, Arizona, U.S.A.

Salvatore Brugaletta Interventional Cardiology Unit, University Hospital of Sant Pau, Barcelona, Spain

Robert A. Byrne ISAResearch Centre, Deutsches Herzzentrum, Munich, Germany

Peter Clemmensen The Heart Centre, Rigshospitalet, University of Copenhagen, Copenhagen, Denmark

Pedro Beraldo de Andrade Santa Casa de Marília, Marília, São Paulo, Brazil

Gregory Ducrocq Centre Hospitalier Bichat-Claude Bernard, Paris, France

William J. French Department of Medicine, Division of Cardiology, Harbor-UCLA Medical Center, Torrance, California, U.S.A.

Bernard J. Gersh Division of Cardiovascular Diseases, Mayo Clinic, Rochester, Minnesota, U.S.A.

Michael Gick Herz-Zentrum Bad Krozingen, Bad Krozingen, Germany

Patrick Goldstein SAMU Régional de Lille CHRU, Lille, France

Cindy L. Grines Cardiovascular Section, William Beaumont Hospital, Royal Oak, Michigan, U.S.A.

Rajiv Gulati Division of Cardiovascular Diseases, Mayo Clinic, Rochester, Minnesota, U.S.A.

Joshua M. Hare Department of Medicine, Cardiovascular Division, University of Miami Miller School of Medicine, and Interdisciplinary Stem Cell Institute, Miami, Florida, U.S.A.

Allan S. Jaffe Cardiovascular Division, Core Clinical Laboratory Services (CCLS), Department of Laboratory Medicine and Pathology, Mayo Clinic and Medical School, Rochester, Minnesota, U.S.A.

Marjan Jahangiri Department of Cardiothoracic Surgery, St. George's Hospital, University of London, London, U.K.

Adnan Kastrati ISAResearch Centre, Deutsches Herzzentrum, Munich, Germany

Steen Dalby Kristensen Department of Cardiology B, Aarhus University Hospital, Skejby, Denmark

Faisal Latif Cardiovascular Section, William Beaumont Hospital, Royal Oak, Michigan, U.S.A.

Alan S. Maisel Department of Cardiovascular Medicine, University of California, San Francisco, California, U.S.A.

Luiz Alberto Mattos Instituto Dante Pazzanese de Cardiologia, Santa Casa de Marília, Marília, São Paulo, Brazil

Jan Minners Herz-Zentrum Bad Krozingen, Bad Krozingen, Germany

Gilles Montalescot Institut de Cardiologie Pitié–Salpêtrièra Hospital, Paris, France

Christopher P. Moriates Department of Medicine, University of California, San Francisco, California, U.S.A.

Franz-Josef Neumann Herz-Zentrum Bad Krozingen, Bad Krozingen, and University of Freiburg, Freiburg, Germany

Thomas Pilgrim Department of Cardiology, Bern University Hospital, Bern, Switzerland

Abhiram Prasad Cardiac Catheterization Laboratory, Mayo Clinic, Rochester, Minnesota, U.S.A.

Manel Sabaté Interventional Cardiology Unit, University Hospital of Sant Pau, Barcelona, Spain

Imran Saeed Department of Cardiothoracic Surgery, St. George's Hospital, University of London, London, U.K.

Kintur Sanghvi Cardiovascular Section, William Beaumont Hospital, Royal Oak, Michigan, U.S.A.

Kari Saunamäki The Heart Centre, Rigshospitalet, University of Copenhagen, Copenhagen, Denmark

Atman P. Shah Department of Medicine, Division of Cardiology, The University of Chicago, Chicago, Illinois, U.S.A.

Kabir J. Singh Department of Cardiology, University of California, San Francisco, California, U.S.A.

Jacob Thorsted Sorensen Department of Cardiology B, Aarhus University Hospital, Skejby, Denmark

Philippe Gabriel Steg   Centre Hospitalier Bichat-Claude Bernard, Paris, France

David P. Taggart   Department of Cardiothoracic Surgery, John Radcliffe Hospital and University of Oxford, Oxford, U.K.

Christian Juhl Terkelsen   Department of Cardiology B, Aarhus University Hospital, Skejby, Denmark

Kristian Thygesen   Department of Medicine and Cardiology, Aarhus University Hospital, Aarhus, Denmark

Barry H. Trachtenberg   Department of Medicine, Cardiovascular Division, University of Miami Miller School of Medicine, Miami, Florida, U.S.A.

Freek W. A. Verheugt   Department of Cardiology, Heartcenter, Onze Lieve Vrouwe Gasthuis, Amsterdam, The Netherlands

Allan J. Wailoo   Health Economics and Decision Science, School of Health and Related Research, University of Sheffield, Sheffield, U.K.

Stephan Windecker   Department of Cardiology, Bern University Hospital, Bern, Switzerland

1 Epidemiology and Historical Perspectives

Peter Clemmensen and Kari Saunamäki

The Heart Centre, Rigshospitalet, University of Copenhagen, Copenhagen, Denmark

EPIDEMIOLOGY

Prevalence and Incidence

The global burden of cardiovascular disease is immense, and it remains the principal cause of mortality worldwide. Coronary heart disease mortality showed a rapid rise after the 2nd World War reaching a peak around 1970. Still it is estimated that 12 millions deaths will be attributable to CHD in the year 2020. Annual coronary event rates differ greatly between countries ranging from 60/100,000 in China to >400/100,000 in the United Kingdom (1).

The epidemiology of primary angioplasty in ST segment elevation AMI is so closely linked to the entire syndrome complex termed acute coronary syndrome that it is best to consider it within this context. We estimate acute coronary syndromes to account for 1.5 million hospitals admission in Europe each year. Between 35% and 48% of these patients present with ST elevation myocardial infarction (STEMI) (2,3).

Clinical Characteristics of STEMI

As outlined in the chapter on definition of AMI (see Chapter 4), ST elevation AMI is a diagnosis based on the characteristic changes in the electrocardiogram (ECG). The prognosis of STEMI in relation to other changes in the presenting ECG is shown in Figure 1. The most important observation is that STEMI is associated with a rather high initial risk of death followed by a rather flat survival curve after six months, whereas the high-risk non-STE presenters continue to have events over the years and thus have a higher mortality already at six months (4).

The median age of STEMI patients is 65 years compared to the 3 to 5 years older non-STE presenters. It is important to appreciate that the patients seen in routine clinical practice differ significantly from the individuals selected to participate in randomized clinical trials, as they are often older, more often female with a higher comorbidity index and more severe cardiac condition upon presentation, including cardiogenic preshock and proper shock. In the GRACE registry only 11% of STEMI patients participated in clinical trials during their hospitalization (5).

Prognosis

In STEMI, approximately 85% of the deaths occur within the first 24 hours after symptom onset. And it is still important to recognize that for every 1000 patients we treat in hospital, there are another 200 individuals who have died suddenly

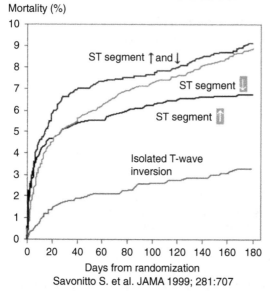

Prognosis of ACS
Admission ECG in the GUSTO-2B trial

Mortality (%)

ST segment ↑ and ↓
ST segment
ST segment
Isolated T-wave inversion

Days from randomization
Savonitto S. et al. JAMA 1999; 281:707

FIGURE 1 The figure depicts the influence of ST segment changes on six-month survival in the GUSTO-2b trial. Note that ST segment elevation is associated with an initial high risk in the early phase and then reaches a plateau around 30 days, whereas patients with non-STE presentation but ST depression have a higher mortality at six months. *Source*: From Ref. 4.

or en route before receiving treatment. In the MONICA populations, the case fatality rate of acute myocardial infarction ranges between 33% and 70% (1) and thus very far from the impressions of clinicians working in high-volume clinics in Western Europe or the United States. In a country like Denmark characterized by a high incidence of ACS and where each inhabitant has a unique person identification number making 100% follow-up possible the 30-day mortality of acute myocardial infarction has decreased among individuals aged 65 years and under, from 10% to 4% in just two decades. The case fatality rate remains high in the elderly increasing from 12% in the 70 to 74 year olds to 26% in the 85+ cohort. Primary PCI is of particular interest in Denmark since the country has almost entirely abandoned fibrinolysis, and there is no age limit for reperfusion. From 2006 to 2007, the five centers treated 5008 patients with a 30-day mortality of 7.6%, rising to 11.0% at one year (6).

Newer registries provide in-depth knowledge of the characteristics and outcomes of the ACS patients. The national Swedish Registry, enrolling around 20,000 patients per year the mean age of STEMI patients is 71 years for males and 76 years for females, compared to 65 years in clinical trials. These facts are important since long-term mortality doubles with every decade of age in the population. There is a remarkable link between implementation of reperfusion therapy and reduced 30-day mortality, favoring primary PCI over thrombolysis. In the Swedish registry, the rate of reperfusion was unchanged

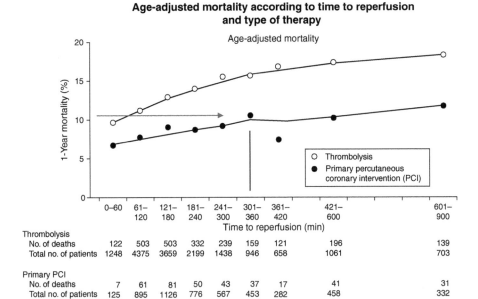

Age-adjusted mortality according to time to reperfusion and type of therapy

Time to reperfusion (min)	0–60	61–120	121–180	181–240	241–300	301–360	361–420	421–600	601–900
Thrombolysis									
No. of deaths	122	503	503	332	239	159	121	196	139
Total no. of patients	1248	4375	3659	2199	1438	946	658	1061	703
Primary PCI									
No. of deaths	7	61	81	50	43	37	17	41	31
Total no. of patients	125	895	1126	776	567	453	282	458	332

FIGURE 2 Note that the one-year mortality after primary PCI in patients presenting up to six hours after symptom onset is similar to the patients treated with thrombolysis with the "golden hour." *Source*: From Ref. 8.

over a 10-year period but the rate of primary PCI and also adjunctive medical therapies increased and resulted in a 50% drop in both in-hospital and 30-day mortality (7,8). Patients treated with primary PCI had significantly lower mortality than patients treated with thrombolysis as shown in Figure 2. The Euro Heart Surveys have shown similar trends with an absolute 6% increase in primary PCI between 2000 and 2004. The same survey depicts how some 39% of the STEMI population is still denied reperfusion therapy and one could speculate that contraindication to lytics still account for a large proportion of the patients since fibrinolysis remains the preferred strategy in approximately 40% of these European populations. In the most recent ACOS registry the reperfusion rate was 73%, and withholding reperfusion therapy doubled the mortality. Patients undergoing primary PCI had significantly lower in-hospital mortality than patients receiving fibrinolysis. Similar trends have been reported from the National Registry of Myocardial Infarction (NRMI) in the United States, collecting data since 1994. There, reperfusion therapy increased from 64% to 72%, favoring primary PCI as early as 2004. Again, mortality decreased over time, reflecting better implementation of reperfusion therapy and adjunctive therapies. Door-to-needle times decreased from 62 minutes in 1990 to 35 minutes in 2004, but still were below 30 minutes as recommended in the current guidelines in only 42% of the patients. In a more recent report from the global GRACE registry primary PCI was favored over fibrinolysis in mid-2002 (Fig. 3), but still one-third of otherwise eligible received no reperfusion (9,10).

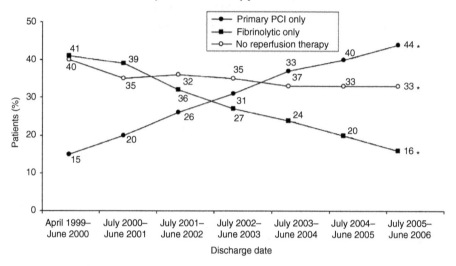

FIGURE 3 Trends in the use of reperfusion therapy for ST segment elevation myocardial infarction. *Source*: From Ref. 10.

HISTORICAL PERSPECTIVE

The description of acute myocardial infarction (AMI) dates back to 1910 by Obrastow and Straschensko (11) and by Herrick in 1912 (12). Then half a century passed and during this time the discussion centered only upon the length of necessary bed rest while a significant proportion of patients died.

"There is hardly anything to gain by active therapy during the first hours after acute coronary occlusion, and if there are signs of pulmonary congestion, strofantine is preferable. When everything else seems to fail, venesection has to be done." This statement was written in the 1956 Nordic Textbook of Internal Medicine by Warburg (13), Professor at the University of Copenhagen.

"My policy is to recommend a minimum of 2 to 3 weeks strict bedrest and after that additional confinement to bed for 3 to 4 weeks part or most of the time." wrote Friedberg (14) in his 1966 textbook. The patients were not even allowed visitors (13).

At that time the main treatment of AMI was bed rest, sedation, and anticoagulation to prevent pulmonary emboli. In-hospital mortality of AMI was about 40% to 50% (13,14).

The concept of coronary care units (CCU) was introduced in the early 1960s and established during the late 1960s. This marked the first major improvement in the survival of the patients in the course of the history of AMI (15). The most important factor was prompt detection and treatment of ventricular fibrillation. Early treatment of heart failure and prophylactic antiarrhythmic treatment might also have contributed to the improved outcome (Table 1). Mortality of the patients was cut to half of that on the previous regime on internal medicine wards (15).

TABLE 1 Overview Over Decline of In-Hospital/30-Day Mortality Induced by New Treatments Over Past 50 Years

Year	1950–1960	1960–1970	1970–1980	1980–1988	1988–1995	1995–2003
Mortality change	–	–50%	–13%	–18%	–23%	–28%
Mortality	40%	20%	17%	14%	11%	8%
Therapy	Bed rest Anticoagulation	CCU Defibrillation Antiarrhythmics	+Beta-blockers	+Thrombolysis	+ASA	+PPCI Clopidogrel Abciximab

The percentage mortality reduction figures are based on published meta-analyses. The baseline mortality figures (general bed ward and CCU) are mean approximates from literature.

During the 1970s the new treatment goal was to limit the size of the myocardial infarction. Beta-blockers came into focus and a new era of cardiovascular megatrials was started. After numerous trials it was concluded that beta-blockers significantly reduced both short- and long-term mortality (16).

The idea of an occluding thrombus and its dissolution had been around since 1950s. By late 1970s and early 1980s there was conclusive evidence that thrombolysis was effective (17). The pivotal trial was publication of the ISIS-2 trial in 1988 that not only proved that thrombolysis was effective but also that treatment with acetyl salicylic acid (ASA) was of equal value and given together their effects were additive (18).

Percutaneous transluminal coronary angioplasty (PTCA) was introduced in the 16th of September 1977 by Andreas Grüntzig. The use of angioplasty started to accelerate in the early 1980s. Patients with stable angina pectoris with single vessel disease were the initial candidates for PTCA.

A few centers started to apply percutaneous coronary intervention (PCI) to patients with AMI. In 1979, Rentrop et al. (19) reported recanalization of acute coronary occlusion by using spiral guidewires. In 1982 to 1983, there were several reports on balloon angioplasty in the setting of AMI with series of 1 to 46 patients. PCI was in most cases done after intracoronary thrombolysis (20–24).

The first evidence that angioplasty was beneficial and not harmful as compared to thrombolysis was published in 1986 by O'Neill et al. in a series of 56 patients randomized to intracoronary thrombolysis versus balloon angioplasty (24). The main findings were that after PCI there was significantly less restenosis and significantly better left ventricular function than after thrombolysis. Later O'Keefe et al. (25) published results on 500 patients treated with PPCI since 1981. The results seemed fairly good without any alarming tendencies.

The following 13 years a substantial number of randomized studies comparing intravenous thrombolysis and primary PCI (PPCI) with or without use of stents/abciximab were made including between 100 and 400 patients in most series. The biggest studies were GUSTO-IIb ($n = 1138$), PRAGUE-2 ($n = 850$), and DANAMI-2 ($n = 1572$). The latter two also included patients who were transported to angioplasty center from their primary hospital.

In a meta-analysis of 23 randomized studies published in 2003 including totally 7739 patients it could be concluded that as compared to thrombolysis primary angioplasty significantly reduced 30-day mortality by 28%, nonfatal reinfarction by 65%, and stroke by 54% (26).

Of special interest is the success of revascularization in the treatment of cardiogenic shock after AMI that has been the number one killer of the patients since cardiac arrest became a manageable condition. Both early and late mortality of shock patients younger than 75 years has been significantly reduced by early revascularization (PCI or bypass grafting) (27).

Thus even when the number of patients in the PPCI trials has been negligible compared to the size of several cardiovascular drug trials the treatment effects are convincingly significant.

The next concept in the therapeutic course for AMI was the idea of reperfusion therapy with thrombolysis and/or IIb/IIIa antagonist followed by transport to angioplasty center (facilitated PPCI). Randomized studies showed that this practice was not helpful (28).

Further attempts to improve the results of primary angioplasty have been thrombectomy and distal protection. The beneficial effects of thrombectomy are encouraging while distal protection studies have been negative (29,30).

The modern acute therapeutic measures have also improved the long-term outcome of the patients that has been further improved by drug therapy with statins and ACE-inhibitors (31,32).

We have made great progress since the days of bed rest and dismal prognosis. The pivotal DANAMI-2 trial is the largest PPCI study to counter the statement of futility of acute treatment by the Danish professor in 1956 quoted in the beginning of this overview.

CONCLUSIONS

The incidence of ischemic heart disease has been declining for 30 years in the western world. With economic growth in the developing countries, these are likely to face a considerable burden of cardiovascular disease in the future.

The mortality of acute coronary syndrome, including STEMI, is historically low, thanks to preventive measures and better treatments. Primary PCI has been one important contributing factor since it has become the preferred reperfusion strategy in the western world. With a 4% 30-day STEMI mortality in the <65 years age group, the focus of the immediate future must be to secure a greater than 80% reperfusion rate and provide this treatment to our increasingly aging population. Primary PCI, which have few contraindications in STEMI, holds the greatest potential to reach this goal.

REFERENCES

1. Tunstall-Pedoe H, Kuulasmaaa K, Mahonen M, et al. Contribution of trends in survival and coronary event rates to changes in coronary heart disease mortality: 10-year results from 37 WHO MONICA project populations. Lancet 1999; 353:1547–1557.
2. Hasdai D, Behar S, Boyko V, et al. Cardiac biomarkers and acute coronary syndromes – the Euro Heart Survey of Acute Coronary Syndromes Experience. Eur Heart J 2003; 24:1189–1194.
3. Stenestrand U, Wallentin L. Early revascularisation and 1-year survival in 14-day survivors of acute myocardial infarction: a prospective cohort study. Lancet 2002; 359:1805–1811.
4. Savonitto S, Ardissino D, Granger CB, et al. Prognostic value of the admission electrocardiogram in acute coronary syndromes. JAMA 1999; 281:707–713.
5. Fox KAA, Goodman SG, Klein W, et al. Management of acute coronary syndromes. Variations in practice and outcome: findings from the Global Registry of Acute Coronary Events (GRACE). Eur Heart J 2002; 23:1177–1189.
6. Danish Heart Register. www.dhreg.dk.

7. Stenestrand U, Wallentin L. Early statin treatment following acute myocardial infarction and 1-year survival. JAMA 2001; 285:430–436.
8. Stenestrand U, Lindbäck J, Wallentin L. RIKS-HIA registry. Long-term outcome of primary percutaneous coronary intervention vs prehospital and in-hospital thrombolysis for patients with ST-elevation myocardial infarction. JAMA 2006; 296:1749–1756.
9. Nallamothu BK, Bates ER, Herrin J, et al. Times to treatment in transfer patients undergoing primary percutaneous coronary intervention in the United States: National Registry of Myocardial Infarction (NRMI)-3/4 analysis. Circulation 2005; 111:761–767.
10. Eagle KA, Nallamothu BK, Mehta RH, et al. Trends in reperfusion therapy for ST-segment elevation myocardial infarction from 1999 to 2006: We are getting better but we have a long way to go. Eur Heart J 2008; 29:609–617.
11. Obrastow WP, Straschensko ND. Zur Kenntnis der Thrombose der Koronararterien des Her zens. Z Klein Med 1910; 71:116–132.
12. Herrick JB. Certain clinical features of sudden obstruction of the coronary arteries. JAMA 1912; 59:2015–2020.
13. Erik Warburg. Cardiovascular Diseases. Nordic Textbook of Internal Medicine. Copenhagen: Gyldendal, 1956.
14. Friedberg CK. Diseases of the Heart. New York: W.B. Saunders, 1966.
15. Julian DG. The history of coronary care units. Br Heart J 1987; 57:497–502.
16. Yusuf S, Peto R, Lewis J, et al. Beta blockade during and after myocardial infarction: an overview of the randomized trials. Progr Cardiovasc Dis 1985; 27:335–371.
17. Fibrinolytic Therapy Trialists Collaborative Group. Indications for fibrinolytic therapy in suspected acute myocardial infarction: collaborative overview of mortality and major morbidity results from all randomized trials of more than 1000 patients. Lancet 1994; 343:311–322.
18. ISIS Collaborative Group. Randomised trial of intravenous streptokinase, oral aspirin, both or neither among 17187 cases of suspected acute myocardial infarction: ISIS-2. Lancet 1988; 2:349–360.
19. Rentrop K, Blanke H, Karsch K, et al. Initial experience with transluminal recanalization of the recently occluded infarct-related coronary artery in acute myocardial infarction – comparison with conventionally treated patients. Clin Cardiol 1979; 2: 92–105.
20. Meyer J, Merx W, Schmitz H, et al. Percutaneous transluminal coronary angioplasty immediately after intracoronary streptolysis of transmural myocardial infarction. Circulation 1982; 666:905–913.
21. Bussmann W, Hopf R, Schneider W, et al. Direct recanalization with transluminal angioplasty in acute myocardial infarction. Dtsch Med Wochen Schr 1983; 108:1383–1386.
22. Phillips S, Kongtahworn C, Skinner J, et al. Emergency coronary artery reperfusion: a choice therapy for evolving myocardial infarction: results in 339 patients. Thoracic and Cardiovascular Surgery 1983; 86:679–688.
23. Hartzler GO, Rutherford BD, McConnahay DR, et al. Percutaneous transluminal coronary angioplasty with and without thrombolytic therapy for treatment of acute myocardial infarction. Am Heart J 1983; 106:965–973.
24. O'Neill W, Timmis GC, Bourdillon PD, et al. A prospective randomized clinical trial of intracoronary streptokinase versus coronary angioplasty for acute myocardial infarction. New Eng J Med 1986; 314:812–818.
25. O'Keefe J, Rutherford B, McConnahay D, et al. Early and late results of coronary angioplasty without antecedent thrombolytic therapy for acute myocardial infarction. Am J Cardiol 1989; 64:1221–1230.
26. Keeley EC, Boura JA, Grines CL. Primary angioplasty versus intravenous thrombolytic therapy for acute myocardial infarction: a quantitative review of 23 randomised trials. Lancet 2003; 361:13–20.
27. Hochman JS, Sleeper LA, White HD, et al. One-year survival following early revascularization for cardiogenic shock. JAMA 2001; 285:190–192.

28. Keeley EC, Boura JA, Grines CL. Comparison of primary and facilitated percutaneous coronary interventions for ST-elevation myocardial infarction: quantitative review of randomised trials. Lancet 2006; 367:579–588.

29. De Luca G, Suryapranata H, Stone G, et al. Adjunctive mechanical devices to prevent distal embolization in patients undergoing mechanical revascularization for acute myocardial infarction: a meta-analysis of randomised trial. Am Heart J 2007; 153: 343–353.

30. Vlaar P, Svilaas T, van der Horst I, et al. Cardiac death and reinfarction after 1 year in the Thrombus Aspiration during Percutaneous coronary intervention in acute myocardial infarction Study (TAPAS): a 1-year follow-up study. Lancet 2008; 371:1915–1920.

31. ACE Inhibitor Myocardial Infarction Collaborative Group. Indications for ACE inhibitors in the early treatment of cute myocardial infarction. Systematic overview of individual data from 100 000 patients in randomized trials. Circulation 1998; 97:2202–2212.

32. Cheung B, Lauder I, Lau C, et al. Meta-analysis of large randomized controlled trials to evaluate the impact of statins on cardiovascular outcomes. Br J Clinical Pharm 2004; 51:640–651.

Prehospital Diagnosis and Management of Acute Myocardial Infarction

Gilles Montalescot

Institut de Cardiologie Pitié–Salpêtrièra Hospital, Paris, France

Patrick Goldstein

SAMU Régional de Lille CHRU, Lille, France

INTRODUCTION

For patients with ST segment elevation myocardial infarction (STEMI), the time elapsed between the onset of pain and initiation of reperfusion has a critical impact on prognosis (1–4). Thus, all current guidelines concur in emphasizing the importance of initiating reperfusion therapy as soon as possible, either by mechanical or by pharmacological means (angioplasty and fibrinolysis, respectively) (5,6). Thus, although angioplasty is generally regarded as being superior to fibrinolysis, it is accepted that fibrinolysis should be initiated if angioplasty cannot be performed promptly and expertly (5,7). Moreover, in patients treated soon after the onset of pain, fibrinolysis or angioplasty is associated with favorable outcomes (8,9).

Both fibrinolysis and angioplasty should be supported by adjunctive therapy with antiplatelet and anticoagulant agents (5,6). As with reperfusion therapy, there is evidence that early initiation of adjunctive therapy is beneficial. Moreover, administration of such treatment in the prehospital setting has been associated with improvements in outcome (10,11).

The time that elapses between the onset of pain and initiation of therapy is affected by three main factors: the time between symptom onset and placement of a call to the emergency services, the speed with which the emergency team arrives at the patient's location, and the speed with which a diagnosis is made and coronary reperfusion and adjuvant medical treatment are initiated. This review discusses strategies that are effective in improving the speed of diagnosis and initiation of therapy in patients with STEMI. STEMI is associated with a higher in-hospital mortality rate than non–ST segment elevation myocardial infarction (NSTEMI) (12), although the latter has a higher long-term mortality.

AMBULANCE-BASED DIAGNOSIS, TRIAGE, AND TREATMENT

Approximately one-third of deaths occur before the patients reach a hospital (13). It thus follows that improvement in prehospital management is likely to be one of the most effective means of lowering mortality rates (6). The critical importance of rapid treatment initiation in STEMI patients means that ambulance-based diagnosis, triage, and, where indicated, treatment should allow patients to achieve the best possible outcome.

Key diagnostic procedures in patients with suspected myocardial infarction (MI) include electrocardiographic examination and assessment of myocardial ischemia (7,14). In most cases, electrocardiography will allow the emergency physician to determine whether the patient is suffering from an Acute Coronary Syndrome (ACS) and, if so, whether it is associated with ST segment elevation. The presence of myocardial ischemia can be determined by measuring serum levels of myoglobin, creatine kinase-MB, and troponins I and T (5,15). Although helpful in diagnosis, it should be noted that detectable increases in these enzymes are not apparent immediately and the absence of a positive result should not delay implementation of reperfusion therapy when ST segment elevation or a suspected new left bundle branch block is present (5,7). Furthermore, in most cases, patients with chest pain call the emergency team (SAMU/MICU) dispatching center during the first three hours (75% of calls), median call time is 60 minutes (16).

As previously noted, rapid reperfusion is the key to reducing morbidity and mortality in patients with STEMI. Patients who are diagnosed with STEMI before arriving at hospital can be admitted directly to the coronary care unit (CCU) therefore, bypassing the need for admission to the emergency room (ER). An observational registry of 369 intensive care units in France found that direct transfer to the CCU, compared with admission via the ER, was associated with more frequent and earlier use of reperfusion therapy and a lower five-day mortality rate in patients, suggesting a survival benefit associated with early initiation of treatment in these patients (17). A key decision in each case is the preferred primary reperfusion technique (fibrinolysis or angioplasty). Angioplasty has traditionally been regarded as being superior to fibrinolysis (5,7,18,19). However, it is now apparent that delayed angioplasty is associated with a higher mortality rate than immediate fibrinolysis (20). Thus, the decision regarding preferred reperfusion strategy—which has to be taken before the patient is admitted to hospital—is generally based on the interval between symptom onset and first medical contact, and on the immediacy of access to angioplasty (5,7,8,18,21–28). American and European guidelines currently recommend the use of angioplasty if it can be performed by an experienced team within 90 to 120 minutes of first medical contact (5,7).

If fibrinolysis is indicated, treatment should be administered as soon as possible. It is here that the importance of ambulance-based diagnosis and decision making becomes most apparent because, if this can be achieved, patients in whom fibrinolysis is indicated must receive reperfusion therapy prior to admission to hospital. Compared with in-hospital thrombolysis, prehospital administration of fibrinolytic agents is associated with a shorter time between symptom onset and initiation of reperfusion, and lower in-hospital, one-month, and one-year mortality rates in patients with STEMI (1,5,9,28–33). Boersma et al. (1) summarized the results of eight randomized clinical trials that reported the effects on outcome of prehospital and in-hospital thrombolysis. Prehospital treatment was associated with a one-hour reduction in the time between symptom onset and initiation of treatment (2.1 hours vs. 3.1 hours) and, in patients who were treated within three hours of symptom onset, this reduction in time to treatment led to a 2.1% reduction in 35-day mortality ($P = 0.002$).

The long-term benefits of prehospital thrombolysis are illustrated by data from 5375 STEMI patients admitted to 75 hospitals that participated in the Swedish Register of Cardiac Intensive Care between 2001 and 2004 (29). As in the summary of randomized trials reported by Boersma et al. (1), prehospital diagnosis and thrombolysis by trained paramedics reduced time to thrombolysis by approximately one hour. More importantly, one-year mortality was reduced by almost 30% (odds ratio, 0.71; 95% confidence interval, 0.55–0.92; $P = 0.008$) (29).

These data show that the short- and long-term outcomes of patients treated with prehospital thrombolysis is better than if the same treatment is administered in hospital. However, recent data show that, if initiated very early, thrombolysis may be more effective than angioplasty. In the comparison of angioplasty and prehospital thrombolysis in acute myocardial infarction (CAPTIM) study, patients randomized to treatment within two hours of symptom onset had a lower 30-day mortality rate if treated using prehospital thrombolysis (2.2%) than if treated by primary angioplasty (5.7%; $P = 0.058$) (27). If further investigation of the relative benefits of prehospital thrombolysis and angioplasty supports these results, current guideline recommendations regarding the relative benefits of angioplasty and thrombolysis in the early post-thrombosis period may need to be revised.

However, fibrinolysis and angioplasty are not mutually exclusive techniques: the two strategies can be used in conjunction in an approach known as "facilitated percutaneous coronary intervention (PCI)." This refers to pharmacological reperfusion therapy prior to PCI with the aim of achieving some recanalization and improvement in myocardial reperfusion, which might be expected to improve clinical outcomes (34). This is because the prognosis of patients with STEMI is known to be critically dependent on fast and effective restoration of blood flow to the infarct-related artery (IRA) and microcirculation (35). The GRACIA-2 study demonstrated the benefit of pre-PCI thrombolytic therapy to improve epicardial and myocardial perfusion and reduce signs of adverse ventricular modeling, when compared with revascularization alone (36). The results of other recent trials, however, appear to question the benefit of using systemic thrombolytics prior to PCI (37–40). For example, in the Facilitated Intervention with Enhanced Reperfusion Speed to Stop Events (FINESSE) trial, pre-PCI pharmacological reperfusion therapy with a half dosage of reteplase/abciximab produced an improvement in patency of the IRA but failed to show a significant effect on short-term outcomes (mortality and short-term postinfarct complications) when used in patients with STEMI who were unlikely to receive PCI within the preferred 90-minute timeframe (38). In contrast, routine PCI after reteplase/abciximab significantly improved the primary endpoint combining mortality, reinfarction, and refractory ischemia in a cohort of high-risk patients aged <75 years with evolving STEMI, when compared with patients receiving optional PCI as a rescue treatment only (41). The results of several recent studies indicate that the time between thrombolysis and transluminal angioplasty (ATL) is critical to the success of facilitated PCI with a treatment window of 3 to 24 hours offering the best results. A recent analysis of registry data from 1714 patients enrolled in the FAST-MI registry, Danchin et al. (42) showed that mortality rates were substantially higher in patients in whom PCI was performed within three hours of thrombolysis (3.7%) than in those in whom the procedure was performed later (1.4–1.6%) (42). Similarly, fibrinolytic therapy followed by PCI from 3 to 12 hours of randomization was associated with significant improvements in six-week left ventricular function when compared with early PCI treatment within three hours of randomization in the GRACIA-2 study (36). Facilitated PCI using pharmacological agents other than fibrinolytics [e.g., glycoprotein (GP) IIb/IIIa inhibitors] is not superior to primary PCI in patients with STEMI (39).

COMPOSITION OF THE MOBILE EMERGENCY TEAM

The characteristics of the health care personnel constituting the patient's first medical contact can have a significant influence on final outcome. For example, Collet et al. (43) used data from the FAST-MI registry to show that, compared with other types of medical contact that may be involved in the initial management of patients with chest pain (e.g., primary care physicians, cardiologists, emergency room physicians), use of a mobile intensive care unit (MICU), which in France comprises an emergency physician or intensivist, an emergency nurse, and a driver, is associated with more rapid transfer to the CCU/catheterization laboratory, higher reperfusion rates, and improved long-term survival. Such success obviously depends on the composition and level of training of the mobile emergency team. The team should be capable of rapid diagnosis, early risk stratification, minimal treatment delay, and administration of aggressive reperfusion (6,44). This can be achieved by trained paramedics working in liaison with specialists based in a CCU (44). Inclusion of a physician in the mobile team has been associated with a delay in time to treatment, but also with improved adherence to protocol-mandated treatments and procedures (45). Moreover, morbidity, mortality, and security outcomes are better in health care systems in which the prehospital team includes a physician (~75% of European countries).

IMMEDIATE (PREHOSPITAL) TREATMENT OF PATIENTS WITH STEMI

Prehospital management of patients with STEMI should include continuous cardioscopic monitoring with a hand-held defibrillator. Two good-caliber peripheral venous lines should be placed, and the patient should receive analgesics (e.g., morphine, diamorphine) and, if necessary, anxiolytics (7). A pulse oximeter should be used and oxygen should be administered, as indicated (7).

Thrombolytics

If thrombolysis is the preferred reperfusion strategy for patients with STEMI, this should be initiated by the emergency team as soon as possible (i.e., in the ambulance or at home) because of the reductions in short- and long-term mortality with which this strategy has been associated (1,3,5,7,8,29–33,46). Thrombolysis is effected by agents that convert the inactive plasma zymogen, plasminogen, to the active fibrinolytic enzyme, plasmin (47). Early thrombolytic agents were associated with a number of problems including susceptibility to inactivation by the physiological plasminogen activator inhibitor, plasminogen activator inhibitor-1 (PAI-1), and a lack of substrate specificity with a consequent propensity to lyse both fibrin and fibrinogen (14,48). Treated patients could thus reach a "systemic lytic state," in which there was substantial risk of hemorrhage (14,49).

Tenecteplase, which is a bioengineered version of the human tissue plasminogen activator, alteplase, represents a molecule in which these problems have largely been overcome. Mutations at three sites in the alteplase molecule have resulted in a 15-fold increase in fibrin specificity, an 80-fold reduction in PAI-1 binding affinity, and a sixfold increase in plasma half-life (50). These alterations in pharmacokinetic and pharmacodynamic properties mean that tenecteplase is currently the thrombolytic agent of choice (11). In addition to a low risk of hemorrhagic complications and resistance to inactivation by PAI-1, tenecteplase has the advantages of easy (bolus) administration, simple calculation of dosage, and low antigenicity (51–59).

Fibrinolytic agents are typically administered in combination with antiplatelet and anticoagulant agents. Such adjunctive treatment is extremely important for two reasons. Firstly, platelets and fibrin play a central role in the pathogenesis of coronary thrombosis (7), and adjunctive treatment will thus minimize the extent of any ongoing atherothrombosis. Secondly, fibrinolytic agents may induce further platelet aggregation by exposing the free thrombin in an existing coronary thrombus (60). Anticoagulant and antiplatelet agents that may be used include aspirin, thienopyridines, unfractionated heparin (UFH), low-molecular-weight heparins (LMWHs), and GP IIb/IIIa inhibitors.

In these patients initially treated by fibrinolytics, several important points of the management should be immediately decided: (*i*) transfer to the nearest hospital or rather to a "heart attack center" even if transfer time is longer. The latter is often the better as the patient would be placed in a center with all catheterization facilities that may be required in emergency in case of reocclusion. (*ii*) Time of catheterization in case of favorable evolution (chest pain resolution and significant ST regression): next day catheterization is probably, as indicated earlier, the optimal and practical time window. (*iii*) In case of reperfusion failure, the chain of care should know how to get rapid rescue PCI in such patients.

Aspirin

Aspirin forms the basis of routine therapy for patients with STEMI. This antiplatelet agent is highly effective in improving patient outcomes (61), and should be administered as soon as possible to all patients in whom it is not contraindicated at a dose of 162 to 325 mg per os (5,7). Aspirin can be prescribed by the emergency dispatching medical center just after the initial call. The thienopyridine, clopidogrel, is the preferred antiplatelet agent in patients who cannot tolerate aspirin (5,7). Aspirin is also part of the basic treatment for NSTEMI patients and should be administered as soon as possible (62,63). An immediate effect is only achieved for doses above 125 mg and the drug does not act against thrombin-induced platelet activation (64).

Although the evidence supporting the routine use of aspirin is overwhelming, this agent affects platelet function via only one mechanism (cyclooxygenase inhibition). The beneficial effects of aspirin may thus be supplemented by administration of agents that act via different mechanisms.

The intravenous form of aspirin available in many countries is more rapidly effective (no delay due to intestinal absorption) and easier to use in emergency, and particularly useful in patients who are agitated, unconscious, in shock or have nausea.

Thienopyridines

The thienopyridines inhibit platelet aggregation induced by adenosine diphosphate. Today, clopidogrel is preferred to ticlopidine because it has fewer side effects (ticlopidine is associated with neutropenia and thrombotic thrombocytopenia), does not require laboratory monitoring, and can be given once daily (5).

Clopidogrel therapy is recommended during the acute phase of treatment and for extended periods after hospital discharge in STEMI patients (5). For example, the American College of Cardiology (ACC)/American Heart Association (AHA) guidelines recommend initiation and maintenance of clopidogrel therapy for periods of up to 12 months in patients who have undergone diagnostic catheterization and in whom PCI is planned (5). These guidelines, which were published in 2004, do not make specific recommendations regarding the use of clopidogrel in patients treated with fibrinolytic agents (except as an alternative to aspirin in those who are aspirin intolerant), but state that the use of clopidogrel in this situation would be clarified by the results of ongoing trials. Relevant results are now available. For example, in the clopidogrel as adjunctive reperfusion therapy-thrombolysis in myocardial infarction 28 (CLARITY-TIMI 28) trial, 3491 STEMI patients who underwent fibrinolysis (plus aspirin and, when appropriate, heparin) received concomitant treatment with clopidogrel (300 mg loading dose followed by 75 mg/day) or placebo (65) (clopidogrel reduced the risk of cardiovascular death, recurrent MI, or recurrent ischemia) leading to the need for urgent revascularization at 30 days from 14.1% to 11.6%, a relative risk reduction of 20% ($P = 0.03$) (65). The rates of major bleeding and intracranial hemorrhage (ICH) were similar in the two groups. Further analysis of data from the CLARITY-TIMI 28 trial suggests that clopidogrel improves late coronary patency and clinical outcomes in fibrinolytic-treated patients by preventing reocclusion of open arteries, rather than by facilitating early perfusion (66,67).

The data discussed above were generated in patients in whom fibrinolysis was the primary reperfusion strategy. However, there is also evidence that clopidogrel is of benefit in fibrinolytic- (and aspirin-) treated STEMI patients who subsequently undergo PCI (68,69). Under these circumstances, patients have lower rates of cardiovascular morbidity and mortality if they are pretreated with clopidogrel (68,69). Clopidogrel has also been administered to fibrinolytic-treated patients in the situation that is the primary focus of this review, that is, prior to arrival at hospital. Using data from a small, prospective, placebo-controlled substudy of the CLARITY-TIMI 28 trial, Verheugt et al. (10) showed that prehospital administration of clopidogrel to STEMI patients treated with fibrinolysis, heparin, and aspirin was associated with substantial improvements in early coronary patency, with no increase in bleeding risk (10). The incidence of an occluded IRA on the predischarge angiogram was 11.8% in the clopidogrel-treated group and 22.3% in the placebo group (odds ratio, 0.52, $P = 0.10$). The results of this preliminary study, which are consistent with those of the overall CLARITY-TIMI 28 cohort (65), show that prehospital administration of clopidogrel is feasible, safe, and beneficial.

The clinical trial data presented above represent a small subset of the body of evidence showing that clopidogrel is associated with significant improvements in outcome, when used in association with both pharmacological and mechanical reperfusion of aspirin-treated STEMI patients (Fig. 1; 65,69–72). However, there has been no clinical trial performed to evaluate clopidogrel in primary PCI of STEMI. Interestingly, the first large set of data published with clopidogrel in PCI of STEMI comes from the STEMI cohort of the large phase 3 TRITON study. An important feature of the Triton-TIMI 38 study design was the prespecified inclusion of patients with STEMI. Patients with STEMI were enrolled within 12 hours after the onset of symptoms if primary PCI was planned or within 14 days after receiving medical treatment for STEMI. (73) Of the 13,608 patients who were enrolled, 3534 patients had STEMI; of these 2438 (69%) and 1094 (31%) patients were treated with primary and secondary PCI, respectively.

Effects of clopidogrel in acute MI

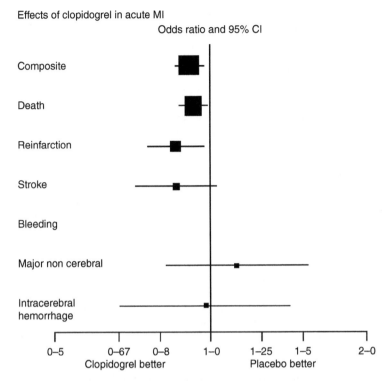

FIGURE 1 Effects of adding clopidogrel to the treatment regimen of aspirin-treated patients with STEMI. The figure shows the effects on a range of endpoints of adding clopidogrel to aspirin monotherapy in patients with suspected acute myocardial infarction enrolled in the Clopidogrel and Metoprolol in Myocardial Infarction Trial (COMMIT). *Source*: From Ref. 66.

Both primary and secondary PCI-treated patients were randomized to receive either prasugrel or clopidogrel on a 1:1 basis.

The baseline characteristics of prasugrel and clopidogrel-treated patients were well matched. There were major differences in the demographics of the primary and secondary PCI groups that reflected differences in patient type, baseline risk, and disease management. Patients with primary PCI, compared with those receiving secondary PCI, had a lower history of previous multivessel PCI (6.5% vs. 11.0%; $P < 0.001$), and more frequent GP IIb/IIIa inhibitor use (64.5% vs. 59.8%; $P < 0.01$) due in part to more frequent bailout use of GP IIb/IIIa inhibitors with clopidogrel (6.1% with clopidogrel vs. 4.4% with prasugrel; $P = 0.06$) (73).

The endpoint of CV death, nonfatal MI, and nonfatal stroke was significantly reduced after 30 days of treatment with prasugrel, compared with clopidogrel: 6.5% versus 9.5%; $P = 0.002$, respectively. The benefit of prasugrel treatment persisted through 15 months, compared with clopidogrel: 10.0% versus 12.4%; $P = 0.02$. These results parallel those of the previously reported overall cohort of the Triton-TIMI 38 study, and demonstrate that, with respect to the prevention of ischemic events, not only does prasugrel have significant benefit over clopidogrel across the overall spectrum of ACSs, but that this is particularly pronounced in patients with STEMI.

The combined endpoint of CV death, MI, and urgent target vessel revascularization (UTVR) at 30 days was a key secondary endpoint of the Triton-TIMI 38 study for both the overall and STEMI cohort analyses. The rate of CV death, MI, and UTVR was significantly reduced in the STEMI cohort after 30 days of treatment with prasugrel, compared with clopidogrel: 6.7% versus 8.8%; $P = 0.02$, respectively. Furthermore, the benefit of prasugrel treatment persisted through 15 months, compared with clopidogrel: 9.6% versus 12.0%; $P = 0.03$, respectively. These results highlight the benefits of prasugrel, compared with clopidogrel, when viewed in the context of an endpoint often used in other STEMI studies (8–12).

Multivariate analyses were performed to identify predictors of CV death, MI, and UTVR in the STEMI cohort at 30 days. These analyses found that common indicators of higher-risk patients were associated with worse outcomes for CV death, MI, and UTVR: GP IIb/IIIa inhibitor use versus no use hazard ratio (HR) = 1.35 ($P = 0.03$); multivessel PCI versus single PCI HR = 1.52 ($P = 0.036$); bare metal stent (BMS) versus drug eluting stent (DES) HR = 1.43 ($P = 0.009$); prior MI versus no prior MI HR = 1.57 ($P = 0.012$); and age ≥ 75 years versus <75 years HR = 1.73 ($P = 0.001$). The only factor that reduced the HR of the key secondary endpoint at 30 days was treatment (prasugrel vs. clopidogrel): HR = 0.73 ($P = 0.015$).

In addition to the reductions in the rates of CV death, MI, and stroke, and CV death, MI, and UTVR, prasugrel, compared with clopidogrel, significantly reduced the single endpoints of all-cause death ($P = 0.04$), MI ($P = 0.01$), and stent thromboses ($P = 0.008$), and the dual endpoint of CV death and MI ($P = 0.004$), after 30 days of treatment. There was also a significant reduction of death in the primary PCI cohort following prasugrel treatment for 30 days, compared with clopidogrel.

Of note, in patients with STEMI, prasugrel and clopidogrel had similar safety profiles with respect to bleeding. Following 15 months of treatment, the rate of TIMI major non-CABG bleeding in prasugrel and clopidogrel-treated patients were comparable: 2.4% versus 2.1%; $P = 0.65$, respectively. Indeed, the 30-day incidence rate of TIMI major non-CABG bleeding was numerically higher in the clopidogrel group, possibly relating to an increased use of bailout therapy with GP IIb/IIIa inhibitors, compared with prasugrel. Furthermore, prasugrel, compared with clopidogrel, did not significantly increase the rate of life-threatening bleeding (1.1% vs. 1.3%, respectively), intracranial bleeding (0.3% vs. 0.2%, respectively), minor non-CABG bleeding (2.7% vs. 2.8%, respectively), minor or major non-CABG bleeding (4.7% vs. 5.1%, respectively), or major or minor CABG or non-CABG bleeding (4.8% vs. 5.9%, respectively).

When taken together, the efficacy and safety profiles after 15 months of treatment with either prasugrel or clopidogrel reveal a significant net clinical benefit for the combined endpoint of CV death, nonfatal MI, nonfatal stroke or TIMI major non-CABG bleeding with prasugrel treatment, compared to clopidogrel: 12.2% versus 14.6%; $P = 0.02$. Furthermore, even when perioperative bleedings were included in the net clinical benefit analysis [CV death, nonfatal MI, nonfatal stroke or major (CABG or non-CABG) bleeding], treatment with prasugrel still provided a net clinical benefit over clopidogrel: 12.5% versus 14.7%; $P = 0.04$.

A trial comparing clopidogrel (600 mg loading dose followed by a 150 mg maintenance dose for 14 days) with prasugrel (60 mg loading dose, 10 mg daily maintenance dose) given as pretreatment in patients ~1 hour before undergoing cardiac catheterization ahead of planned PCI, demonstrated more potent inhibition of platelet aggregation for prasugrel-treated patients (74).

Clopidogrel High Dose in CURRENT-OASIS 7

The objective of the CURRENT-OASIS 7 trial was to determine whether a high dose regimen of clopidogrel (600 mg loading dose, followed by 150 mg o.d. from day 2 to day 7, then 75 mg daily) was superior to a standard dose regimen of clopidogrel (300 mg LD followed by 75 mg daily) in preventing cardiovascular death, MI, or stroke in patients with non–ST segment elevation acute coronary syndromes who are treated with an early invasive strategy within 24 hours. An amendment to the protocol extended the recruitment to primary PCI of STEMI. The safety of the clopidogrel high dose regimen was also compared to the standard dose regimen in terms of TIMI major bleeding. This part of the study is double-blind. [Results presented at the European Society of Cardiology (ESC) 2009 Congress by Dr. Shamir Mehta, Barcelona, Spain].

No significant difference was observed for the primary objective in the overall cohort of 25,087 patients who received the higher loading and maintenance doses compared to standard dosing [0.95 (0.84–1.07)]. Although the trial failed to meet its primary endpoint that theoretically limits further subgroup analysis, the benefit of double-dose clopidogrel appears to outweigh the risk in ACS patients undergoing PCI. There was a significant interaction for PCI versus no PCI (as well as for aspirin). In focusing on the 17,232 patients who underwent PCI, there was a significant 15% reduction in cardiovascular, death, MI, and stroke, only driven by a reduction in the risk of MI. In addition, there was a significant 42% reduction in the risk of definite stent thrombosis. In contrast, the 7855 patients who did not undergo PCI because no significant Coronary Artery Disease (CAD) was identified or because they had severe CAD requiring CABG surgery or just medical treatment; there was no significant difference in the primary composite endpoint of death, MI, or stroke between the two clopidogrel doses groups.

The bleeding risk was difficult to evaluate and varied according to the definitions. There was no difference with the standard and doubled clopidogrel doses when the stringent TIMI major bleeding definition was used (primary safety objective). However, there was a significant increase in bleeding when the CURRENT major and severe bleeding definition was used, and this was driven by an increased need for red blood cell transfusions. There was no difference in fatal bleeding, ICH, or CABG-related major bleeding.

Interestingly, while the success of clopidogrel at a standard dose regimen (against placebo) in CURE was driven by the benefit obtained in a population mostly medically treated, this type of patients did not benefit from higher doses of clopidogrel in CURRENT. It suggests that the dose of clopidogrel should not be the same for PCI and non-PCI patients. The higher platelet inhibition and the good clinical results obtained with prasugrel and ticagrelor in the recent TRITON and PLATelet inhibition and patient Outcomes (PLATO) studies confirm the need for more aggressive treatment in ACS patients undergoing stenting.

Ticagrelor, a Reversible P2Y$_{12}$ Antagonist

Ticagrelor is an oral, reversible, direct-acting inhibitor of the adenosine diphosphate receptor P2Y$_{12}$ that has a more rapid onset and more pronounced platelet inhibition than clopidogrel and comparable platelet inhibition to prasugrel. In a multicenter, double-blind, randomized trial, ticagrelor (180-mg loading dose, 90 mg twice daily thereafter) was compared with clopidogrel (300-to-600-mg loading dose, 75 mg daily thereafter) for the prevention of cardiovascular events in 18,624 patients admitted to the hospital with an acute coronary syndrome, with or without ST segment elevation. The composite of death from vascular causes, MI, or stroke occurred in 9.8% of patients receiving ticagrelor as compared with 11.7% of those receiving clopidogrel ($P < 0.001$). Death from vascular causes was reduced (4.0% vs. 5.1%, $P = 0.001$) but not stroke (1.5% vs. 1.3%, $P = 0.22$). No significant difference in the rates of major bleeding was found between the ticagrelor and clopidogrel groups (11.6% and 11.2%, respectively; $P = 0.43$) using new definitions specific to this trial, but ticagrelor was associated with a higher rate of major bleeding not related to coronary artery bypass grafting (4.5% vs. 3.8%, $P = 0.03$), including more instances of fatal intracranial bleeding and fewer of fatal bleeding of other types. Altogether, ticagrelor as compared with clopidogrel has a favorable risk/benefit ratio. The results in primary PCI of STEMI are expected soon.

Anticoagulants

Heparin preparations (e.g., UFH and LMWHs) have multiple inhibitory effects on the coagulation cascade (5). Current guidelines recommend that intravenous heparin should be administered to all patients who receive fibrinolytic therapy with alteplase, reteplase, or tenecteplase (5,7), and to those treated with nonselective fibrinolytic agents (streptokinase, anistreplase, urokinase) who are at high risk of systemic emboli (5). The routine use of heparin in conjunction with nonselective fibrinolytic agents is not recommended because these agents are themselves anticoagulants (5).

In spite of widespread use of heparin in patients receiving fibrinolytic therapy, the optimal duration of heparin coadministration in this situation has not been established. The ACC/AHA guidelines recommend that intravenous heparin should be administered for 48 hours, and that subsequent use should be guided by the clinical characteristics of the patient (5). Gradually reducing the dose of heparin (rather than discontinuing treatment abruptly) may help to decrease the risk of "heparin rebound" and recurrent thrombosis (5). Support for the use of heparin in combination with aspirin in patients with NSTEMI is provided by a meta-analysis of six randomized clinical trials (75). UFH is included in the strategic recommendations for early conservative management of NSTEMI patients proposed by the AHA. In addition, LMWH and UFH are recommended in those low-risk patients who evolve to an intermediate and high-risk status that requires an invasive strategy, with LMWH being the preferred option to UFH unless bypass surgery is planned within the proceeding 24 hours (63).

The specific heparin regimen that should be used in fibrinolysis-treated patients depends to some extent on the patient's age and on the presence or absence of comorbid conditions. UFH is the most widely studied heparin preparation, and its use as a first-line antithrombin agent in patients receiving fibrinolysis is recommended by current guidelines (5,7). However, LMWHs have a number of theoretical advantages over UFH (5,76). These include greater factor Xa inhibition (and therefore better prevention of thrombin generation), more predictable kinetics, a more stable therapeutic response, lower protein binding, less platelet activation, and a lower rate of heparin-induced thrombocytopenia (7,77). Moreover, in contrast to the situation in patients receiving UFH therapy, there is no need to monitor activated partial thromboplastin time in LMWH-treated patients (7,77).

Clinical trials have shown that these theoretical advantages translate into improvements in clinical outcome (78). The LMWH/fibrinolytic regimen that has been studied most extensively is enoxaparin/tenecteplase (5) and the favorable results achieved have led to enoxaparin becoming the heparin preparation of choice in the majority of ACS patients. For example, in the recent ExTRACT-TIMI 25 trial, 20,506 STEMI patients who were scheduled to undergo fibrinolysis were randomized to receive enoxaparin (throughout the index hospitalization) or UFH (weight-based, for at least 48 hours) (79). Enoxaparin was administered at a reduced dose in patients >75 years of age because of evidence that "full dose" enoxaparin increases the risk of ICH in this age group (11). The results of the ExTRACT-TIMI 25 trial showed that enoxaparin was associated with a significant reduction in the risk of death or nonfatal recurrent MI at 30 days (12.0% vs. 9.9%; 17% reduction in relative risk; $P < 0.001$), and with significantly greater net clinical benefit. This latter outcome was measured as a composite of death, nonfatal reinfarction, and nonfatal ICH (enoxaparin, 10.1%; UFH, 12.2%; $P < 0.001$) (79). There was no excess of ICH in the enoxaparin group (UFH, 0.7%; enoxaparin, 0.8%). A second, more recent study has confirmed that the excess risk of major bleeding associated with full-dose enoxaparin in elderly, fibrinolysis-treated STEMI patients can be managed by reducing the dose (80). Guidelines published before these results became available recommend that LMWH should not be used as an alternative to UFH in patients >75 years of age (5). However, these recommendations may require revision in the light of recent evidence, and significant renal dysfunction remains the only major contraindication to enoxaparin administration in fibrinolysis-treated patients (5). Enoxaparin or UFH is recommended in the AHA guidelines for management of low-risk patients presenting with unstable angina/NSTEMI in the emergency department (63).

The reversible, direct thrombin inhibitor bivalirudin was not included in the OASIS trials but in other studies, including the Acute Catheterization and Urgent Intervention Triage Strategy (ACUITY) trial, bivalirudin demonstrated a reduction in 30-day bleeding rates in moderate to high-risk patients with NSTEMI ACS undergoing urgent PCI, compared with UFH and GP IIb/IIIa inhibitor treatment. This was in addition to a comparable ischemic and mortality benefit assessed at 1 year in these patients (81,82). Moreover, in a recent comparison of heparin plus a GP IIb/IIIa inhibitor or bivalirudin alone in PCI-treated patients with STEMI [the harmonizing outcomes with revascularization and stents in acute myocardial infarction (HORIZONS-AMI) study], bivalirudin was associated with significantly lower 30-day rates of major bleeding, cardiac death, all-cause mortality, and net adverse clinical events (83).

Glycoprotein IIb/IIIa Inhibitors

In contrast to aspirin, GP IIb/IIIa inhibitors block the final pathway of platelet aggregation, and agents of this class should be regarded as standard adjuvant therapy in patients destined for angioplasty (5,7). When used in combination with fibrinolytic agents, GP IIb/IIIa inhibitors improve reperfusion and reduce the risk of early ischemic complications, but these advantages are offset by an increase in the risk of hemorrhage (84,85). Moreover, although GP IIb/IIIa inhibitors reduce the risk of early infarction, this has not been associated with improvements in 30-day or one-year survival (84–86). As a result, the routine use of GP IIb/IIIa inhibitors in patients destined to receive fibrinolytic agents is not recommended by the current European guidelines (7), and the ACC/AHA guidelines restrict the potential use of this treatment combination to the subset of STEMI patients who have an anterior MI, are <75 years of age, and have no risk factors for bleeding (5). If GP IIb/IIIa inhibitors are used in combination with a thrombolytic agent, the dose of fibrinolytic should be reduced by 50% (5).

GP IIb/IIIa inhibitors have been administered in the prehospital setting prior to PCI (87–89). These studies have shown that this strategy is safe and feasible (87,88). The Abciximab before direct angioplasty and stenting in myocardial infarction regarding acute and long-term follow-up (ADMIRAL) study investigated the clinical benefit of early administration of the GP IIb/IIIa inhibitor abciximab versus placebo in patients with STEMI undergoing primary coronary stent implantation. Early GP IIb/IIIa inhibition was associated with improved coronary patency and left ventricular function, as well as significant reductions in the combined clinical outcome of death, reinfarction, and urgent revascularization of the target vessel measured at 30 days and six months after the procedure (90). Data available from 87% of patients at 3-year follow-up confirmed these results. According to an intent-to-treat analysis, abciximab treatment resulted in an absolute survival benefit of 3.1% (95% CI: −3.9%; 10.1%) compared with placebo at 3 years, which was comparable with an absolute benefit of 3.2% (95% CI: −1.7%; 8.1%) measured at 30 days (91). A further meta-analysis of six clinical trials (three with abciximab and three with tirofiban) confirmed the significant benefit of early GP IIb/IIIa inhibition on coronary patency. The rate of TIMI grade 2 and 3 flow before angioplasty increased in the early treatment group (receiving GP IIb/IIIa inhibitors before entry into the catheterization laboratory), compared with the late group (92). However, in a small study that compared prehospital and ER administration of abciximab in PCI-treated patients with STEMI, there were no significant differences between groups in TIMI flow grade before revascularization, grade after revascularization, or outcome (87). A similar result was achieved in the recent FINESSE study that found no significant difference in outcome at 90 days in PCI-treated STEMI patients who received early treatment with abciximab plus half-dose reteplase (combination-facilitated PCI), early treatment with abciximab (abciximab-facilitated PCI), or abciximab administered immediately before the procedure (primary PCI) (38). The proportion of patients who achieved a TIMI flow grade of 3 was significantly higher before PCI in the combination-facilitated PCI group than in the other two groups, but this difference was not maintained after the procedure (38).

Recent findings from the Ongoing Tirofiban in Myocardial Infarction Evaluation 2 study (ON-TIME-2) have demonstrated that prehospital initiation of tirofiban in combination with aspirin, clopidogrel, and UFH improves ST resolution before and after PCI compared with placebo in acute MI patients treated in the ambulance or referral center. There was a significant reduction in the primary endpoint of residual ST segment deviation (>3 mm) one hour after PCI in tirofiban-treated patients, compared with placebo. The combined occurrence of the secondary endpoints of death, recurrent MI, UTVR or thrombotic bailout at 30 days follow-up was also improved with early tirofiban treatment without an increase in bleeding risk (93).

CONCLUSIONS

Ambulance-based diagnosis, triage, and treatment of ACS patients are widely used in countries like France (94) and additional measures are in place to aid the establishment of common practice and dialogue between cardiologists and emergency physicians. Similar approaches have been made in other European countries. There is thus an opportunity for substantial improvements in the prehospital management of MI patients.

It is likely that the growing body of evidence demonstrating the benefits of ambulance-based diagnosis, triage, and treatment of ACS patients will lead to gradual acceptance of this approach (Fig. 2). Moreover, if economic evaluations of this strategy demonstrate cost savings, this might speed its integration into national health care recommendations. However, if it is to be effective,

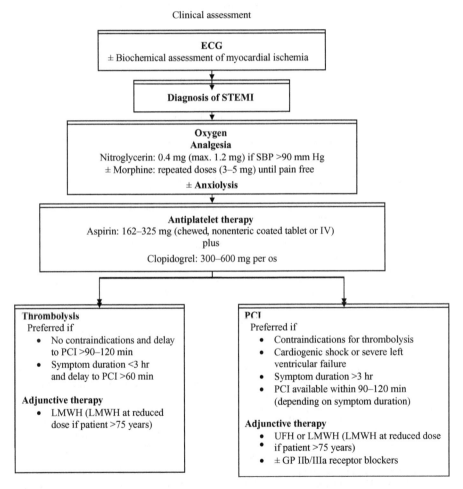

FIGURE 2 Treatment algorithm for patients presenting with signs/symptoms of acute coronary syndrome. *Abbreviations*: ECG, electrocardiogram; GP, glycoprotein; IV, intravenous; LMWH, low-molecular-weight heparin; PCI, percutaneous coronary intervention; SBP, systolic blood pressure; UFH, unfractionated heparin.

prehospital treatment must be introduced on a regional or national basis and must involve integration and coordination of procedures practiced by emergency call centers, mobile emergency units, community-based physicians, and hospital emergency departments. The French initiative demonstrates that current barriers to the introduction of prehospital treatment can be overcome, with beneficial consequences for patients.

Whatever the mode of reperfusion in STEMI optimal medical therapy should be initiated in the prehospital setting in all patients. Thus, antiplatelet agents (aspirin and/or clopidogrel) and heparin (usually LMWH)—which are indicated in all STEMI patients—can be administered in the ambulance and early treatment with such agents should be considered as part of routine practice for patients with STEMI. Fibrinolysis should also be initiated in this setting, if indicated. All treatment decisions should be guided by the strong, well-documented relationship between speed of reperfusion and improved outcome that exists for both fibrinolysis and primary PCI.

REFERENCES

1. Boersma E, Maas AC, Deckers JW, et al. Early thrombolytic treatment in acute myocardial infarction: reappraisal of the golden hour. Lancet 1996; 348:771–775.
2. Dracup K, Alonzo AA, Atkins JM, et al. The physician's role in minimizing prehospital delay in patients at high risk for acute myocardial infarction: recommendations from the National Heart Attack Alert Program. Working Group on Educational Strategies to Prevent Prehospital Delay in Patients at High Risk for Acute Myocardial Infarction. Ann Intern Med 1997; 126:645–651.
3. Fibrinolytic Therapy Trialists' (FTT) Collaborative Group. Indications for fibrinolytic therapy in suspected acute myocardial infarction: collaborative overview of early mortality and major morbidity results from all randomised trials of more than 1000 patients. Lancet 1994; 343:311–322.
4. Gruppo Italiano per lo Studio della Streptochinasi nell'Infarto Miocardico (GISSI). Effectiveness of intravenous thrombolytic treatment in acute myocardial infarction. Lancet 1986; 1:397–402.
5. Antman EM, Anbe DT, Armstrong PW, et al; American College of Cardiology/American Heart Association Task Force on Practice Guidelines (Writing Committee to Revise the 1999 Guidelines for the Management of Patients with Acute Myocardial Infarction). ACC/AHA guidelines for the management of patients with ST-elevation myocardial infarction—executive summary: a report of the American College of Cardiology/American Heart Association Task Force on Practice Guidelines (Writing Committee to Revise the 1999 Guidelines for the Management of Patients with Acute Myocardial Infarction). Circulation 2004; 110:588–636.
6. Arntz HR, Bossaert L, Filippatos GS; European Resuscitation Council. European Resuscitation Council guidelines for resuscitation 2005. Section 5. Initial management of acute coronary syndromes. Resuscitation 2005; 67(suppl 1):S87–S96.
7. Van de Werf F, Ardissino D, Betriu A, et al; Task Force on the Management of Acute Myocardial Infarction of the European Society of Cardiology. Management of acute myocardial infarction in patients presenting with ST-segment elevation. The Task Force on the Management of Acute Myocardial Infarction of the European Society of Cardiology. Eur Heart J 2003; 24:28–66.
8. Bonnefoy E, Lapostolle F, Leizorovicz A, et al; Comparison of Angioplasty and Prehospital Thromboysis in Acute Myocardial Infarction Study Group. Primary angioplasty versus prehospital fibrinolysis in acute myocardial infarction: a randomised study. Lancet 2002; 360:825–829.

9. Kalla K, Christ G, Karnik R, et al; Vienna STEMI Registry Group. Implementation of guidelines improves the standard of care: the Viennese registry on reperfusion strategies in ST-elevation myocardial infarction (Vienna STEMI registry). Circulation 2006; 113:2398–2405.

10. Verheugt FW, Montalescot G, Sabatine MS, et al. Prehospital fibrinolysis with dual antiplatelet therapy in ST-elevation acute myocardial infarction: a substudy of the randomized double blind CLARITY-TIMI 28 trial. J Thromb Thrombolysis 2007; 23:173–179.

11. Wallentin L, Goldstein P, Armstrong PW, et al. Efficacy and safety of tenecteplase in combination with the low-molecular-weight heparin enoxaparin or unfractionated heparin in the prehospital setting: the Assessment of the Safety and Efficacy of a New Thrombolytic Regimen (ASSENT)-3 PLUS randomized trial in acute myocardial infarction. Circulation 2003; 108:135–142.

12. Steg PG, Goldberg RJ, Gore JM, et al; GRACE Investigators. Baseline characteristics, management practices, and in-hospital outcomes of patients hospitalized with acute coronary syndromes in the Global Registry of Acute Coronary Events (GRACE). Am J Cardiol 2002; 90:358–363.

13. Löwel H, Meisinger C, Heier M, et al. Sex specific trends of sudden cardiac death and acute myocardial infarction: results of the population-based KORA/MONICA-Augsburg register 1985 to 1998 [article in German]. Dtsch Med Wochenschr 2002; 127:2311–2316.

14. Wallentin L. Reducing time to treatment in acute myocardial infarction. Eur J Emerg Med 2000; 7:217–227.

15. Kost GJ, Tran NK. Point-of-care testing and cardiac biomarkers: the standard of care and vision for chest pain centers. Cardiol Clin 2005; 23:467–490.

16. Lapandry C, Laperche T, Lambert Y, et al. Prise en charge préhospitalière des syndromes coronaires aigus ST + en Ile-de-France. Le registre E-must. Arch Mal Coeur Vaiss 2005; 98:1137–1142.

17. Steg PG, Cambou J-P, Goldstein P, et al. Bypassing the emergency room reduces delays and mortality in ST elevation myocardial infarction: the USIC 2000 registry. Heart 2006; 92:1378–1383.

18. Andersen HR, Nielsen TT, Rasmussen K, et al; DANAMI-2 Investigators. A comparison of coronary angioplasty with fibrinolytic therapy in acute myocardial infarction. N Engl J Med 2003; 349:733–742.

19. Weaver WD, Simes RJ, Betriu A, et al. Comparison of primary coronary angioplasty and intravenous thrombolytic therapy for acute myocardial infarction: a quantitative review. JAMA 1997; 278:2093–298.

20. Nallamothu BK, Bates ER. Percutaneous coronary intervention versus fibrinolytic therapy in acute myocardial infarction: is timing (almost) everything? Am J Cardiol 2003; 92:824–826.

21. Bassand JP, Danchin N, Filippatos G, et al. Implementation of reperfusion therapy in acute myocardial infarction. A policy statement from the European Society of Cardiology. Eur Heart J 2005; 26:2733–2741.

22. Danchin N. Should intravenous thrombolysis keep a place in the treatment of acute ST-elevation myocardial infarction? Eur Heart J 2006; 27:1131–1133.

23. Ferrier C, Belle L, Labarere J, et al. Comparison of mortality according to the revascularisation strategies and the symptom-to-management delay in ST-segment elevation myocardial infarction [article in French]. Arch Mal Coeur Vaiss 2007; 100:13–19.

24. Nallamothu BK, Antman EM, Bates ER. Primary percutaneous coronary intervention versus fibrinolytic therapy in acute myocardial infarction: does the choice of fibrinolytic agent impact on the importance of time-to-treatment? Am J Cardiol 2004; 94:772–774.

25. Nallamothu BK, Bates ER, Herrin J, et al; NRMI Investigators. Times to treatment in transfer patients undergoing primary percutaneous coronary intervention in the United States: National Registry of Myocardial Infarction (NRMI)-3/4 analysis. Circulation 2005; 111:761–767.

26. Pinto DS, Kirtane AJ, Nallamothu BK, et al. Hospital delays in reperfusion for ST-elevation myocardial infarction: implications when selecting a reperfusion strategy. Circulation 2006; 114:2019–2025.

27. Steg PG, Bonnefoy E, Chabaud S, et al; Comparison of Angioplasty and Prehospital Thrombolysis in acute Myocardial infarction (CAPTIM) Investigators. Impact of time to treatment on mortality after prehospital fibrinolysis or primary angioplasty: data from the CAPTIM randomized clinical trial. Circulation 2003; 108:2851–2856.

28. Stenestrand U, Lindbäck J, Wallentin L; RIKS-HIA Registry. Long-term outcome of primary percutaneous coronary intervention vs prehospital and in-hospital thrombolysis for patients with ST-elevation myocardial infarction. JAMA 2006; 296:1749–1756.

29. Björklund E, Stenestrand U, Lindbäck J, et al. Pre-hospital thrombolysis delivered by paramedics is associated with reduced time delay and mortality in ambulance-transported real-life patients with ST-elevation myocardial infarction. Eur Heart J 2006; 27:1146–1152.

30. Danchin N, Blanchard D, Steg PG, et al; USIC 2000 Investigators. Impact of prehospital thrombolysis for acute myocardial infarction on 1-year outcome: results from the French Nationwide USIC 2000 Registry. Circulation 2004; 110:1909–1915.

31. European Myocardial Infarction Project Group. Prehospital thrombolytic therapy in patients with suspected acute myocardial infarction. N Engl J Med 1993; 329:383–389.

32. GREAT Group. Feasibility, safety, and efficacy of domiciliary thrombolysis by general practitioners: Grampian region early anistreplase trial. BMJ 1992; 305:548–553.

33. Morrison LJ, Verbeek PR, McDonald AC, et al. Mortality and prehospital thrombolysis for acute myocardial infarction: a meta-analysis. JAMA 2000; 283:2686–2692.

34. Zimarino M, Sacchetta D, Renda G, et al. Facilitated PCI: rationale, current evidence, open questions and future directions. J Cardiovasc Pharmacol 2008; 51:3–10.

35. Gersh BJ, Stone GW, White HD, et al. Pharmacological facilitation of primary percutaneous coronary intervention for acute myocardial infarction: is the slope of the curve the shape of the future? JAMA 2005; 293:979–986.

36. Abraham JM, Gibson CM, Pena G, et al. Association of angiographic perfusion score following percutaneous coronary intervention for ST-elevation myocardial infarction with left ventricular remodeling at 6 weeks in GRACIA-2. J Thromb Thrombolysis 2009; 27(3):253–258.

37. Assessment of the Safety and Efficacy of a New Treatment Strategy with Percutaneous Coronary Intervention (ASSENT-4 PCI) Investigators. Primary versus tenecteplase-facilitated percutaneous coronary intervention in patients with ST-segment elevation acute myocardial infarction (ASSENT-4 PCI): randomised trial. Lancet 2006; 367:569–578.

38. Ellis SG, Tendera M, de Belder MA,et al. Facilitated PCI in patients with ST-elevation myocardial infarction. N Engl J Med 2008; 358:2205–2217.

39. Keeley EC, Boura JA, Grines CL. Comparison of primary and facilitated percutaneous coronary interventions for ST-elevation myocardial infarction: quantitative review of randomised trials. Lancet 2006; 367:579–588.

40. Kiernan TJ, Ting HH, Gersh BJ. Facilitated percutaneous coronary intervention: current concepts, promises, and pitfalls. Eur Heart J 2007; 28:1545–1553.

41. DiMario C, Dudek D, Piscione F, et al. Immediate angioplasty versus standard therapy with rescue angioplasty after thrombolysis in the combined Abciximab REteplase Stent Study in Acute Myocardial Infarction (CARESS-in-AMI): an open, prospective, randomized, multicentre trial. Lancet 2008; 371:559–568.

42. Danchin N, Belle L, Goldstein P, et al; for the FAST-MI Investigators. Combined prehospital thrombolysis and high use of early PCI in STEMI patients is associated with mortality outcomes comparing favourably with those of primary PCI: data from the French FAST-MI registry [abstract]. Eur Heart J 2007; 28(abstract suppl): 571–572.

43. Collet JP, Cambou JP, Goldstein P, et al; Danchin N for the working group of FAST-MI. Type of first medical contact and transfer organization rather than the number of

medical contacts prior to admission affect survival of STEMI patients. Insight from the FAST-MI registry [abstract]. Eur Heart J 2007; 28(abstract suppl):825.

44. Liem SS, Van Der Hoeven BL, et al. MISSION!: optimization of acute and chronic care for patients with acute myocardial infarction. Am Heart J 2007; 153:14.e1–e11.

45. Welsh RC, Chang W, Goldstein P, et al; ASSENT-3 PLUS Investigators. Time to treatment and the impact of a physician on prehospital management of acute ST elevation myocardial infarction: insights from the ASSENT-3 PLUS trial. Heart 2005; 91:1400–1406.

46. Franzosi MG, Santoro E, De Vita C, et al. Ten-year follow-up of the first megatrial testing thrombolytic therapy in patients with acute myocardial infarction: results of the Gruppo Italiano per lo Studio della Sopravvivenza nell'Infarto-1 study. The GISSI Investigators. Circulation 1998; 98:2659–2665.

47. Bell WR Jr. Evaluation of thrombolytic agents. Drugs 1997; 54(suppl 3):11–16.

48. Ouriel K. Comparison of safety and efficacy of the various thrombolytic agents. Rev Cardiovasc Med 2002; 3(suppl 2):S17–S24.

49. Mueller HS, Roberts R, Teichman SL, et al. Thrombolytic therapy in acute myocardial infarction: Part I. Med Clin North Am 1988; 72:197–226.

50. Tanswell P, Modi N, Combs D, et al. Pharmacokinetics and pharmacodynamics of tenecteplase in fibrinolytic therapy of acute myocardial infarction. Clin Pharmacokinet 2002; 41:1229–1245.

51. Assessment of the Safety and Efficacy of a New Thrombolytic (ASSENT-2) Investigators; Van De Werf F, Adgey J, Ardissino D, et al. Single-bolus tenecteplase compared with front-loaded alteplase in acute myocardial infarction: the ASSENT-2 double-blind randomised trial. Lancet 1999; 354:716–722.

52. Cannon CP. Thrombolysis medication errors: benefits of bolus thrombolytic agents. Am J Cardiol 2000; 85:17C–22C.

53. Cannon CP, McCabe CH, Gibson CM, et al. TNK-tissue plasminogen activator in acute myocardial infarction. Results of the Thrombolysis in Myocardial Infarction (TIMI) 10A dose-ranging trial. Circulation 1997; 95:351–356.

54. Cannon CP, Gibson CM, McCabe CH, et al. TNK-tissue plasminogen activator compared with front-loaded alteplase in acute myocardial infarction: results of the TIMI 10B trial. Thrombolysis in Myocardial Infarction (TIMI) 10B Investigators. Circulation 1998; 98:2805–2814.

55. Dunn CJ, Goa KL. Tenecteplase: a review of its pharmacology and therapeutic efficacy in patients with acute myocardial infarction. Am J Cardiovasc Drugs 2001; 1:51–66.

56. Gibson CM, Marble SJ. Issues in the assessment of the safety and efficacy of tenecteplase (TNK-tPA). Clin Cardiol 2001; 24:577–584.

57. Guerra DR, Karha J, Gibson CM. Safety and efficacy of tenecteplase in acute myocardial infarction. Expert Opin Pharmacother 2003; 4:791–798.

58. Van de Werf F, Cannon CP, et al. Safety assessment of single-bolus administration of TNK tissue-plasminogen activator in acute myocardial infarction: the ASSENT-1 trial. The ASSENT-1 Investigators. Am Heart J 1999; 137:786–791.

59. Van de Werf F, Barron HV, Armstrong PW, et al; ASSENT-2 Investigators. Assessment of the Safety and Efficacy of a New Thrombolytic. Incidence and predictors of bleeding events after fibrinolytic therapy with fibrin-specific agents: a comparison of TNK-tPA and rt-PA. Eur Heart J 2001; 22:2253–2261.

60. Topol EJ. Toward a new frontier in myocardial reperfusion therapy: emerging platelet preeminence. Circulation 1998; 97:211–218.

61. ISIS-2 (Second International Study of Infarct Survival) Collaborative Group. Randomised trial of intravenous streptokinase, oral aspirin, both, or neither among 17,187 cases of suspected acute myocardial infarction: ISIS-2. Lancet 1988; 2:349–360.

62. Task Force for Diagnosis and Treatment of Non-ST-Segment Elevation Acute Coronary Syndromes of European Society of Cardiology; Bassand JP, Hamm CW, Ardissino D, et al. Guidelines for the diagnosis and treatment of non-ST-segment elevation acute coronary syndromes. Eur Heart J 2007; 13:1598–660.

63. Gibler WB, Cannon CP, Blomkains AL, et al. Practical implementation of the guidelines for unstable angina/non-ST-segment elevation myocardial infarction in the emergency department: a scientific statement from the American Heart Association Council on Clinical Cardiology (Sub-committee on Acute Cardiac Care). Council on Cardiovascular nursing, and Quality of Care and Outcomes Research interdisciplinary Working Group, in Collaboration with the Society of Chest Pain Centers. Circulation 2005; 111:2699–2710.

64. Assez N, Rouyer F, Lapostolle F, et al. Syndromes coronariens aigus non ST+. Congres national d' anesthesia et de reanimation 2007. Les Essentiels. Elsevier Masson SAS, 2007.

65. Sabatine MS, Cannon CP, Gibson CM, et al; CLARITY-TIMI 28 Investigators. Addition of clopidogrel to aspirin and fibrinolytic therapy for myocardial infarction with ST-segment elevation. N Engl J Med 2005a; 352:1179–1189.

66. Sabatine MS. Something old, something new: beta blockers and clopidogrel in acute myocardial infarction. Lancet 2005; 366:1587–1589.

67. Scirica BM, Sabatine MS, Morrow DA, et al. The role of clopidogrel in early and sustained arterial patency after fibrinolysis for ST-segment elevation myocardial infarction: the ECG CLARITY-TIMI 28 Study. J Am Coll Cardiol 2006; 48:37–42.

68. Gibson CM, Murphy SA, Pride YB, et al; TIMI Study Group. Effects of pretreatment with clopidogrel on nonemergent percutaneous coronary intervention after fibrinolytic administration for ST-segment elevation myocardial infarction: a Clopidogrel as Adjunctive Reperfusion Therapy-Thrombolysis in Myocardial Infarction (CLARITY-TIMI) 28 study. Am Heart J 2008; 155:133–139.

69. Sabatine MS, Cannon CP, Gibson CM, et al; Clopidogrel as Adjunctive Reperfusion Therapy (CLARITY)-Thrombolysis in Myocardial Infarction (TIMI) 28 Investigators. Effect of clopidogrel pretreatment before percutaneous coronary intervention in patients with ST-elevation myocardial infarction treated with fibrinolytics: the PCI-CLARITY study. JAMA 2005b; 294:1224–1232.

70. Chen ZM, Jiang LX, Chen YP, et al; COMMIT (ClOpidogrel and Metoprolol in Myocardial Infarction Trial) Collaborative Group. Addition of clopidogrel to aspirin in 45,852 patients with acute myocardial infarction: randomised placebo-controlled trial. Lancet 2005; 366:1607–1621.

71. Dogan A, Ozgul M, Ozaydin M, et al. Effect of clopidogrel plus aspirin on tissue perfusion and coronary flow in patients with ST-segment elevation myocardial infarction: a new reperfusion strategy. Am Heart J 2005; 149:1037–1042.

72. Zeymer U, Gitt AK, Jünger C, et al; Acute COronary Syndromes (ACOS) Registry Investigators. Effect of clopidogrel on 1-year mortality in hospital survivors of acute ST-segment elevation myocardial infarction in clinical practice. Eur Heart J 2006; 27:2661–2666.

73. Montalescot G, Wiviott SD, Braunwald E, et al; TRITON-TIMI 38 investigators. Prasugrel compared with clopidogrel in patients undergoing percutaneous coronary intervention for ST-elevation myocardial infarction (TRITON-TIMI 38): double-blind, randomised controlled trial. Lancet. 2009; 373(9665):723–731

74. Wiviott SD, Trenk D, Frelinger AL, et al. Prasugrel compared with high loading-and maintenance-dose clopidogrel in patients with planned percutaneous coronary intervention: the Prasugrel in Comparison to Clopidogrel for Inhibition of Platelet Activation and Aggregation-Thrombolysis in Myocardial Infarction 44 trial. Circulation 2007a; 116:2923–2932.

75. Oler A, Whooley MA, Oler J, et al. Adding heparin to aspirin reduces the incidence of myocardial infarction and death in patients with unstable angina. A meta-analysis. JAMA 1996; 276:811–815.

76. Montalescot G, Collet JP, Lison L, et al. Effects of various anticoagulant treatments on von Willebrand factor release in unstable angina. J Am Coll Cardiol 2000; 36:110–114.

77. Cohen M. The role of low-molecular-weight heparin in the management of acute coronary syndromes. Curr Opin Cardiol 2001; 16:384–389.
78. Eikelboom JW, Quinlan DJ, Mehta SR, et al. Unfractionated and low-molecular-weight heparin as adjuncts to thrombolysis in aspirin-treated patients with ST-elevation acute myocardial infarction: a meta-analysis of the randomized trials. Circulation 2005; 112:3855–3867.
79. Antman EM, Morrow DA, McCabe CH, et al; ExTRACT-TIMI 25 Investigators. Enoxaparin versus unfractionated heparin with fibrinolysis for ST-elevation myocardial infarction. N Engl J Med 2006; 354:1477–1488.
80. White HD, Braunwald E, Murphy SA, et al. Enoxaparin vs. unfractionated heparin with fibrinolysis for ST-elevation myocardial infarction in elderly and younger patients: results from ExTRACT-TIMI 25. Eur Heart J 2007; 28:1066–1071.
81. Singh S, Molnar J, Arora R. Efficacy and safety of bivalirudin versus heparins in reduction of cardiac outcomes in acute coronary syndrome and percutaneous coronary interventions. J Cardiovasc Pharmacol Ther 2007; 12:283–291.
82. Stone GW, McLaurin BT, Cox DA, et al. Bivalirudin for patients with acute coronary syndromes. N Engl J Med 2006; 355:2203–2216.
83. Stone GW, Witzenbichler B, Guagliumi G, et al. Bivalirudine during primary PCI in acute myocardial infarction. N Engl J Med 2008; 358:2218–2230.
84. Assessment of the Safety and Efficacy of a New Thrombolytic Regimen (ASSENT)-3 Investigators. Efficacy and safety of tenecteplase in combination with enoxaparin, abciximab, or unfractionated heparin: the ASSENT-3 randomised trial in acute myocardial infarction. Lancet 2001; 358:605–613.
85. Topol EJ; GUSTO V Investigators. Reperfusion therapy for acute myocardial infarction with fibrinolytic therapy or combination reduced fibrinolytic therapy and platelet glycoprotein IIb/IIIa inhibition: the GUSTO V randomised trial. Lancet 2001; 357:1905–1914.
86. Lincoff AM, Califf RM, Van de Werf F, et al; Global Use of Strategies to Open Coronary Arteries Investigators (GUSTO). Mortality at 1 year with combination platelet glycoprotein IIb/IIIa inhibition and reduced-dose fibrinolytic therapy vs conventional fibrinolytic therapy for acute myocardial infarction: GUSTO V randomized trial. JAMA 2002; 288:2130–2135.
87. Arhan A, Ecollan P, Madonna-Py B, et al. Assessment of early administration of abciximab in acute ST-segment elevation myocardial infarction in the emergency room. Presse Med 2006; 35:45–50.
88. Glatt B, Luycx-Bore A, Guyon P, et al. Pre-hospitalization treatment with Abciximab in the preparation of patients for primary angioplasty in the acute phase of myocardial infarct. Immediate and long-term (one month) results [article in French]. Arch Mal Coeur Vaiss 1999; 92:1301–1308.
89. Svensson L, Aasa M, Dellborg M, et al. Comparison of very early treatment with either fibrinolysis or percutaneous coronary intervention facilitated with abciximab with respect to ST recovery and infarct-related artery epicardial flow in patients with acute ST-segment elevation myocardial infarction: the Swedish Early Decision (SWEDES) reperfusion trial. Am Heart J 2006; 151:798.e1–e7.
90. Montalescot G, Barragan P, Wittenberg O, et al. Platelet glycoprotein IIb/IIIa inhibition with coronary stenting for acute myocardial infarction. N Eng J Med 2001; 344:1895–1903.
91. The ADMIRAL Investigators. Three-year duration of benefit from abciximab in patients receiving stents for acute myocardial infarction in the randomized double-blind ADMIRAL study. Eur Heart J 2005; 26:2520–2523.
92. Montalescot G, Borentain M, Payot L, et al. Early vs late administration of glycoprotein IIb/IIIa inhibitors in primary percutaneous coronary intervention of acute ST-segment elevation myocardial infarction: a meta-analysis. JAMA 2004; 292:362–366.

93. Hamm CW, van t'Hof A, ten Berg JM, et al. ONgoing-Tirofiban in Myocardial Infarction Evaluation :ON-TIME 2 trial. Presented at the 57th scientific session of American College of Cardiology; March 29th–April 1st 2008; Chicago.
94. SAMU de France. Société francophone de médecine d'urgence, and Société française de cardiologie. Prise en charge de l'infarctus du myocarde à la phase aiguë en dehors des services de cardiologie. Conférence de consensus; November, 2006; Paris, France.

3 Presentation of AMI—Symptoms, Examination, Biomarkers, and Atypical Presentations

Christopher P. Moriates
Department of Medicine, University of California, San Francisco, California, U.S.A.

Kabir J. Singh
Department of Cardiology, University of California, San Francisco, California, U.S.A.

Alan S. Maisel
Department of Cardiovascular Medicine, University of California, San Francisco, California, U.S.A.

CLASSIC PRESENTATIONS OF AMI

Though the symptoms and signs of myocardial ischemia can often be nonspecific, familiarity with the more common, "classic" presentations is critical for virtually all physicians. A focused history and physical examination, with particular attention towards risk factors, are central components to the evaluation of patients presenting with chest pain and/or dyspnea.

History and Symptoms

The classic chest pain associated with an acute myocardial infarction (AMI) is often described as a "pressure," "heaviness," "tightness," "aching," or "squeezing." However, other pain patterns are also common. In a multicenter chest pain study, 22% had sharp, stabbing pain, 13% had pleuritic pain, and 7% had reproducible pain (1). The severity of the pain varies but can be severe to intolerable. It generally lasts for more than 30 minutes, differentiating itself from angina, which should relieve relatively quickly with rest (<2–10 minutes). The pain is often retrosternal and/or on the left side of the chest, although patients may commonly present with referred pain to the neck, jaw, shoulder, or arms. Chest pain radiation is strongly associated with myocardial ischemia (2). Chest pain radiating to the left arm is approximately 1.5 times as likely to occur in patients with AMI as compared to those with noncardiac chest pain; and radiation to the right arm/shoulder is more than twice as likely to occur in patients with AMI (Table 1) (3). The response to nitroglycerin does not assist in diagnosis, with a sensitivity of 35% and a specificity of 59% for AMI (4, 5).

Circadian Variation

It has been shown that there is a marked circadian variation in the frequency of onset of AMI, with a peak incidence occurring between 6 a.m. and noon. There appears to be a threefold increase in onset of AMI at peak (9 a.m.) as compared with trough (11 p.m.) periods (6). There has also been evidence of increased

TABLE 1 Sensitivity, Specificity, Positive and Negative Likelihood Ratios, and Odds Ratios for Signs and Symptoms of AMI in Pooled Studies of Selected Patient Groups

Symptom	Sensitivity (95% CI)	Specificity (95% CI)	LR+ (95% CI)	LR− (95% CI)	OR (95% CI)
Pain in left arm and/or shoulder	54 (50.2–56.9)	65 (56.4–72.8)	1.49 (1.20–1.85)	0.76 (0.66–0.88)	2.00 (1.39–2.88)
Pain in right arm and/or shoulder	32 (25.1–40.8)	86 (78.4–91.2)	2.35 (1.44–3.84)	0.81 (0.66–1.00)	3.09 (1.63–5.85)
Pain in neck	24 (18.3–30.2)	75 (71.6–77.7)	0.99 (0.83–1.17)	1.00 (0.95–1.07)	0.98 (0.78–1.23)
Pain in back	25 (22.0–28.2)	71 (66.4–75.6)	0.84 (0.62–1.14)	1.07 (0.96–1.19)	0.78 (0.52–1.19)
Epigastric pain	5 (2.1–10.8)	91 (85.0–95.4)	0.73 (0.61–0.87)	1.04 (1.02–1.05)	0.69 (0.57–0.85)
Oppressive pain	77 (71.3–81.2)	35 (28.7–41.3)	1.79 (1.07–1.30)	0.70 (0.52–0.86)	1.77 (1.25–2.51)
Vomiting and/or nausea	29 (12.5–51.5)	81 (76.6–85.1)	1.42 (0.76–2.64)	0.82 (0.66–1.03)	1.73 (0.71–4.12)
Sweating	41 (22.9–60.5)	85 (69.2–94.7)	2.44 (1.42–4.20)	0.72 (0.56–0.91)	3.81 (1.88–7.70)

Abbreviations: LR+, positive likelihood ratio; LR−, negative likelihood ratio; OR, odds ratio; CI, confidence interval.
Source: Adapted from Ref. 3.

sudden cardiac death and "silent" infarctions during this same time period, with at least a 70% higher risk of sudden cardiac death during the peak period versus the average risk during other times of the day (7). Proposed mechanisms include morning rises in plasma catecholamines and/or cortisol, and increases in platelet aggregability.

ATYPICAL PRESENTATIONS OF AMI

AMI often presents atypically or even asymptomatically ("Silent MI"). Atypical chest pain may be not as severe or prolonged or may involve areas other than the chest, such as the arms, epigastrium, shoulder, or neck. It also may be of an atypical quality, such as burning, sharp, positional, or pleuritic. It is clear that atypical symptoms do not rule out acute coronary syndrome (ACS), and in fact some researchers have found that up to 30% of patients with ACS do not have chest pain at all (8). Sudden dyspnea has been observed to be the sole presenting feature in 4% to 14% of patients with AMI (9). Other observed atypical symptoms of AMI include dizziness/syncope, epigastric discomfort, fatigue, palpitations, or midback pain (10). Atypical presentations may be more prevalent in certain groups, including the elderly, diabetics, and women.

Unrecognized ("Silent") MI

Unrecognized, or so-called "silent," myocardial infarctions (MI) are often found as diagnostic Q-waves on subsequent ECGs, without a history of preceding ischemic symptoms. Multiple large cohort studies have found that the rate of unrecognized AMIs represent approximately 22% to 44% of all MIs (11). It is estimated that approximately half of affected patients actually had absolutely no symptoms whatsoever, whereas the other half of the patients experienced nonspecific symptoms that at the time were not thought to be due to AMI (11). It has been suggested that diabetes mellitus, hypertension, and advanced age may be associated with higher incidences of unrecognized AMIs, however, the data is conflicting.

Presentation in the Elderly

Elderly patients appear to often present with atypical symptoms. Patients with diagnosed ST-segment elevation myocardial infarction (STEMI) above the age of 85 have significantly lower occurrences of chest pain at presentation when compared to patients younger than 65 years (56.8% versus 89.9%, respectively) (12).

Presentation in Women

It has been well established that women with ACS tend to be older than men with such syndromes and are more likely to have a prior history of hypertension, diabetes, angina, and congestive heart failure. They also are less likely to be smokers and less likely to have had a prior MI than their male counterparts (13).

In both men and women, chest pain and dyspnea are the most frequently reported symptoms. In one series, after adjustment for age and diabetes, women were observed to be more likely to present with nausea and/or vomiting (OR 2.43), and indigestion (OR 2.13) than men (14).

PHYSICAL EXAMINATION IN AMI

The physical examination of a patient with chest pain is very important, particularly in evaluating for nonischemic causes of chest pain. For instance, the diagnosis of an aortic dissection or pulmonary embolism would lead the clinician down very different therapeutic routes. It may be true that the physical examination is better for ruling out other causes of chest pain, rather than ruling in an AMI, since the physical examination in AMI can vary dramatically. The physical examination in a patient suspected to have ACS should focus on the vital signs, cardiac and chest examinations, as well as sequelae of CAD risk factors such as obesity or evidence of peripheral vascular disease.

Vitals
Immediate attention should be directed toward the vital signs. Though there are numerous variables that affect the vital signs, and there are not any specific findings that point to an AMI (indeed the vitals may often be completely normal), the careful consideration of the vital signs is an important initial step in the triage of any patient with an AMI.

Heart Rate and Rhythm
Sinus tachycardia at 100–110 bpm is the most common abnormality observed in AMI, most likely due to a combination of pain and anxiety. Premature ventricular contractions are very common in patients suffering an AMI, and in fact have been shown to be present in more than 95% of patients within the first four hours of ischemia (15). Depending on the area of myocardium injured, marked bradycardia and/or irregular rhythms are possible. Ischemia can lead to ventricular fibrillation or ventricular tachycardia, commonly within the first 48 hours following an AMI. Supraventricular arrhythmias may also occur, potentially secondary to a number of different factors including ischemia, drugs, or autonomic nervous system activation.

Blood Pressure
The baseline blood pressure of the patient should be taken into consideration when assessing the current blood pressure. Patients presenting with AMI are usually normotensive, however, an adrenergic response to the pain and anxiety may lead to hypertension. An inferior AMI may cause a Bezold-Jarisch reflex, which can result in vagal stimulation, leading to hypotension. A large AMI may lead to cardiogenic shock, resulting in systolic blood pressure below 90 mm Hg with organ hypoperfusion.

Respiratory Rate
The respiratory rate is often slightly elevated secondary to the patient's anxiety and pain. In left ventricular failure (LVF), pulmonary edema develops and the respiratory rate usually correlates with the severity of failure.

General Appearance
The typical patient presenting with an AMI will appear anxious, distressed, and restless. If the infarction results in failure, the sympathetic autonomic nervous system may be activated, resulting in a cold sweat and skin pallor. If the AMI results in cardiogenic shock, the patient will likely present lying listless with cool, clammy skin, bluish or mottled extremities, facial pallor, cyanosis, and possibly confusion or disorientation.

Neck
Examination of the neck in a patient with AMI should focus on the jugular venous distention (JVD) and the carotid pulse. The JVD is typically normal in AMI, however, it may be elevated in cases of cardiogenic shock or tamponade. The carotid pulse may provide a clue to underlying cardiac injury, with a weak carotid pulse suggesting reduced stroke volume. It is also important to note any carotid bruits that suggest systemic atherosclerosis.

Chest
The chest examination should evaluate for evidence of heart failure, as well as to rule out other causes of acute chest pain, including pneumonia, pneumothorax, or pulmonary embolism. In LV failure, pulmonary edema may result in rales or diffuse wheezing.

Cardiac
The cardiac examination may be normal in AMI, even in cases of extensive myocardial damage. However, there are many instances when a thorough cardiac examination may reveal a critical finding necessitating immediate management.

Palpation
Most commonly, palpation of the precordium does not reveal any abnormalities; however, a transmural STEMI can lead to a palpable presystolic pulsation as a result of a vigorous left atrium contraction filling the left ventricle with decreased compliance.

Auscultation
The heart sounds (S1, S2) are frequently muffled or soft immediately following an AMI. An S4 gallop is very common in patients with an AMI, and is considered to be universally present in patients in sinus rhythm with an STEMI. An S3 gallop usually reflects severe left ventricular dysfunction with increased left ventricular filling pressures.

Systolic murmurs are sometimes present following an AMI and may be transient or persistent. New onset systolic murmurs following an AMI are often the result of acute mitral regurgitation (MR) due to dysfunction of the valve apparatus. A pericardial friction rub is present in approximately 7% to 20% of patients with AMI (15). It is especially heard in patients with large transmural AMI.

The Killip Class
In 1967, Killip created a system to risk stratify patients presenting with AMI based on physical examination findings (Table 2) (16). To date, this remains one of the most accurate prognostic tools. The use of the well-known Killip classification system has been validated to predict mortality in patients treated with thrombolytic agents and those treated with primary percutaneous coronary intervention. Furthermore, a study of more than 26,000 patients with non-ST-elevation ACS found that the Killip classification provided powerful and independent prognostic information for both 30-day and six-month all-cause mortality (Fig. 1), and in fact claimed that Killip class III/IV is the "most powerful predictor of short-term and long-term mortality in non-ST-elevation ACS" (17).

TABLE 2 The Killip Classification System

Killip class	Physical findings	Mortality
I	No heart failure	6%
II	Mild heart failure: rales at bases, S3 gallop, or elevated JVP	17%
III	Heart failure: acute pulmonary edema	38%
IV	Cardiogenic shock (SBP <90 mm Hg, cyanosis, oliguria, sweating)	81%

Abbreviations: JVP, Jugular venous pressure; SBP, Systolic blood pressure.
Source: From Ref. 16.

ECG DIAGNOSIS OF AMI

The electrocardiogram (ECG) is considered the single most important data in the initial evaluation of suspected AMI and should be obtained within five to ten minutes after presentation (18). Approximately 50% to 60% of patients with AMI will have diagnostic ECG changes. Still, the findings may be nonspecific; thus, the pretest probability of an individual patient having coronary artery disease must be taken into account when interpreting the ECG. The careful evaluation of the ST segment will influence decisions regarding management.

While it is possible for an ECG to be completely normal in a patient with significant myocardial ischemia and evolving infarction, there is a "classic" ECG evolution that occurs in acute STEMI. Typically the first changes to develop are "hyperacute" T waves, which are followed by ST elevations with possible reciprocal ST depressions. Generally, this is followed by the appearance of

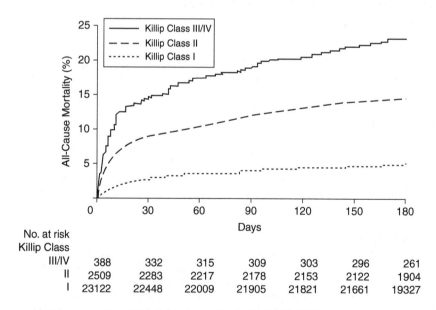

p < 001 for comparison of Killip Class I vs. Class II vs. Class III/IV.

FIGURE 1 Kaplan-Meier curve of all-cause mortality in patients with non-ST-elevation acute coronary syndromes according to Killip Classification. Data is from a combined analysis of 26,090 patients with non-ST-elevation ACS. *Source*: From Ref. 17.

TABLE 3 ECG Findings for the Diagnosis of Acute Coronary Syndromes

Occluded vessel	Myocardial territory	ECG Changes		Sensitivity	Specificity	PPV	NPV
		ST elevation	ST depression				
Proximal left anterior descending	Anterior wall	VI, V2, V3	II, III, aVF	34	98	93	68
Distal left anterior descending	Anterior wall and apex	VI, V2, V3	II, III, aVF	66	73	78	62
Circumflex	Lateral wall	I, aVL, V5, V6	VI, V2, V3	83	96	91	93
Right coronary artery	Posterior lateral segment, inferior segment, posterior septum	III>II	I, aVL, or both	90	71	94	70

Source: Adapted from Ref. 31.

abnormal Q waves within 24 hours. Eventually, the progression leads to T-wave inversions and ST-segment normalization. Subendocardial ischemia classically leads to ST-segment depression and/or T-wave inversion. Table 3 shows different ECG findings in ACS.

BIOMARKERS IN AMI
Serum biomarkers have become an essential tool in the evaluation of patients with chest pain. Elevations of biomarkers indicating myocardial necrosis are now required for the diagnosis of AMI, and a variety of other biomarkers carry additional diagnostic and prognostic information.

Markers of Myocardial Necrosis
The biomarkers of cardiac myocyte necrosis include the troponins I and T (TnI/TnT), creatine kinase (CK) and its myocardium-specific subtype CK-MB, and myoglobin. The unique kinetics (Fig. 2), strengths, and limitations of each biomarker in the diagnosis of ACS makes a multimarker strategy optimal and is routine clinical practice.

Troponins
A rise and fall of troponins (either TnT or TnI), in the setting of clinical symptoms or pathologic ECG changes, is required for the diagnosis of AMI. Cardiac-specific isotypes are released from myocytes in response to necrosis, making these proteins both highly sensitive and specific for cardiac injury. Initial elevations in troponins are typically seen within four to six hours of initial injury; they peak within 12 to 24 hours and remain elevated for approximately one to two weeks. The sustained duration of troponin elevation assists in the diagnosis of a delayed presentation of AMI. Serial assays were shown to provide incremental diagnostic information in the large Global Use of Strategies to Open occluded coronary arteries (GUSTO) IIa study. In that study, the majority of patients that ultimately demonstrated a positive troponin had a negative test at presentation. Moreover, those with negative troponin levels on serial testing had a zero percent 30-day mortality (19).

Troponin elevations also guide treatment and offer prognostic information. The use of low-molecular-weight heparin, glycoprotein IIb-IIIa antagonists, and early interventional strategy in ACS have all been shown to benefit patients with

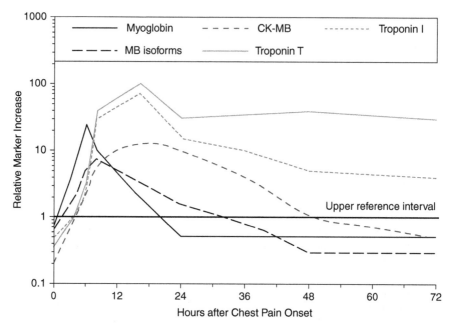

FIGURE 2 Time course of various markers of cardiac myocyte necrosis following symptom onset. *Source*: From Ref. 22.

troponin elevations, with only marginal or no benefit shown in those with a normal level. Troponins also implicate an increased short-term risk of MI and death. In one meta-analysis surveying 21 studies with a total of 18,982 patients with ACS, an elevated troponin was associated with an increased risk of 30-day mortality or MI (odds ratio [OR] 2.86, 95% confidence interval [CI] 2.35–3.47) (20). This association was even more robust in patients presenting with ST-elevation MI (OR 4.93, 95% CI 3.77–6.45).

Creatine Kinase and CK-MB

Creatine kinase (CK) is present in many organs and in high concentration in striated muscle, so it is not a specific marker. The subtype CK-MB is more specific to myocardium, however, it is present in skeletal muscle and can be elevated in conditions other than myocardial ischemia. Therefore, elevations in CK or CK-MB should always be further evaluated with the more specific troponins. CK and CK-MB both become detectable at about 4–12 hours after the onset of myocardial necrosis, peak at 18–24 hours, and fall to normal within 36–48 hours. The relatively rapid clearance and moderate specificity make CK and CK-MB useful markers for the diagnosis of early or peri-procedural re-infarction. Elevated CK-MB levels, regardless of total CK, carry an increased relative risk of 25% to 49% for worse outcomes (21). However, patients with isolated CK-MB elevation, in the absence of troponin elevation, were found to not be associated with significantly different risk than patients with both markers negative (22).

Myoglobin
Myoglobin is generally the earliest detectable biomarker of cardiac necrosis, with rising concentrations as early as one to three hours following onset. However, myoglobin is a ubiquitous heme protein, and is therefore nonspecific. Myoglobin concentration peaks within six hours and returns to baseline within about 24 hours. The greatest value of myoglobin measurement is its strong negative predictive value, which has been found to be as high as 97.3% (23).

Markers of Hemodynamic Stress
Natriuretic peptides (NPs), well known for their role in the diagnosis and management of heart failure, may have a role in the setting of ACS. Both B-type natriuretic peptide (BNP) and the amino-terminal fragment of its precursor, NT-proBNP, have been shown in multiple studies to be independent predictors of short- and long-term mortality (24). In a substudy of the GUSTO-IV trial including 6,809 ACS patients, quartiles of NT-proBNP predicted both short-term and one-year mortality (25). This predictive value was superior to other established prognostic markers, including troponin T and renal function. Furthermore, among patients with non-ST-elevation MI or unstable angina, NTproBNP elevation also identified patients who had a mortality benefit from PCI (26). Multiple studies, including TACTICS-TIMI-18, have shown the NPs to predict the onset of new heart failure after ACS (27). Perhaps surprisingly, most studies have found that NPs have not identified patients at risk for recurrent infarction. Though it is clear that NPs offer substantial prognostic information in the setting of ACS, above and beyond other recognized prognostic markers, their exact role in the management of ACS patients has yet to be determined.

Markers of Ischemia
Biomarkers for ischemia, as a harbinger of impending necrosis, would prove extraordinarily useful in early diagnosis of ACS, possibly allowing for intervention prior to myocardial damage. Of the ischemia markers currently under investigation, ischemia-modified albumin (IMA) and heart-type fatty acid biding protein (H-FABP) are among the most promising.

IMA is a modified form of human serum albumin generated during ischemia, possibly via oxidative free radicals (28). IMA accounts for 1% to 2% of total albumin concentration in the normal population as compared to 6% to 8% in patients with ischemia. Several studies have shown IMA to increase within minutes of ischemia, remain elevated for 6 to 12 hours, and normalize within 24 hours. In one meta-analysis including 1800 patients, IMA, in conjunction with ECG and troponin, demonstrated a sensitivity of 94.4% and NPV of 97.1% in diagnosis of AMI at initial presentation, representing a substantial improvement over troponin and ECG alone in early diagnosis (29).

H-FABP is a protein that has a kinetic profile similar to that of myoglobin, though it potentially has improved specificity. Early studies suggest that FABP may have improved sensitivity over troponin within 2 hours of presentation, though is substantially less specific.

Markers of Inflammation and Oxidative Stress
Plaque rupture with subsequent thrombus formation is hypothesized to be a primary event in the pathophysiology of ACS. Though the factors that contribute

to plaque instability have yet to be elucidated, a close association between markers of inflammation and cardiovascular risk has been observed, suggesting that chronic inflammation may play an important role.

C-reactive Protein (CRP) is an acute phase reactant and a well-recognized marker of systemic inflammation. Patients presenting with non-ST-elevation ACS have been observed to have higher CRP levels than those with stable or variant angina, and elevations of CRP have been shown to correlate with the number of angiographically significant stenoses. Further, increases in CRP are associated worse short- and long-term prognosis independent of troponin levels in ACS patients.

Myeloperoxidase (MPO) is a pro-oxidative and pro-inflammatory enzyme released by neutrophils. It is found in abundance in ruptured plaque, and levels in the circulation have been associated with plaque instability (30). MPO levels increase within two hours of symptom onset, and return to baseline within one week of presentation. Chest pain patients with decreased neutrophil MPO content (indicating recent MPO activity) have been found to have increased short-term mortality. Importantly, this phenomenon has been observed to be strongest in those with undetectable troponin, the excess mortality risk is realized within 72 hours of presentation, and neutrophil MPO content returns to within normal range within a week of presentation. Taken together, MPO may find utility as a marker of plaque instability implying substantial short-term risk, even in the absence of frank infarct.

REFERENCES

1. Lee TH, Cook EF, Weisberg M, et al. Acute chest pain in the emergency room. Identification and examination of low-risk patients. Arch Intern Med 1985; 145:65–69.
2. Goodacre S, Locker T, Morris F, et al. How useful are clinical features in the diagnosis of acute, undifferentiated chest pain? Acad Emerg Med 2002; 9:203–208.
3. Bruyninckx R, Aertgeerts B, Bruyninckx P, et al. Signs and symptoms in diagnosing acute myocardial infarction and acute coronary syndrome: a diagnostic meta-analysis. Br J Gen Pract 2008; 58:105–111.
4. Gibbons RJ. Nitroglycerin: should we still ask? Ann Intern Med 2003; 139:1036–1037.
5. Shry EA, Dacus J, Van De Graaff E, et al. Usefulness of the response to sublingual nitroglycerin as a predictor of ischemic chest pain in the emergency department. Am J Cardiol 2002; 90:1264–1266.
6. Muller JE, Stone PH, Turi ZG, et al. Circadian variation in the frequency of onset of acute myocardial infarction. N Engl J Med 1985; 313:1315–1322.
7. Willich SN, Levy D, Rocco MB, et al. Circadian variation in the incidence of sudden cardiac death in the Framingham Heart Study population. Am J Cardiol 1987; 60:801–806.
8. Coronado BE, Pope JH, Griffith JL, et al. Clinical features, triage, and outcome of patients presenting to the ED with suspected acute coronary syndromes but without pain: a multicenter study. Am J Emerg Med 2004; 22:568–574.
9. McCarthy BD, Wong JB, Selker HP. Detecting acute cardiac ischemia in the emergency department: a review of the literature. J Gen Intern Med 1990; 5:365–373.
10. Funk M, Naum JB, Milner KA, et al. Presentation and symptom predictors of coronary heart disease in patients with and without diabetes. Am J Emerg Med 2001; 19:482–487.
11. Sheifer SE, Manolio TA, Gersh BJ. Unrecognized myocardial infarction. Ann Intern Med 2001; 135:801–811.
12. Alexander KP, Newby LK, Armstrong PW, et al. Acute coronary care in the elderly, part II: ST-segment-elevation myocardial infarction: a scientific statement for healthcare professionals from the American Heart Association Council on Clinical

Cardiology: in collaboration with the Society of Geriatric Cardiology. Circulation 2007; 115:2570–2789.

13. Hochman JS, Tamis JE, Thompson TD, et al. Sex, clinical presentation, and outcome in patients with acute coronary syndromes. Global Use of Strategies to Open Occluded Coronary Arteries in Acute Coronary Syndromes IIb Investigators. N Engl J Med 1999; 341:226–232.

14. Milner KA, Funk M, Richards S, et al. Gender differences in symptom presentation associated with coronary heart disease. Am J Cardiol 1999; 84:396–399.

15. Zipes DP, Libby P, Bonow RO, et al. Braunwald's Heart Disease: A Textbook of Cardiovascular Medicine, 7th ed. Philadelphia, PA: Elsevier Saunders, 2004.

16. Killip T III, Kimball JT. Treatment of myocardial infarction in a coronary care unit. A two year experience with 250 patients. Am J Cardiol 1967; 20:457–464.

17. Khot UN, Jia G, Moliterno DJ, et al. Prognostic importance of physical examination for heart failure in non-ST-elevation acute coronary syndromes: the enduring value of Killip classification. JAMA 2003; 290:2174–2181.

18. Lee TH, Goldman L. Evaluation of the patient with acute chest pain. N Engl J Med 2000; 342:1187–1195.

19. Newby LK, Christenson RH, Ohman EM, et al. Value of serial troponin T measures for early and late risk stratification in patients with acute coronary syndromes. The GUSTO-IIa Investigators. Circulation 1998; 98:1853–1859.

20. Ottani F, Galvani M, Nicolini FA, et al. Elevated cardiac troponin levels predict the risk of adverse outcome in patients with acute coronary syndromes. Am Heart J 2000; 140:917–927.

21. Galla JM, Mahaffey KW, Sapp SK, et al. Elevated creatine kinase-MB with normal creatine kinase predicts worse outcomes in patients with acute coronary syndromes: results from 4 large clinical trials. Am Heart J 2006; 151:16–24.

22. Newby LK. Markers of cardiac ischemia, injury, and inflammation. Prog Cardiovasc Dis 2004; 46:404–416.

23. Laurino JP, Bender EW, Kessimian N, et al. Comparative sensitivities and specificities of the mass measurements of CK-MB2, CK-MB, and myoglobin for diagnosing acute myocardial infarction. Clin Chem 1996; 42:1454–1459.

24. Farmakis D, Filippatos G, Tubaro M, et al. Natriuretic peptides in acute coronary syndromes: prognostic value and clinical implications. Congest Heart Fail 2008; 14:25–29.

25. James SK, Lindahl B, Siegbahn A, et al. N-terminal pro-brain natriuretic peptide and other risk markers for the separate prediction of mortality and subsequent myocardial infarction in patients with unstable coronary artery disease: a Global Utilization of Strategies To Open occluded arteries (GUSTO)-IV substudy. Circulation 2003; 108:275–281.

26. James SK, Lindback J, Tilly J, et al. Troponin-T and N-terminal pro-B-type natriuretic peptide predict mortality benefit from coronary revascularization in acute coronary syndromes: a GUSTO-IV substudy. J Am Coll Cardiol 2006; 48:1146–1154.

27. Morrow DA, de Lemos JA, Sabatine MS, et al. Evaluation of B-type natriuretic peptide for risk assessment in unstable angina/non-ST-elevation myocardial infarction: B-type natriuretic peptide and prognosis in TACTICS-TIMI 18. J Am Coll Cardiol 2003; 41:1264–1272.

28. Pantazopoulos I, Papadimitriou L, Dontas I, et al. Ischaemia modified albumin in the diagnosis of acute coronary syndromes. Resuscitation 2009; 80:306–310.

29. Peacock F, Morris DL, Anwaruddin S, et al. Meta-analysis of ischemia-modified albumin to rule out acute coronary syndromes in the emergency department. Am Heart J 2006; 152:253–262.

30. Loria V, Dato I, Graziani F, Biasucci LM. Myeloperoxidase: a new biomarker of inflammation in ischemic heart disease and acute coronary syndromes. Mediators Inflamm 2008; 2008:135625.

31. Zimetbaum PJ, Josephson ME. Use of the electrocardiogram in acute myocardial infarction. N Engl J Med 2003; 348: 933–940.

The Definition of Myocardial Infarction

Kristian Thygesen

Department of Medicine and Cardiology, Aarhus University Hospital, Aarhus, Denmark

Joseph S. Alpert

University of Arizona College of Medicine, Tucson, Arizona, U.S.A.

Allan S. Jaffe

Cardiovascular Division, Core Clinical Laboratory Services (CCLS), Department of Laboratory Medicine and Pathology, Mayo Clinic and Medical School, Rochester, Minnesota, U.S.A.

DEFINITION OF MYOCARDIAL INFARCTION

Myocardial infarction (MI) is defined pathologically as myocardial cell death due to prolonged ischemia. In the clinical setting these conditions are met when the following criteria are present: Detection of a rise and/or fall of cardiac biomarkers with at least one value above the 99th percentile of the upper reference limit (URL) together with evidence of myocardial ischemia as recognized by at least one of the following: symptoms of ischemia, ECG changes of new ischemia or development of pathological Q waves, or imaging evidence of new loss of viable myocardium or new regional wall motion abnormality (Table 1) (1).

CLASSIFICATION OF MYOCARDIAL INFARCTION

MI can be a spontaneous event related to plaque rupture, fissuring, or dissection of an atherosclerotic plaque or as recently described, nodular plaque rupture, which is classified as MI type 1. Alternatively, MI can result from increased myocardial oxygen demand combined with inadequate myocardial supply of oxygen and nutrients. This could be the result of anemia, arrhythmia, and hyper- or hypotension. Vasoconstriction or arterial spasm, causing a marked reduction in myocardial blood flow can also lead to severe myocardial ischemia and MI. This second group of entities is termed MI type 2 (Table 2) (1).

One circumstance in which biomarkers are not of value in the diagnosis of MI is when the patient with a typical presentation for myocardial ischemia/infarction dies prior to the time when it is possible to detect blood biomarker elevations either because blood samples for troponin determination were not obtained or the patient succumbed soon after the onset of symptoms before troponin values could become elevated. Such patients are designated as having a MI type 3 (Table 2) (1).

Elevated troponin values (greater than $3 \times$ 99th percentile URL) following PCI are designated as an acute MI resulting from myocardial ischemia (MI type 4a). A second category of type 4 MI can be caused by stent thrombosis,

TABLE 1 Definition for Myocardial Infarction (1)

Any one of the following criteria meets the diagnosis for MI

Acute myocardial infarction
1. Detection of elevated values of cardiac biomarkers (preferably troponin) above the 99th percentile of the upper reference limit (URL) together with evidence of myocardial ischemia with at least one of the following:
    a. Ischemic symptoms
    b. ECG changes indicative of new ischemia (new ST-T changes or new LBBB)
    c. Development of pathological Q waves in the ECG
    d. Imaging evidence of new loss of viable myocardium or new regional wall motion abnormality
2. Sudden unexpected cardiac death, including cardiac arrest, with symptoms suggestive of myocardial ischemia, accompanied by new ST elevation, or new LBBB, or definite new thrombus by coronary angiography, but death occurring before blood samples could be obtained, or at a time before the appearance of cardiac biomarkers in the blood
3. For PCI in patients with normal baseline values, elevations of cardiac biomarkers above the 99th percentile URL are indicative of periprocedural myocardial necrosis. By convention, increases of biomarkers greater than 3 $\times$ 99th percentile URL have been designated as defining PCI-related MI
4. For CABG in patients with normal baseline values, elevations of cardiac biomarkers above the 99th percentile URL are indicative of periprocedural myocardial necrosis. By convention, increases of biomarkers greater than 5 $\times$ 99th percentile URL plus either new pathological Q waves or new LBBB, or angiographically documented new graft or native coronary artery occlusion, or imaging evidence of new loss of viable myocardium have been designated as defining CABG-related MI
5. Pathological findings postmortem of an acute MI

Prior myocardial infarction
1. Development of new pathological Q waves with or without symptoms
2. Imaging evidence of a region of loss of viable myocardium that is thinned and fails to contract in the absence of a nonischemic cause
3. Pathological findings postmortem of a healed or healing MI

TABLE 2 Clinical Classification of Different Types of Myocardial Infarction (1)

Type 1: Spontaneous MI related to ischemia due to a primary coronary event such as plaque erosion and/or rupture, fissuring, or dissection

Type 2: MI secondary to ischemia due to either increased oxygen demand or decreased supply, e.g., coronary artery spasm, coronary embolism, anemia, arrhythmias, hypertension, or hypotension

Type 3: Sudden unexpected cardiac death, including cardiac arrest, often with symptoms suggestive of myocardial ischemia, accompanied by presumably new ST elevation, or new LBBB, or evidence of fresh thrombus in a coronary artery by angiography and/or at autopsy, but death occurring before blood samples could be obtained, or at a time before the appearance of cardiac biomarkers in the blood

Type 4a: MI associated with PCI

Type 4b: MI associated with stent thrombosis as documented by angiography or at autopsy

Type 5: MI associated with CABG

and is termed MI type 4b. The criteria for the diagnosis of this type of acute MI are similar to those for types 1 and 2 (a rising pattern of troponin values with at least one sample above the 99th percentile URL). Moreover, elevations of troponin measurements (greater than 5 × 99th percentile URL) at the time of CABG should suggest evaluation for an MI type 5 that requires additional criteria as well (Table 2). Elevations of troponin at baseline are associated with greater elevations post procedurally. Accordingly, the guidelines for type 4a and type 5 require a normal baseline value (1).

CARDIAC BIOMARKERS

Cardiac troponins I and T are the preferred markers for the diagnosis of myocardial injury since these have nearly absolute myocardial tissue specificity, as well as high sensitivity, reflecting even microscopic zones of myocardial necrosis. Optimal precision at the 99th percentile URL for each assay should be defined as a coefficient of variation ≤10% (2). If troponin assays are not available, the best alternative is the MB fraction of CK measured by mass assay. As with troponin, an increased CKMB mass value is defined as a measurement above the 99th percentile URL using gender appropriate normal ranges (3). However, given its greater sensitivity and specificity, troponin is greatly preferred for the diagnosis of MI.

Both cTnI and cTnT, assuming good assays and appropriate cutoff values, perform comparably in terms of their diagnostic accuracy. The one difference between these two troponin assays occurs in renal failure patients where there are greater numbers of elevations of cTnT compared with cTnI. These elevations are usually stable over time (4). Pathologic studies suggest that these elevated values denote cardiac abnormalities in these patients with renal insufficiency (5). Moreover, they are highly prognostic (4) and thus, patients with renal insufficiency who have elevated levels of cTnT require further clinical evaluation, although not necessarily acutely. Although there is a relationship between cTnT elevations and coronary artery disease in these patients, not all elevations are due to coronary artery disease (6). If this group displays the characteristic rise and/or fall of cTnT values, albeit from an abnormal baseline, these renal patients are having acute events and should be assessed as having MI if there are signs and/or symptoms of ischemia (7).

A variety of disease entities can injure myocardium (e.g., trauma, myocarditis, chemotherapeutic agents, etc.) thereby leading to elevated blood values of troponin. These other entities are not the result of acute ischemic heart disease and careful clinical evaluation is essential to prevent these patients from being labeled as having had an acute MI (Table 3).

ELECTROCARDIOGRAPHY

The ECG criteria for the diagnosis of acute myocardial ischemia that may lead to infarction are listed in Table 4 (1). The measurement of ST elevation should be done at the J point to determine the magnitude of the ST elevation. J point elevation in men decreases with increasing age; however, that is not observed in women. Importantly, with infarction, J point elevation is less in women than in men (8).

As shown in Table 5, Q waves or QS complexes are usually pathognomonic of a prior MI in the absence of QRS confounders (9). ST or T wave deviations

TABLE 3   Elevations of Troponin in the Absence of Overt Ischemic Heart Disease (1)

Cardiac contusion, including ablation, pacing, cardioversion, or endomyocardial biopsy
Congestive heart failure—acute and chronic
Aortic dissection, aortic valve disease or hypertrophic cardiomyopathy
Tachy- or bradyarrhythmias, or heart block
Apical ballooning syndrome
Rhabdomyolysis with cardiac injury
Pulmonary embolism, severe pulmonary hypertension
Renal failure
Acute neurological disease, including stroke, or subarachnoid hemorrhage
Infiltrative diseases, e.g., amyloidosis, hemochromatosis, sarcoidosis, and scleroderma
Inflammatory diseases, e.g., myocarditis or myocardial extension of endo-/pericarditis
Drug toxicity, e.g., adriamycin, 5-fluorouracil, herceptin, snake venoms
Critically ill patients, especially with respiratory failure, or sepsis
Burns, especially if affecting >30% of body surface area

alone are nonspecific findings. However, when these abnormalities occur in the same leads as the Q waves, the likelihood of MI is increased (1).

IMAGING TECHNIQUES
Imaging techniques can be useful in the diagnosis of MI because of the ability to detect wall motion abnormalities in the presence of elevated cardiac biomarkers. If for some reason biomarkers have not been measured or may have normalized, demonstration of new loss of myocardial viability alone in the absence of a nonischemic cause would meet criteria for MI. Echocardiography is the imaging technique of choice for detecting complications of acute MI including myocardial free wall rupture, acute ventricular septal defect, and mitral regurgitation secondary to papillary muscle rupture or ischemia. However, echocardiography cannot distinguish regional wall motion abnormalities due to myocardial ischemia from infarction (1).

DEFINITION OF REINFARCTION
If a recurrent MI is suspected from clinical signs or symptoms following the initial MI, an immediate measurement of the employed cardiac marker (preferably troponin) is recommended. A second sample should be obtained three to six hours later. Recurrent infarction is diagnosed if there is a 20% or more increase of the value in the second sample (1,10).

   The ECG diagnosis of reinfarction following the initial MI may be confounded by the initial evolutionary ECG changes. Reinfarction should be considered when ST elevation ≥0.1 mV occurs in a patient previously with lesser

TABLE 4   ECG Manifestations of Acute Myocardial Ischemia (in the Absence of LVH and LBBB) (1)

ST elevation
   New ST elevation at the J point in two contiguous leads with the cut-off points: ≥0.2 mV in
   men or ≥0.15 mV in women in leads V_2–V_3 and/or ≥0.1 mV in other leads
ST depression and T wave changes
   New horizontal or downsloping ST depression ≥0.05 mV in two contiguous leads; and/or
   T inversion ≥0.1 mV in two contiguous leads with prominent R wave or R/S ratio >1

TABLE 5   ECG Changes Associated with Prior Myocardial Infarction (1)

- Any Q wave in leads V_2–V_3 $\geq$0.02 sec or QS complex in leads V_2 and V_3
- Q wave $\geq$0.03 sec and $\geq$0.1 mV deep or QS complex in leads I, II, aVL, aVF or V_4 –V_6 in any two leads of a contiguous lead grouping (I, aVL, V_6; V_4–V_6; II, III, aVF)
- R wave $\geq$0.04 sec in V_1–V_2 and R/S $\geq$1 with a concordant positive T wave in the absence of a conduction defect

degrees of ST elevation or if new pathognomonic Q waves develop in two contiguous leads, particularly when associated with ischemic symptoms of 20 minutes or longer. ST depression or LBBB alone should not be considered valid MI criteria (1).

Myocardial Infarction Associated with Revascularization Procedures

Periprocedural MI is different from the spontaneous infarction, because the former is associated with the instrumentation that is required during mechanical revascularization procedures either by PCI or CABG (11).

During PCI, myocardial necrosis may result from recognizable periprocedural events, alone or in combination, such as side-branch occlusion, disruption of collateral flow, distal embolization, coronary dissection, slow flow or no reflow phenomenon, and microvascular plugging. Embolization of intracoronary thrombus or atherosclerotic particulate debris cannot be entirely prevented despite current antiplatelet adjunctive therapy or protection devices. Such events induce extensive inflammation of noninfarcted myocardium surrounding small islets of myocardium necrosis. A separate subcategory of MI is related to stent thrombosis as documented by angiography and/or autopsy (1,11,12).

During CABG, numerous additional factors can lead to periprocedural necrosis. These include direct myocardial trauma from sewing needles or manipulation of the heart, coronary dissection, global or regional ischemia that cannot be totally obviated by techniques of cardiac protection, microvascular events related to reperfusion, myocardial damage induced by oxygen free radical generation, or failure to reperfuse areas of the myocardium that are not subtended by graftable vessels (11,13,14).

Diagnostic Criteria for Myocardial Infarction with PCI

In the setting of PCI, the balloon inflation during a procedure almost always results in ischemia whether or not accompanied by ST-T changes. The occurrence of procedure-related cell necrosis can be detected by measurement of cardiac biomarkers before or immediately after the procedure, and again at 6 to 12 and 18 to 24 hours (15,16). Elevations of biomarkers above the 99th percentile URL after PCI, assuming a normal baseline troponin value, are indicative of post procedural myocardial necrosis. If the baseline value is elevated, it is impossible to distinguish the injury associated with the procedure and that associated with the inciting event that leads to the elevation. If there are chronic elevations, criteria for reinfarction can be employed. There is currently no solid scientific basis for defining a biomarker threshold for the diagnosis of periprocedural MI. Pending further data, and by arbitrary convention, it is suggested to designate increases greater than 3 × 99th percentile URL as PCI-related MI type 4a. However, in the event of stent thrombosis as documented by angiography and/or autopsy in association with a troponin value above the 99th percentile URL, it is suggested to designate this subcategory as PCI-related MI type 4b (1).

Diagnostic Criteria for Myocardial Infarction with CABG
Any increase of cardiac biomarkers after CABG indicates myocyte necrosis, which is related to impaired outcome (14,17). One cannot distinguish between rises of biomarkers related to the details of anesthesia, cardioprotection, and technical aspects of the surgery from those related to graft or native coronary abnormalities. Thus, biomarkers cannot stand alone for the diagnosis of infarction. In view of the adverse impact on survival observed in patients with significant biomarker elevations, it is suggested, by arbitrary convention, that biomarker values greater than the $5 \times$ 99th percentile URL during the first 72 hours following CABG should prompt a search for other associated criteria such as appearance of new pathological Q waves or new LBBB, or angiographically documented new graft or native coronary artery occlusion, or imaging evidence of new loss of viable myocardium. If such criteria are met, the patient should be considered to have suffered a CABG-related MI type 5 (1).

REFERENCES
1. Thygesen K, Alpert JS, White HD, Joint ESC/ACCF/AHA/WHF Task Force for the Redefinition of Myocardial Infarction. Universal definition of myocardial infarction. Eur Heart J 2007; 28:2525–2538; Circulation 2007; 116:2634–2653; J Am Coll Cardiol 2007; 50:2173–2195.
2. Apple FS, Jesse RL, Newby LK, et al. National Academy of Clinical Biochemistry and IFCC Committee for Standardization of Markers Cardiac Damage Laboratory Medicine Practice Guidelines: analytical issues for biochemical markers of acute coronary syndromes. Circulation 2007; 115:e352–e355.
3. Panteghini M, Pagani F, Yeo KT, et al. Evaluation of imprecision for cardiac troponin assays at low-range concentrations. Clin Chem 2004; 50:327–332.
4. Apple F, Murakami M, Pearce L, et al. Predictive value of cardiac troponin I and T for subsequent death in end-stage renal disease. Circulation 2002; 106:2941–2945.
5. Ooi DS, Isotalo PA, Veinot JP. Correlation of antemortem serum creatine kinase, creatine kinase-MB, troponin I, and troponin T with cardiac pathology. Clin Chem 2000; 46:338–344.
6. Hayashi T, Obi Y, Kimura T, et al. Cardiac troponin T predicts occult coronary artery stenosis in patients with chronic kidney disease at the start of renal replacement therapy. Nephrol Dial Transplant 2008; 23:2936–2942.
7. Le Ehy, Klootwijk PJ, Weimar W, et al. Significance of acute versus chronic troponin T elevation in dialysis patients. Nephron Clin Pract 2004; 98:c87–c92.
8. Mcfarlane PW. Age, sex, and the ST amplitude in health and disease. J Electrocardiol 2001; 34:S35–S41.
9. Pahlm US, Chaitman BR, Rautaharju PM, et al. Comparison of the various electrocardiographic scoring codes for estimating anatomically documented sizes of single and multiple infarcts of the left ventricle. Am J Cardiol 1998; 81:809–815.
10. Thygesen K, Alpert JS, Jaffe AS, et al. Diagnostic application of the universal definition of myocardial infarction in the intensive care unit. Curr Opin Crit Care 2008; 14:543–548.
11. Herrman J. Peri-procedural myocardial injury: 2005 update. Eur Heart J 2005; 26:2493–2519.

12. Akkerhuis KM, Alexander JH, Tardiff BE, et al. Minor myocardial damage and prognosis: are spontaneous and percutaneous coronary intervention-related events different? Circulation 2002; 105:554–556.

13. Holmvang L, Jurlander B, Rasmussen C, et al. Use of biochemical markers of infarction for diagnosing perioperative myocardial infarction and early graft occlusion after coronary artery bypass surgery. Chest 2002; 121:103–111.

14. Croal BL, Hillis GS, Gibson PH, et al. Relationship between postoperative cardiac troponin I levels and outcome of cardiac surgery. Circulation 2006; 114:1468–1475.

15. Miller WL, Garratt KN, Burrit MF, et al. Baseline troponin level: Key to understanding the importance of post-PCI troponin elevations. Eur Heart J 2006; 27:1061–1069.

16. Prasad A, Rihal CS, Lennon RJ, et al. Significance of periprocedural myonecrosis on outcomes after percutaneous coronary intervention. Circ Cardiovasc Interv 2008; 1:10–19.

17. Muehlschlegel JD, Perry TE, Liu KY, et al; CABG Genomics Investigators. Troponin is superior to electrocardiogram and creatinine kinase MB for predicting clinically significant myocardial injury after coronary artery bypass grafting. Eur Heart J 2009; 30:1574–1583.

5 Optimal Reperfusion Therapy: Clinical Trial Evidence of Primary Angioplasty and (Prehospital) Fibrinolysis

Freek W. A. Verheugt

Department of Cardiology, Heartcenter, Onze Lieve Vrouwe Gasthuis, Amsterdam, The Netherlands

Reperfusion therapy has become the gold standard for the early management of acute ST segment elevation myocardial infarction. The benefit of this strategy rises exponentially, the earlier the therapy is initiated. The highest number of lives saved by reperfusion therapy is within the first hour after symptom onset: a window of opportunity aptly termed the *golden hour* (1). Clearly and logically, the mechanism of this benefit relates to maximizing myocardial salvage by early restoration of adequate coronary blood flow, resulting in preservation of left ventricular function and thereby enhancing both early and long-term survival.

According to the principle of the infarct wave front by Reimer and Jennings a brief interruption of blood flow is associated with a small infarct size (2). The temporal dependence of the beneficial effect of coronary reperfusion has also been characterized by multiple metrics including positron emission tomography (3). Irrespective of the methodology, however, the relationship between duration of symptoms and infarct size remains consistent.

The exponential form of the curve illustrating the benefit of reperfusion therapy upon mortality and myocardial salvage has major implications for the timing of treatment. The impact of delay in time to treatment lessens as the duration of ischemia lengthens. Consequently, reducing delays will have a much more positive return in patients presenting early versus those presenting late (4). These considerations have provided strong incentive for the initiation of very early reperfusion therapy including the use of fibrinolysis at home or in the ambulance (5).

PREHOSPITAL REPERFUSION THERAPY

In 1985, prehospital triage and treatment of patients with ST segment elevation myocardial infarction was started in Jerusalem, Israel (6). The authors demonstrated the presence of minimal myocardial damage after the early administration of streptokinase. Nine years later, in a larger and randomized home fibrinolysis study prehospital treatment achieved significantly less Q wave infarctions, which may be correlated with a greater number of smaller infarctions (7). The same trial also demonstrated accelerated and more extensive ST segment resolution with prehospital treatment suggesting enhanced myocardial perfusion (8). Subsequently, the large In-TIME-2 study showed that with each additional hour of symptom onset to the start of fibrinolytic reperfusion therapy the chance of achieving complete ST-segment resolution decreases by 6% (9). In an ASSENT-2 substudy, including 13,100 patients, the earlier the lytic therapy was initiated, the higher the likelihood of ST-segment resolution on the ECG. Moreover, earlier therapy was inversely related to one-year mortality (10).

Hence, the ultimate objective of reperfusion therapy is early and effective treatment, which can only be established by prehospital treatment.

OPTIMAL PREHOSPITAL DIAGNOSIS

Clearly, medical history and appropriate electrocardiographic recording are necessary for the proper diagnosis of ST elevation acute myocardial infarction. Transtelephonic or computer diagnosis can be used for this purpose and seems to be equivalent in accuracy (11). Also, the ambulance staff is important in the quality of prehospital triage. Usually, ambulances are staffed with nurses with or without physicians. Importantly, nurses seem to work faster than physicians in the diagnosis of ST elevation myocardial infarction and proper administration of a fibrinolytic agent (12) (Fig. 1). This is useful in reducing the treatment delay. In general, treatment delay can be shortened by about 55 minutes using prehospital fibrinolysis versus in-hospital fibrinolysis, which significantly reduces hospital mortality by 17% (13) (Fig. 2). Both high risk and lower risk patients benefit from prehospital fibrinolysis (Fig. 3)

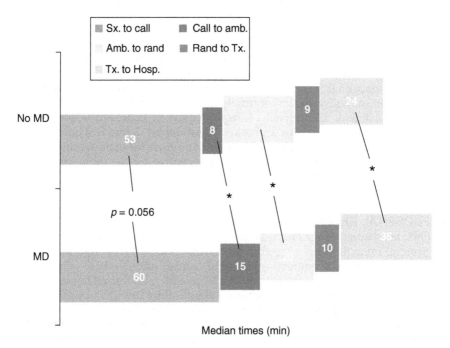

FIGURE 1 Time to fibrinolytic therapy in ambulances with (1045 patients) and without (594 patients) physicians on board. *Abbreviations*: Sx., symptom onset; Amb., ambulance; rand., randomization; Tx., start of fibrinolysis; Hosp., hospital. *Source*: From Ref. 12.

Study	No. of patients	Quality score	OR (95% CI)	Favors prehospital thrombolysis · Favors in-hospital thrombolysis
MITI,[14] 1993	360	0.91	0.69 (0.30–1.57)	
EMIP,[15] 1993	5469	0.85	0.86 (0.72–1.03)	
GREAT,[16] 1991	311	0.78	0.56 (0.25–1.23)	
Roth et al,[17] 1990	116	0.65	0.80 (0.17–3.77)	
Schofer et al,[18] 1990	78	0.63	0.46 (0.04–5.31)	
Castaigne et al,[19] 1989	100	0.48	0.74 (0.14–3.86)	
Overall	**6434**		0.83 (0.70–0.98)	

FIGURE 2 Meta-analysis of early mortality of prehopital versus in-hospital fibrinolysis in ST elevation myocardial infarction. *Source*: From Ref. 13.

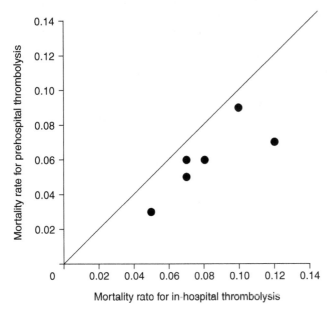

FIGURE 3 Relation of early mortality of prehopital versus in-hospital fibrinolysis in various risk categories in ST elevation myocardial infarction. *Source*: From Ref. 13.

PREHOSPITAL DRUG ADMINISTRATION

Both streptokinase and alteplase have been used in the prehospital setting but resulted in medication errors in more than 10% of cases that was associated with more than doubling of the 24-hour and 30-day mortality rate (20). The most common medication error is miscalculation of dosing according to body weight. Especially, patients with a low body weight may be overdosed resulting in a high number of intracranial hemorrhages (20). The introduction of bolus lytic therapy has facilitated the use of prehospital fibrinolysis, although the safety with regard to intracranial bleeding has been questioned (21). However, in later observations the safety looks excellent in patients under the age of 75 years (22). The first trial with a bolus lytic given in the prehospital setting was ER TIMI-19 study in 315 patients in the Boston area showing a 30-minute reduction in treatment delay compared with in-hospital lytic therapy (23). In the ASSENT-3 PLUS trial, a bolus lytic was given to 1639 patients showing an excellent safety combined with unfractionated heparin but in the elderly patients treated with enoxaparin the intracranial hemorrhage rate was unacceptable (24). In the primary angio-plasty era (see below), the CAPTIM trial in France was carried out in 845 patients showing that prehospital fibrinolytic therapy is not inferior to primary PCI pro-vided the patients are triaged in the ambulance (25). In the patients treated within two hours mortality was nearly significantly lower in the prehospital fibrinoly-sis group compared to those treated with primary PCI (26). After five years this mortality benefit was still statistically significantly different (27) (Fig. 4). Thus, the use of modern bolus lytic therapy in the prehospital setting is an attractive one, because of speed and ease of administration that may challenge the benefit of primary PCI in ST elevation acute myocardial infarction. However, the data from the CAPTIM trial should be confirmed in a larger trial comparing the best of two worlds: prehospital fibrinolysis and primary PCI preferably triaged in the ambulance. Prehospital diagnosis and subsequent immediate transfer to a PCI center result in shorter time delays than triage of these patients in non-PCI cen-ters (28). Therefore, a new CAPTIM-like trial should be set up to compare prehos-pital fibrinolysis versus primary PCI triaged in the ambulance with immediate

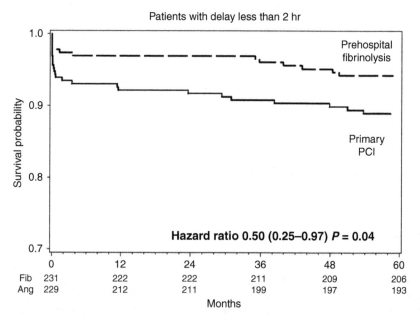

FIGURE 4 Mortality at five-year follow-up of the patients randomized within two hours after symptom onset in the CAPTIM trial. *Source*: From Ref. 27.

transfer to a PCI center in both arms. This is currently evaluated in the STREAM study.

Other agents than fibrinolytics can be utilized in the prehospital setting to speed up coronary reperfusion. Platelet glycoprotein IIb/IIIa blockers have been tested and show better preangioplasty coronary patency in ST elevation acute coronary syndrome than placebo (29). However, the results in clinical outcome are conflicting (30,31).

Finally, it has been shown that fibrinolytic therapy should be a routine invasive strategy, usually angioplasty of the infarct-related artery, within 24 hours after lysis. Recurrent ischemia and infarction, but not mortality is reduced by this strategy (32), which is now part of the European guidelines of acute ST segment elevation myocardial infarction (33).

PRIMARY ANGIOPLASTY

The clear alternative to fibrinolytic therapy in the reperfusion strategy of ST segment elevation acute myocardial infarction is primary coronary angioplasty. This therapy has a clinical benefit over the optimal fibrinolytic strategy: front-loaded rt-PA or tenecteplase (34). Early and long-term reduction in mortality over fibrinolysis has been shown in numerous trials, but in registries and observational studies the long-term benefit has not been proven (35).

The procedure should be performed in patients with less than 12 hours symptoms and must be performed within 120 minutes after first medical contact by an experienced cath lab team (33). The major drawback of primary angioplasty is its limited availability and treatment delay. The delay is caused by preparation of the catheterization laboratory and mobilization of personnel to perform the procedure. Moreover, when patients have to be transferred for primary angioplasty, the delay can be considerable. The initial cost of primary angioplasty seems higher than that of fibrinolytic therapy, but the patency achieved is superior to fibrinolytic therapy: up to 90% (36). The risk of fibrinolytic therapy is higher than that of primary angioplasty, since cerebral bleeding is absent with primary angioplasty. During the treatment delay, patients may be treated with a fibrinolytic to speed up reperfusion prior to angioplasty (*facilitated angioplasty*). However, as stated above the trials evaluating this therapy show better preangioplasty patency, but no benefit over plain primary angioplasty and bleeding is significantly increased (37). Also lower doses of fibrinolytic agents alone or in combination with platelet glycoprotein receptor antagonists failed to improve outcome.

CONCLUSION

Primary angioplasty is the optimal approach to restore coronary patency in STEMI provided it is performed within 120 minutes after first medical contact by an experienced cath lab team. The best results of reperfusion therapy of ST elevation acute coronary syndromes can be obtained by prehospital triage at home or in the ambulance. The introduction of ECG computer diagnosis and bolus formulation of fibrinolytic agents has further facilitated proper and timely prehospital treatment of ST elevation acute coronary syndromes. This strategy has shown to be not inferior to primary angioplasty with prehospital triage in a single trial. However, more studies are needed to confirm these results.

REFERENCES

1. Boersma E, Maas AC, Deckers JW, et al. Early thrombolytic therapy in acute myocardial infarction: reappraisal of the golden hour. Lancet 1996; 348:771–775.
2. Reimer KA, Lowe JE, Rasmussen MM, et al. The wavefront phenomenon of ischemic cell death. 1. Myocardial infarct size versus duration of coronary occlusion in dogs. Circulation 1977; 56:786–794.
3. Bergmann SR, Lerch RA, Fox KAA, et al. Temporal dependence of beneficial effects of coronary thrombolysis characterized by positron emission tomography. Am J Med 1982; 73:573–580.
4. Gersh BJ, Stone GW, White HD, et al. Pharmacological facilitation of primary percutaneous coronary intervention for acute myocardial infarction: is the slope of the curve the shape of the future? JAMA 2005; 293:979–986.
5. Huber K, De Caterina R, Kristensen SD, et al. Prehospital reperfusion therapy: a strategy to improve therapeutic outcome in patients with ST-elevation myocardial infarction. Eur Heart J 2005; 26:2063–2074.
6. Koren G, Weiss AT, Hasin Y, et al. Prevention of myocardial damage in acute myocardial infarction by early treatment with intravenous streptokinase. N Engl J Med 1985; 313:1384–1389.
7. Rawles J. Halving of mortality at 1 year by domiciliary thrombolysis in the Grampian Region Early Anistreplase Trial. J Am Coll Cardiol 1994; 23:1–5.
8. Trent R, Adams J, Rawles J. Electrocardiographic evidence of reperfusion occurring before hospital admission. Eur Heart J 1994; 15:895–897.
9. Antman EM, Cooper HA, Gibson CM, et al. Determinants of improvement of epicardial flow and myocardial perfusion for ST-elevation myocardial infarction. Eur Heart J 2002; 23:928–933.
10. Fu Y, Goodman S, Wei-Ching C, et al. Time to treatment influences the impact of ST-segment resolution on one-year prognosis. Circulation 2001; 104:2653–2659.
11. Lamfers EJP, Hooghoudt TEH, Uppelschoten A, et al. Prehospital versus hospital fibrinolytic therapy using automated versus cardiologist ECG diagnosis of myocardial infarction: abortion of myocardial infarction and unjustified fibrinolytic therapy. Am Heart J 2004; 147:509–515.
12. Welsh RC, Chang W, Goldstein P, et al. Time to treatment and the impact of a physician on prehospital management of acute ST-elevation myocardial infarction: insights from the ASSENT-3 PLUS trial. Heart 2005; 91:1400–1406.
13. Morrison LJ, Verbeek PR, McDonald AC, et al. Mortality and prehospital thrombolysis for acute myocardial infarction. JAMA 2000; 283:2686–2692.
14. Weaver WD, Cerquiera M, Hallstrom AP, et al. Prehospital-initiated vs hospital-initiated thrombolytic therapy. The Myocardial Infarct Triage and Intervention Trial. JAMA 1993; 270:1211–1216.
15. The European Myocardial Infarction Project Group. Prehospital thrombolytic therapy in patients with suspected acute myocardial infarction. N Engl J Med 1993; 329:383–389.
16. GREAT Group. Feasibility, safety and efficacy of domiciliary thrombolysis by general practitioners: Grampian region early anistreplase trial. Br Med J 1992; 305:548–553.
17. Roth A, Barbash GI, Hod H, et al. Should thrombolytic therapy be administered in the mobile intensive care unit in patients with evolving myocardial infarction? a pilot study. J Am Coll Cardiol 1990; 15:932–936.
18. Schofer J, Buttner J, Geng G, et al. Prehospital thrombolysis in acute myocardial infarction. Am J Cardiol 1990; 66:1429–1433.
19. Castaigne AD, Herve C, Duval-Moulin AM, et al. Prehospital use of APSAC: results of a placebo controlled study. Am J Cardiol 1989; 64:30A–33A.
20. Cannon CP. Exploring the issues of appropriate dosing in the treatment of acute myocardial infarction: potential benefits of bolus fibrinolytic agents. Am Heart J 2000; 140:154–160.

21. Metha SR, Eikelboom JW, Yusuf S. Risk of intracranial hemorrhage with bolus versus infusion thrombolytic therapy: a meta-analysis. Lancet 2000; 356:449–454.
22. ASSENT-3 Investigators. Efficacy and safety of tenecteplase with enoxaparin, abciximab or unfractionated heparin: the ASSENT-3 randomised trial in acute myocardial infarction. Lancet 2001; 358:605–613.
23. Morrow DA, Antman EM, Sayah AJ, et al. Evaluation of the time saved by pre-hospital initiation of reteplase for ST-elevation myocardial infarction: results of the Early Retevase-Thrombolysis in Myocardial Infarction (ER-TIMI)-19 trial. J Am Coll Cardiol 2002; 40:71–77.
24. Wallentin L, Goldstein P, Armstrong PW, et al. Efficacy and safety of tenecteplase in combination with the low-molecular weight heparin enoxaparin, or unfractionated heparin in the pre-hospital setting: the ASSENT-3 PLUS randomized trial in acute myocardial infarction. Circulation 2003; 108:135–142.
25. Bonnefoy E, Lapostolle F, Leizorovicz A, et al. Primary angioplasty versus prehospital fibrinolysis in acute myocardial infarction. Lancet 2002; 360:825–829.
26. Steg PG, Bonnefoy E, Chabaud S, et al. Impact of time to treatment on mortality after prehospital fibrinolysis or primary angioplasty: data from the CAPTIM randomized clinical trial. Circulation 2003; 103:2851–2856.
27. Bonnefoy E, Steg PG, Boutitie F, et al. Comparison of primary angioplasty and pre-hospital fibrinolysis in acute myocardial infarction (CAPTIM) trial: a 5 year follow-up. Eur Heart J 2009; 30:1598–1606.
28. Terkelsen GJ, Lassen JF, Norgaard BL, et al. Reduction of treatment delay in patients with ST-elevation myocardial infarction: impact of prehospital diagnosis and direct referral to primary percutaneous coronary intervention. Eur Heart J 2005; 26: 770–777.
29. Montalescot G, Borentain M, Payot L, et al. Early vs late administration of glyco-protein IIb/IIIa inhibitors in primary percutaneous coronary intervention of acute ST-segment elevation myocardial infarction: a meta-analysis. JAMA 2004; 292:362–366.
30. Ellis SG, Tendera M, De Belder MA, et al. Facilitated PCI in patients with ST-elevation myocardial infarction. N Engl J Med 2008; 358:2205–2217.
31. Van 't Hof AWJ, Ten Berg JM, Heestermans T, et al. Prehospital initiation of tirofiban in patients with ST-elevation myocardial infarction undergoing primary angioplasty (On-TIME-2): a multicentre, double-blind, randomised trial. Lancet 2008; 372:537–546.
32. Verheugt FWA. Routine angioplasty after fibrinolysis: how early should "early" be? N Engl J Med 2009; 360:2779–2281.
33. Van de Werf F, Bax J, Betriu A, et al. Management of acute myocardial infarction in patients presenting with persistent ST-segment elevation. Eur Heart J 2008; 29;2909–2945.
34. Keeley EC, Boura JA, Grines CL. Primary coronary angioplasty versus intravenous fibrinolytic therapy for acute myocardial infarction: a quantitative review of 23 randomised trials. Lancet 2003; 361:13–20.
35. Huynh T, Perron S, O'Loughlin J, et al. Comparison of primary percutaneous coronary intervention and fibrinolytic therapy in ST-segment elevation myocardial infarction: Bayesian hierarchical meta-analyses of randomized controlled trials and observational studies. Circulation 2009; 119:3101–3109.
36. Grines CL, Serruys PW, O'Neil WW. Fibrinolytic therapy: is it a treatment of the past? Circulation 2003; 107:2538–2542.
37. Keeley EC, Boura JA, Grines CL. Comparison of primary and facilitated percutaneous coronary intervention for ST-elevation myocardial infarct: quantitative review of randomized trials. Lancet 2006; 367:579–588.

6 | Adjunctive Pharmacologic Therapies

Gregory Ducrocq and Philippe Gabriel Steg

Centre Hospitalier Bichat-Claude Bernard, Paris, France

Primary PCI for ST elevation myocardial infarction (STEMI) is an effective technique to restore coronary artery patency and improve clinical outcomes in patients with STEMI (1). However, to achieve these goals, primary PCI must be associated with adjunctive pharmacological therapies.

ANTITHROMBOTIC ADJUNCTIVE THERAPIES

STEMI is mainly caused by occlusive thrombus triggered by rupture or erosion of the fibrous cap of a culprit atheromatous plaque. The formation of this thrombus is determined by the combination of platelet aggregation and activation of the coagulation cascade culminating in the generation of thrombin and fibrin. Both platelets and thrombin generation can be targeted by pharmacologic treatment (Fig. 1). Antithrombotic therapies in the context of STEMI therefore combine anti-coagulant (antithrombin) and antiplatelet therapies (Fig. 2).

Antiplatelet Therapy

Aspirin

Aspirin acts through inhibition of thromboxane A_2 generation.

The Second International Study of Infarct Survival (ISIS-2) (2) has shown the efficacy of aspirin for treatment of acute MI, with an absolute risk reduction in 35-day mortality of 2.4% and a relative risk reduction of 23%, compared to placebo. This trial, published in 1988, was a thrombolysis study and aspirin has never been formally evaluated in the specific setting of primary PCI. However, given the strong evidence for the benefit of aspirin in this setting, ESC guidelines (3) recommend the utilization of aspirin in primary PCI class I, level of evidence B.

In practice, aspirin should be given to all patients as soon as possible after the diagnosis is deemed probable. It should be started at a dose of 150 to 325 mg in a chewable form (enteric coated aspirin should not be given because of slow onset of action). An alternative approach, especially if oral ingestion is not possible is intravenous (IV) administration of aspirin at a dose of 250 to 500 mg, although no specific data are available on the relative merits of this strategy. A lower dose (75–160 mg) is given orally thereafter for life.

Clopidogrel

Clopidogrel is a thienopyridine antagonist of the $P2Y_{12}$ ADP platelet receptor. There is abundant evidence of its usefulness as an adjunctive antiplatelet therapy on top of aspirin in patients undergoing stenting in a context of elective angioplasty or NSTEMI (4,5). In the context of STEMI, the CLARITY TIMI 28 study

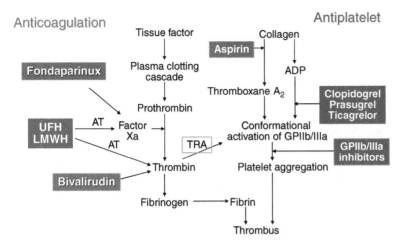

FIGURE 1 Targets of antithrombotic adjunctive therapies.

(6) showed a benefit of adding clopidogrel to aspirin in patients treated with thrombolysis. In addition, the COMMIT trial (7) randomized more than 45,000 patients with suspected myocardial infarction to clopidogrel or placebo, and demonstrated a survival benefit of approximately 9% in relative terms in patients taking clopidogrel. However, no randomized study has evaluated clopidogrel in the context of STEMI treated with primary PCI. Therefore, while guidelines concur in giving a class I recommendation to its use, the level of evidence is C (3).

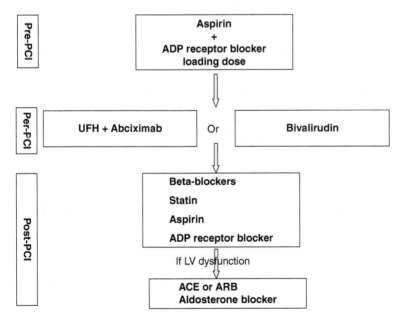

FIGURE 2 Algorithm of adjunctive pharmacologic therapies in primary PCI.

Clopidogrel is a prodrug that must be metabolized into an active compound in order to achieve its antiplatelet effect. This requires up to several days in order to achieve its full effect. In order to shorten this delay, loading doses of 300 mg (4) and more recently 600 mg have been advocated (8). However, the definitive evidence of a clinical benefit from using such high loading doses is still lacking and is the subject of the OASIS 7/CURRENT trial (9).

Clopidogrel should be given as soon as possible to all patients with STEMI undergoing PCI. It is also recommended to start clopidogrel treatment with a loading dose. The optimal loading dose is still debated. Since biological studies (8) have shown that high loading doses achieve a more rapid and stronger inhibition of platelet aggregation it seems logical to start with a 600 mg rather than a 300 mg loading dose. This should be followed by a daily dose of 75 mg (although a higher maintenance dose of 150 mg for one week is also being tested in CURRENT OASIS 7) (9).

New P2Y$_{12}$ Receptor Antagonists

Because of the slow onset of action, variable, and moderate level of platelet inhibition produced by clopidogrel (10) there is active research into newer compounds to produce stronger, quicker, and more reliable inhibition of P2Y$_{12}$ than clopidogrel. Prasugrel is the first such compound to have been tested in large clinical trials. It is a thienopyridine that allows a faster and stronger inhibition of platelet aggregation compared to clopidogrel (11). The faster effect is of particular importance in the context of primary PCI where there is a need for rapid inhibition of platelet function. The Triton TIMI 38 trial (12) has shown that this greater efficacy translates into reduced rates of ischemic events in patients with moderate-to-high risk acute coronary syndromes with scheduled PCI but carries an increased risk of major bleeding, when a loading dose of 60 mg and a maintenance dose of 10 mg/day are compared to a 300 mg load of clopidogrel and a maintenance dose of 75 mg. Importantly, this balance results into a lack of reduction in overall mortality. A subgroup analysis of the TRITON trial (13) focusing on the prespecified subgroup of STEMI patients showed a benefit of prasugrel in reducing ischemic events (cardiovascular death, nonfatal myocardial infarction or nonfatal stroke) without apparent excess in bleeding (10.0% vs. 12.4% at 15 months; HR = 0.79). It is not entirely clear whether this different balance of risk and benefit reflects different pathophysiological mechanisms among STEMI patients (such as greater background platelet activation) or merely a chance finding from a subset analysis (although the latter was prespecified). Another noticeable finding is that most (but not all) of the benefit of prasugrel over clopidogrel was achieved within the early days of therapy. Prasugrel is therefore a promising alternative to clopidogrel in the setting of primary PCI for STEMIs. Other new agents are being explored in the treatment of ACS, particularly ticagrelor (formerly AZD 6140), an oral and reversible P2Y$_{12}$ antagonist, which is being compared to clopidogrel in the large PLATO trial in acute coronary syndromes (14).

IIb/IIIa Receptor Antagonists

Platelet glycoprotein IIb/IIIa antagonists block the IIb/IIIa platelet receptor, which is the final pathway of platelet aggregation. Most studies of GP IIb/IIIa blockade in STEMI have used abciximab rather than the two other IIb/IIIa antagonists (tirofiban and eptifibatide). A systematic review of randomized trials assessing the value of periprocedural administration of IV abciximab in addition to aspirin and heparin in the setting of STEMI showed that abciximab reduced 30-day mortality by 32% without affecting the risk of hemorrhagic stroke and major bleeding (15). Therefore, abciximab carries a IIa A recommendation in the ESC guidelines (3).

The optimal timing for initiation of abciximab is still debated. A meta-analysis (16) showed that early administration of abciximab (prior to transfer to the catheterization laboratory) was associated with improved coronary patency compared with late administration (at the time of PCI). However, in the large FINESSE trial (17), upstream use of abciximab did not have a significant impact on the patency of infarct-related vessels or on clinical outcomes compared to the administration in the catheterization laboratory. Therefore, early administration of abciximab upstream of primary PCI is currently not recommended.

In practice, abciximab is given IV as a bolus of 0.25 mg/kg at the time of PCI, and then 0.125 µg/kg per minute infusion (maximum 10 µg/min) for 12 hours.

The use of the small molecules eptifibatide or tirofiban instead of abciximab is another subject of debate. In the On-TIME 2 trial ($n = 984$), prehospital initiation of high bolus dose tirofiban in association with aspirin, clopidogrel (600 mg), and heparin improved ST segment resolution but was not associated with more patency of the infarct vessel or a significant net clinical benefit when compared to placebo (17). The EVA-AMI trial ($n = 400$) compared eptifibatide to abciximab on top of conventional treatment and showed similar ST segment resolution with both treatments. However, despite these encouraging results, large outcome data are still missing and the use of these small molecules instead of abciximab is not recommended in the STEMI setting (ESC recommendation IIb) (3).

Antithrombin Therapy

Unfractionated Heparin (UFH)

Unfractioned heparin is a polysaccharide binding to the enzyme inhibitor antithrombin (AT) causing a conformational change resulting in activation. The activated AT then inactivates thrombin (factor IIa) and factor Xa. There is no placebo-controlled randomized trial of heparin in PCI for STEMI due to the strong belief that anticoagulation is an absolute requirement during the procedure and heparin is the standard antithrombotic therapy during PCI in STEMI (ESC recommendation I C[3]).

Heparin is given as an IV bolus at a usual starting dose of 100 U/kg weight (60 U/kg if GP IIb/IIIa antagonists are used).

It is recommended to perform primary PCI under activated clotting time (ACT) guidance: heparin should be given at a dose able to maintain an ACT of 250 to 350 seconds (200–250 if GP IIb/IIIa antagonists are used). However, the actual value of ACT monitoring is uncertain, and there is data to suggest that in the contemporary era, in which combination antiplatelet therapy and stents are used, there is no need for higher dose heparin and for ACT monitoring (18).

Low-Molecular-Weight Heparins (LMWH)

LMWH consist of only short chains of polysaccharide that selectively inhibit Xa factor via AT (ratio of antifactor Xa activity to antithhrombin actitivity >1.5).

Despite interesting data in elective PCI (19), LMWH have been studied in a limited number of STEMI patients undergoing PCI. The FINESSE study (17) included a LMWH substudy with encouraging data for LMWH: in this trial, there was a significant reduction of TIMI major bleeding in the LMWH group (2.9% vs. 4.6% for the UFH group; $P = 0.043$) as well as a reduction of mortality at 90 days (3.8% in the LMWH group vs. 5.6% in the UFH group). However, it is important to note that the utilization of LMWH versus UFH was not randomized in this trial, therefore the results may be confounded. Thus, in contrast to thrombolysis, there is still little evidence to support LMWH use instead of UFH in the setting of primary PCI STEMI. The ATOLL trial is currently randomizing patients between IV enoxaparin and UFH in the setting of primary PCI and should settle the safety and efficacy of LMWH in this specific setting.

Bivalirudin

Bivalirudin directly inhibits thrombin by specifically reversibly binding to the catalytic site and the anion-binding exosite of circulating and clot- or thrombus-bound thrombin.

In the harmonizing outcomes with revascularization and stents in acute myocardial infarction (HORIZONS-AMI) trial, 3602 patients undergoing PCI were randomly assigned to receive either bivalirudin with provisional use of GP IIb/IIIa inhibitor or heparin (or enoxaparin) plus a GP IIb/IIIa inhibitor (20). The primary endpoint, the composite of a 30-day incidence of major adverse cardiac events or major bleeding was significantly reduced by bivalirudin due to a 40% reduction in major bleeding. Importantly, all cause mortality at 30 days was 1% lower ($P < 0.47$) but acute stent thrombosis occurred more frequently ($P < 0.001$). Those encouraging data led to a class IIa B recommendation in ESC guidelines (3). However, arterial access site has a dramatic impact on bleeding access site and since the benefit of bivalirudin is driven by a reduction in bleeding events in HORIZON-AMI trial (20), it would be interesting to confirm the benefit of bivalirudin in a radial access trial. In clinical practice, bivalirudin is given an IV bolus of 0.75 mg/kg followed by an infusion of 1.75 mg/kg/hr not titrated to ACT and usually terminated at the end of the procedure. The benefit of starting therapy "upstream" of PCI in the ambulance and to continue infusion with a tapered dose of 0.25 mg/kg/hr will be tested in the upcoming EUROMAX randomized trial.

Fondaparinux

Fondaparinux is a pentasaccharide binding on AT. It is a selective inhibitor of factor Xa. In the OASIS 6 randomized trial, fondaparinux has been compared with heparin or placebo in 12,092 STEMI patients treated with fibrinolytic agents or PCI or no reperfusion therapy (21). In the PCI subset, fondaparinux was associated with a nonsignificant 1% higher incidence of death or recurrent infarction at 30 days. These findings together with the more frequent occurrence of catheter thrombosis when fondaparinux is used as sole anticoagulant for PCI suggest that fondaparinux should not be used in patients undergoing primary PCI (ESC recommendation III B[3]).

OTHER ADJUNCTIVE THERAPIES

Beta-blockers

The benefit of long-term beta-blockers after STEMI is well established. A meta-analysis including 82 randomized trials (22) showed reduction in death in "long-term trials" of 23%.

The benefit of beta-blockers in the acute phase is more debated. The same meta-analysis (22) showed only a 4% reduction in "short-term trials." It is important to note that most of the trials evaluating long-term beta-blockers after STEMI were performed in the prereperfusion era. However, in the reperfusion era, observational studies have consistently shown that STEMI patients who did not receive beta-blockers were at higher risk of death and adverse events (23).

Early IV administration of beta-blockers is also debated. Two randomized trials of IV beta-blockade in patients receiving fibrinolysis (24,25) were too small to allow firm conclusions. A posthoc analysis of the use of atenolol in the GUSTO-I trial and a systematic review did not support the routine early IV use of beta-blockers (26).

In the COMMIT CCS 2 trial IV metoprolol followed by oral administration until discharge or up to four weeks in 45,852 patients with suspected myocardial infarction (27) did not improve survival when compared to placebo. Fewer patients had reinfarction or VF with metoprolol but this was counterbalanced by a significant increase in cardiogenic shock. Early IV use of beta-blockers is clearly contraindicated in patients with clinical signs of hypotension or congestive heart failure. Early use may be associated with a modest benefit in low-risk, hemodynamically stable patients. In most patients, however, it is prudent to wait for the patient to stabilize before starting an oral beta-blocker.

ESC recommendations (3) are therefore IA for oral beta-blockers and IIbA for IV beta-blockers.

In clinical practice, oral beta-blockers should be orally administered in the absence of contra indication after patient stabilization. A cardiac frequency at rest <60 BPM and >50 BPM is a good reflect on the efficacy of beta-blockers.

Nitrates

Sublingual nitroglycerin should be used as a diagnostic test in case of chest pain with ST segment elevation every five minutes for a total of three doses. Indeed, nitrates may have particular utility in patients with coronary spasm presenting as a STEMI.

Intravenous nitroglycerin is indicated for relief of ongoing ischemic discomfort, control of hypertension or management of pulmonary congestion.

The GISSI-3 trial (28) tested in 19,394 STEMI patients a systematic strategy of 24 hours intravenous followed by transdermal use of nitrates. No significant reduction in mortality was observed with this strategy. Similarly, the ISIS-4 trial (29) evaluated oral mononitrate administered acutely and continued for one month. In this study, this strategy also failed to show a benefit on mortality.

The routine use of nitrates in the initial phase of a STEMI has not shown a benefit on mortality and is, therefore, not recommended (ESC recommendation IIb[3]). Moreover, nitrates in all forms should be avoided in patients with initial systolic blood pressure less than 90 mm Hg or known or suspected right ventricle infarction.

Angiotensin-Converting Enzyme (ACE) Inhibitors and Angiotensin Receptor Blockers

The benefit of early administration of angiotensin-converting enzyme (ACE) inhibitors in STEMI is now well established. In the ISIS-4 (29) trial, 58,000 patients with STEMI were randomly assigned to captopril started 24 hours from onset of STEMI or placebo. In this trial, captopril allowed a 7% reduction in overall five-week mortality with a larger benefit in patients with heart failure or with anterior MI. Similarly, in the GISSI-3 (28) trial, lisinopril produced a significant reduction in mortality over placebo. A systematic overview (30) of trials of ACE inhibition in STEMI including nearly 100,000 patients showed a 7% proportional reduction with most of the benefit observed in the first week. In the same meta-analysis, the benefit was greater in high-risk patients (Killip class 2 or 3, heart rate ≥ 100 BPM, anterior localization). Therefore, opinions still differ as to whether to give ACE inhibitors to all patients or to high-risk patients only and ESC guidelines (3) recommend ACE inhibitors on first day for all patients in whom it is not contraindicated with a class IIa A and for high-risk patients with a class IA.

In patients who do not tolerate an ACE inhibitor, angiotensin receptor blocker (ARB) should be considered. Two trials have evaluated ARBs as an alternative to ACE inhibitors in the context of STEMI. The OPTIMAAL trial (31), evaluating losartan over captopril in 5477 post-STEMI patients with left ventricular dysfunction failed to show noninferiority. Conversely, the VALIANT (32) trial randomized patients between valsartan (4909 pts), valsartan plus captopril (4885 pts) or captopril (4909 pts). Mortality was similar in the three groups; however, discontinuations were more frequent in the groups receiving captopril. Therefore, valsartan, 160 mg twice daily represents an alternative to ACE inhibitors in patients intolerant to ACE inhibitors (recommendation class Ib[3])

Aldosterone Blockade
In the EPHESUS trial (33), 6642 post-STEMI patients with LV dysfunction were randomized between eplerenone or placebo on top of conventional treatment. Mortality was significantly reduced in patients taking eplerenone (15% relative reduction). There was however a significant increase in serious hyperkalemia in this group. Aldosterone blockade has therefore a class IB indication (3) in patients with LV dysfunction.

Statins
Several trials have unequivocally demonstrated the benefits of long-term use of statins in the prevention of new ischemic events and mortality in secondary prevention after STEMI (34). Early administration (during hospital phase) has also shown to produce early benefits. The MIRACL trial (35) randomized 3086 patients for atorvastatin 80 mg or placebo within 96 hours after admission. The primary composite endpoint of death, nonfatal MI, resuscitated cardiac arrest or recurrent severe myocardial ischemia was reduced from 17.4% to 14.8%.

The benefits of early post ACS use of statins appear greater when using intensive versus standard lipid-lowering therapy. A recent meta-analysis (36) of randomized controlled trials that compared different intensities of statin therapy, with a total of 29,395 patients with coronary artery diseases showed that intensive regimens further reduced LDLc levels and reduced the risk of myocardial infarction and stroke in overall population. Moreover, all cause mortality was reduced among patients with acute coronary syndromes treated with more intensive stain regimens (OR 0.75; 95% CI; 0.61–0.93). The PROVE-IT-TIMI 22 trial compared intensive lipid-lowering therapy (atorvastatin 80 mg) to moderate lipid-lowering therapy (pravastatin 40 mg). The intensive lowering arm allowed a 16% reduction in the hazard ratio of the composite endpoint. Benefit

TABLE 1 Antithrombotic Agents and Primary PCI

	Mechanism of action	Posology	Timing of initiation	ESC recommendation (class/level of evidence)
Antiplatelet agents				
Aspirin	Inhibition of thromboxane A_2 generation	150–325 mg in a chewable form or 250–500 mg IV, then 75–160 mg/day	First medical contact	IB
Thienopyridines	Antagonist of the $P2Y_{12}$ ADP platelet receptor			
Clopidogrel		300 or 600 mg loading dose, then 75 mg/day	First medical contact	IC
Prasugrel		60 mg loading dose, then 10 mg/day	First medical contact	None
Ticagrelor		180 mg loading dose then 90 mg twice daily	First medical contact	None
IIb/IIIa inhibitors				
Abciximab		IV bolus of 0.25 mg/kg, then 0.125 μg/kg per minute infusion (maximum 10 μg/min) for 12 hr	Precath	IIa A
Eptifibatide				IIb C
Tirofiban				IIb B
Antithrombin agents				
Unfractioned heparin	Polysaccharide activating antithrombin (inactivation of factor IIa and factor Xa)	100 U/kg weight (60 U/kg if GP IIb/IIIa antagonists are used)	Precath	I C
Low-molecular-weight heparins	Xa factor selective inhibitor via AT (ratio of antifactor Xa activity to antithrombin activity >1.5)	0.5 mg/kg IV bolus	Precath	None
Bivalirudin	Direct thrombin inhibitor	IV bolus of 0.75 mg/kg followed by an infusion of 1.75 mg/ kg/hr	Precath	IIa B
Fondaparinux	Selective inhibitor of factor Xa			III B

was observed within 30 days of initiation in all subgroups, even in patients with LDL-C less than 100 mg/dL.

Overall, there is strong data to support the early use of intensive statin regimens in STEMI patients.

In clinical practice, high dose statins (atorvastatin 80 mg) should be started in all patients, in the absence of contraindication, irrespective of cholesterol levels and as soon as possible.

ESC guidelines (3) recommend to target LDL cholesterol levels <100 mg/dL (I A), although many clinicians actually aim for levels below 70 mg/dL.

CONCLUSION

Despite a few controversies, adjunctive pharmacologic therapies for primary PCI are now well standardized and established on solid evidence-based data (Table 1). This topic represents, however, an intensive research field aiming to optimize the utilization of the available drugs and to develop new molecules. This intense development makes adjunctive pharmacologic therapies in primary PCI a very evolving field with the necessity to permanently adapt our clinical practice to new clinical data.

REFERENCES

1. Keeley EC, Boura JA, Grines CL. Primary angioplasty versus intravenous thrombolytic therapy for acute myocardial infarction: a quantitative review of 23 randomised trials. Lancet 2003; 361:13–20.
2. ISIS-2 (Second International Study of Infarct Survival) Collaborative Group. Randomised trial of intravenous streptokinase, oral aspirin, both, or neither among 17,187 cases of suspected acute myocardial infarction: ISIS-2. Lancet 1988; 2:349–360.
3. Van de Werf F, Bax J, Betriu A, et al. Management of acute myocardial infarction in patients presenting with persistent ST-segment elevation: the Task Force on the Management of ST-Segment Elevation Acute Myocardial Infarction of the European Society of Cardiology. Eur Heart J 2008; 29:2909–2945.
4. Steinhubl SR, Berger PB, Mann JT III, et al. Early and sustained dual oral antiplatelet therapy following percutaneous coronary intervention: a randomized controlled trial. JAMA 2002; 288:2411–2420.
5. Mehta SR, Yusuf S, Peters RJ, et al. Effects of pretreatment with clopidogrel and aspirin followed by long-term therapy in patients undergoing percutaneous coronary intervention: the PCI-CURE study. Lancet 2001; 358:527–533.
6. Sabatine MS, Cannon CP, Gibson CM, et al. Addition of clopidogrel to aspirin and fibrinolytic therapy for myocardial infarction with ST-segment elevation. N Engl J Med 2005; 352:1179–1189.
7. Chen ZM, Jiang LX, Chen YP, et al. Addition of clopidogrel to aspirin in 45,852 patients with acute myocardial infarction: randomised placebo-controlled trial. Lancet 2005; 366:1607–1621.
8. Montalescot G, Sideris G, Meuleman C, et al. A randomized comparison of high clopidogrel loading doses in patients with non-ST-segment elevation acute coronary syndromes: the ALBION (Assessment of the Best Loading Dose of Clopidogrel to Blunt Platelet Activation, Inflammation and Ongoing Necrosis) trial. J Am Coll Cardiol 2006; 48:931–938.
9. Mehta SR, Bassand JP, Chrolavicius S, et al. Design and rationale of CURRENT-OASIS 7: a randomized, 2 × 2 factorial trial evaluating optimal dosing strategies for clopidogrel and aspirin in patients with ST and non-ST-elevation acute coronary syndromes managed with an early invasive strategy. Am Heart J 2008; 156:1080–1088.e1.
10. Bonaca M, Steg PG, Feldman LJ, et al. Antithrombotics in acute coronary syndromes. J Am Coll Cardiol 2009; 54:969–984.

11. Brandt JT, Payne CD, Wiviott SD, et al. A comparison of prasugrel and clopidogrel loading doses on platelet function: magnitude of platelet inhibition is related to active metabolite formation. Am Heart J 2007; 153:66.e9–e16.
12. Wiviott SD, Braunwald E, McCabe CH, et al. Prasugrel versus clopidogrel in patients with acute coronary syndromes. N Engl J Med 2007; 357:2001–2015.
13. Montalescot G, Wiviott SD, Braunwald E, et al. Prasugrel compared with clopidogrel in patients undergoing percutaneous coronary intervention for ST-elevation myocardial infarction (TRITON-TIMI 38): double-blind, randomised controlled trial. Lancet 2009; 373:723–731.
14. James S, Akerblom A, Cannon CP, et al. Comparison of ticagrelor, the first reversible oral P2Y(12) receptor antagonist, with clopidogrel in patients with acute coronary syndromes: rationale, design, and baseline characteristics of the PLATelet inhibition and patient Outcomes (PLATO) trial. Am Heart J 2009; 157:599–605.
15. De Luca G, Suryapranata H, Stone GW, et al. Abciximab as adjunctive therapy to reperfusion in acute ST-segment elevation myocardial infarction: a meta-analysis of randomized trials. JAMA 2005; 293:1759–1765.
16. Montalescot G, Borentain M, Payot L, et al. Early vs late administration of glycoprotein IIb/IIIa inhibitors in primary percutaneous coronary intervention of acute ST-segment elevation myocardial infarction: a meta-analysis. JAMA 2004; 292:362–366.
17. Ellis SG, Tendera M, de Belder MA, et al. Facilitated PCI in patients with ST-elevation myocardial infarction. N Engl J Med 2008; 358:2205–2217.
18. Brener SJ, Moliterno DJ, Lincoff AM, et al. Relationship between activated clotting time and ischemic or hemorrhagic complications: analysis of 4 recent randomized clinical trials of percutaneous coronary intervention. Circulation 2004; 110:994–998.
19. Montalescot G, White HD, Gallo R, et al. Enoxaparin versus unfractionated heparin in elective percutaneous coronary intervention. N Engl J Med 2006; 355:1006–1017.
20. Stone GW, Witzenbichler B, Guagliumi G, et al. Bivalirudin during primary PCI in acute myocardial infarction. N Engl J Med 2008; 358:2218–2230.
21. Yusuf S, Mehta SR, Chrolavicius S, et al. Effects of fondaparinux on mortality and reinfarction in patients with acute ST-segment elevation myocardial infarction: the OASIS-6 randomized trial. JAMA 2006; 295:1519–1530.
22. Freemantle N, Cleland J, Young P, et al. Beta blockade after myocardial infarction: systematic review and meta regression analysis. BMJ 1999; 318:1730–1737.
23. Juliard JM, Charlier P, Golmard JL, et al. Age and lack of beta-blocker therapy are associated with increased long-term mortality after primary coronary angioplasty for acute myocardial infarction. Int J Cardiol 2003; 88:63–68.
24. Roberts R, Rogers WJ, Mueller HS, et al. Immediate versus deferred beta-blockade following thrombolytic therapy in patients with acute myocardial infarction. Results of the Thrombolysis in Myocardial Infarction (TIMI) II-B Study. Circulation 1991; 83:422–437.
25. Van de Werf F, Janssens L, Brzostek T, et al. Short-term effects of early intravenous treatment with a beta-adrenergic blocking agent or a specific bradycardiac agent in patients with acute myocardial infarction receiving thrombolytic therapy. J Am Coll Cardiol 1993; 22:407–416.
26. Pfisterer M, Cox JL, Granger CB, et al. Atenolol use and clinical outcomes after thrombolysis for acute myocardial infarction: the GUSTO-I experience. Global Utilization of Streptokinase and TPA (alteplase) for Occluded Coronary Arteries. J Am Coll Cardiol 1998; 32:634–640.
27. Chen ZM, Pan HC, Chen YP, et al. Early intravenous then oral metoprolol in 45,852 patients with acute myocardial infarction: randomised placebo-controlled trial. Lancet 2005; 366:1622–1632.
28. Gruppo Italiano per lo Studio della Sopravvivenza nell' infarto Miocardico. GISSI-3: effects of lisinopril and transdermal glyceryl trinitrate singly and together on 6-week mortality and ventricular function after acute myocardial infarction. Lancet 1994; 343:1115–1122.
29. ISIS-4 (Fourth International Study of Infarct Survival) Collaborative Group. ISIS-4: a randomised factorial trial assessing early oral captopril, oral mononitrate, and

intravenous magnesium sulphate in 58,050 patients with suspected acute myocardial infarction. Lancet 1995; 345:669–685.

30. ACE Inhibitor Myocardial Infarction Collaborative Group. Indications for ACE inhibitors in the early treatment of acute myocardial infarction: systematic overview of individual data from 100,000 patients in randomized trials. Circulation 1998; 97:2202–2212.

31. Dickstein K, Kjekshus J. Effects of losartan and captopril on mortality and morbidity in high-risk patients after acute myocardial infarction: the OPTIMAAL randomised trial. Optimal Trial in Myocardial Infarction with Angiotensin II Antagonist Losartan. Lancet 2002; 360:752–760.

32. Pfeffer MA, McMurray JJ, Velazquez EJ, et al. Valsartan, captopril, or both in myocardial infarction complicated by heart failure, left ventricular dysfunction, or both. N Engl J Med 2003; 349:1893–1906.

33. Pitt B, Remme W, Zannad F, et al. Eplerenone, a selective aldosterone blocker, in patients with left ventricular dysfunction after myocardial infarction. N Engl J Med 2003; 348:1309–1321.

34. Sacks FM, Pfeffer MA, Moye LA, et al. The effect of pravastatin on coronary events after myocardial infarction in patients with average cholesterol levels. Cholesterol and Recurrent Events Trial investigators. N Engl J Med 1996; 335:1001–1009.

35. Schwartz GG, Olsson AG, Ezekowitz MD, et al. Effects of atorvastatin on early recurrent ischemic events in acute coronary syndromes: the MIRACL study: a randomized controlled trial. JAMA 2001; 285:1711–1718.

36. Josan K, Majumdar SR, McAlister FA. The efficacy and safety of intensive statin therapy: a meta-analysis of randomized trials. CMAJ 2008; 178:576–584.

Primary Percutaneous Coronary Intervention: Role of Stenting versus Balloon Angioplasty and Drug-Eluting Stents versus Bare Metal Stents: Trial Evidence and Current Concepts

Robert A. Byrne and Adnan Kastrati

ISAResearch Centre, Deutsches Herzzentrum, Munich, Germany

Epicardial arterial occlusion secondary to coronary thrombosis has long been recognized as the predominant mechanism underlying the clinical presentation of acute ST segment elevation myocardial infarction (STEMI) (1). Expeditious restoration of normal coronary flow is the goal of medical intervention, in order that the metabolic needs of the jeopardized myocardium may be resupplied as rapidly as possible and the extent of irreversible myocardial damage be minimized. Mechanical flow restoration in the setting of STEMI was first reported by Rentrop et al. in 1979 (2). Since then primary angioplasty has emerged as the reperfusion modality of choice. Specifically, a primary angioplasty reperfusion strategy has proven superior to thrombolytic therapy in terms of both early and late survival—findings driven by higher rates of achieved vessel patency (TIMI 3 flow), enhanced stability of vessel reopening (reduced incidence of reinfarction), and lower rates of stroke (3,4).

BALLOON ANGIOPLASTY VERSUS ROUTINE STENTING IN AMI

Despite its clinical superiority in comparison with thrombolytic therapy, balloon angioplasty in the setting of STEMI remains associated with some significant limitations: recurrent ischemia or reocclusion within the first month occurs not infrequently and late vessel renarrowing (restenosis) may be detected in up to 40% of cases.

By the mid-1980s, bare metal stent implantation had emerged as a means of stabilizing early outcomes—sealing both fissured plaques and balloon-generated dissection planes. In addition, the larger postprocedural minimal luminal diameter observed with stenting, coupled with the elimination of vessel recoil and constrictive remodeling, improved patency durability over the longer term. On the other hand, the advisability of implanting a metal prosthesis in an aggressively prothrombotic milieu was not without concerns. It was against this background that the Stent Primary Angioplasty in Myocardial Infarction (Stent PAMI) trial was undertaken (5).

The Stent PAMI and CADILLAC Trials

The Stent PAMI investigators randomized 900 STEMI patients to undergo either balloon angioplasty ($n = 448$) or Palmaz–Schatz stent implantation ($n = 452$) at the time of primary percutaneous intervention for STEMI. The primary endpoint was clinical—a composite of death, reinfarction, disabling stroke, and target vessel revascularization at six months. The results demonstrated a significant reduction in this endpoint with stenting as compared to angioplasty (12.6% vs. 20.1%; $P < 0.01$). This difference was due entirely to differential rates of target vessel revascularization (7.7% vs. 17.0%; $P < 0.001$) between the groups; rates of reinfarction were almost identical. Angiographic analysis revealed a larger minimal luminal diameter (2.56 ± 0.44 mm vs. 2.12 ± 0.45; $P < 0.001$), less residual stenosis ($11.1 \pm 11.6\%$ vs. $25.1 \pm 11.9\%$; $P < 0.001$), and fewer residual dissections (11.9% vs. 30.8%; $P < 0.001$) in the stent group immediately postprocedure. Surveillance angiography at 6.5 months demonstrated maintenance of larger minimal luminal diameter (1.81 ± 0.70 mm vs. 1.57 ± 0.75 mm; $P < 0.001$) and lower diameter stenosis in the stent group ($35.6 \pm 22.2\%$ vs. $44.7 \pm 23.5\%$; $P < 0.001$), which translated into lower rates of binary restenosis (20.3% vs. 33.5%; $P < 0.001$).

However, in contrast to findings from studies of angioplasty versus thrombolysis, no signal of reduced mortality was seen in the stenting arm. On the contrary, much of the debate relating to this study centered on a trend toward higher mortality in the stent group, at both one month (3.5% vs. 1.8%; $P = 0.15$) and six months (4.2% vs. 2.7%; $P = 0.27$). A possible explanation was suggested by an unexpected lower incidence of postprocedure TIMI grade 3 flow in the stent group (89.4% vs. 94.2%; $P = 0.10$), which was observed in spite of less frequent residual dissection in this arm of the study. This concerning finding may have been caused by a longer symptom-to-admission duration in the stent group (predisposing to increased no reflow) or more likely an increase in distal embolization of platelet-rich microthrombi in the stent group due to thrombus extrusion through the stent struts, a scenario possibly exacerbated by thrombus dislodgement during delivery of the somewhat bulky Palmaz–Schatz stent device.

The aforementioned concerns were directly addressed by the same investigators in the subsequent Controlled Abciximab and Device Investigation to Lower Late Angioplasty Complications (CADILLAC) trial (6). In acknowledging the potential for increased distal embolization with an elective stenting strategy and the possibility for attenuation of this complication by adjunctive glycoprotein inhibitor administration, the 2×2 factorial design compared stenting with angioplasty with or without abciximab in a similar patient cohort to that recruited for the Stent PAMI study. In addition, stenting was carried out with a modern low-profile stent (MultiLink; Guidant). Of 2082 randomized patients, 518 were treated with angioplasty alone, 528 with angioplasty plus abciximab, 512 with stenting alone, and 524 with stenting plus abciximab. In general the risk profile of the enrolled patients was modest, for example, median age across the groups was young (59–60 years) and median ejection fraction was >55%. Concentrating on the outcomes in non-abciximab-treated patients, the primary endpoint of death, reinfarction, disabling stroke, and target lesion revascularization was reduced by a very similar margin in this study (20.0% vs. 11.5%; $P < 0.001$), again driven predominantly by lower rates of repeat revascularization (15.7% vs. 8.3%; $P < 0.001$) with no differences in rates of reinfarction (1.8% vs. 1.6%). These results were consistent across all subgroups analyzed. In contrast to Stent PAMI, in this case a favorable trend in differential mortality was seen in the direction of stenting as compared to PTCA (3.0% vs. 4.5%). The issue of differences in postprocedure TIMI grade 3 flow appeared to have been resolved in this study (94.5% stent alone vs. 94.7% angioplasty alone). Whether the discrepancy with outcomes observed in the earlier study was due to the lower crossing profile of the MultiLink stent or perhaps improved operator experience remains a matter of conjecture. In terms of the adjunctive administration of abciximab, this was associated with a reduced incidence of subacute thrombosis and recurrent ischemia (though not reinfarction) early after intervention. However, no differences were seen in terms of TIMI flow postprocedure, late reocclusion of the infarct artery or late cardiac events after PTCA or stenting.

Additional Trials on Stenting Versus Primary Angioplasty

Outside of these two large-scale multicenter studies, concordant findings had already been observed in a number of smaller randomized trials. In the Zwolle trial ($n = 227$), a strategy of coronary stenting was associated with lower rates of reinfarction (1% vs. 7%; $P = 0.036$) and TLR (4% vs. 17%; $P = 0.016$) as compared with plain balloon angioplasty in a selected population of patients with lesions deemed *a priori* to be suitable for stenting (7). Both the Florence Randomized Elective Stenting in Acute Coronary Occlusions (FRESCO) ($n = 150$) and the Gianturco–Roubin in Acute Myocardial Infarction (GRAMI) ($n = 104$) randomized trials also reported significantly reduced composite rates of death, reinfarction, or target vessel revascularization in selected patients treated with elective stenting versus primary angioplasty (8,9). Interestingly, a subsequent larger study ($n = 1683$) from the Zwolle group undertaken on an unselected patient cohort (with randomization performed before angiography) failed to replicate such benefits in terms of either reinfarction or indeed target vessel revascularization, which raises some question on the impact of patient selection in randomized control trials (10).

The results of these studies were underscored by a 6922 patient meta-analysis compiled by De Luca et al (11). They confirmed that in comparison to primary angioplasty stenting reduced repeat revascularization (risk ratio 0.56; 95% CI, 0.49–0.65) (Fig. 1) but had no effect on mortality (risk ratio 0.97; 95% CI, 0.78–1.21) or reinfarction (risk ratio 0.93; 95% CI, 0.72–1.20). Limitations of these conclusions include significant variation within study crossover rates and the possible confounding role of thienopyridine cotreatment in patients treated with stent implantation.

Taken together Stent-PAMI, CADILLAC, and these other studies provided a sound evidence base for the incorporation of routine implantation of a bare metal stent at the time of mechanical reperfusion for STEMI. By doing so the rate of repeat revascularization might be substantially reduced. The lack of mortality benefit is not surprising. In contemporary practice, both strategies of primary angioplasty and primary stenting are associated with (*i*) similar rates of TIMI grade 3 flow at the end of the procedure; and (*ii*) comparable rates of reinfarction (driven primarily by similar rates of subacute abrupt vessel closure). Both these factors may be regarded as the dominant predictors of survival following intervention for STEMI. On the other hand, although instances of TLR are not universally benign (with up to 40% of clinical restenosis events associated with troponin positivity), the proportion of such events associated with prognostically

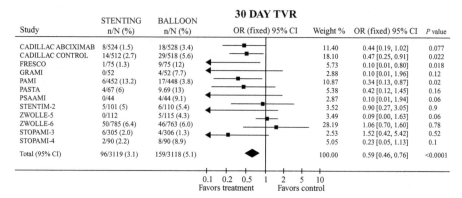

FIGURE 1 Target vessel revascularization at 30 days and 6 to 12 months following stenting versus primary angioplasty in acute myocardial infarction. *Source*: From Ref. 11.

significant myocardial necrosis may be expected to be small and unlikely to exert a sizable effect on mortality rates.

DRUG-ELUTING STENTS IN AMI

Drug-eluting stent (DES) therapy has represented a very significant development in the evolution of catheter-based revascularization. By successfully inhibiting neointimal hyperplasia, randomized control trials have shown that DES reduces the rate of TLR in comparison to BMS by 60% to 70% (12). This benefit also appears to extend to the treatment of so-called "off-label" indications (including implantation in the setting of acute myocardial infarction) – which currently comprise over 50% of interventions – although the magnitude of relative risk reduction may be somewhat smaller (13). Initial widespread enthusiasm for DES was dampened somewhat by concerns regarding late outcomes. Specifically, in comparison to bare metal stents an excess of stent thrombosis and restenosis late (>1 year) after intervention (14,15). In general, these concerns have been allayed by extended follow-up of large patient numbers demonstrating durable safety and efficacy out to four to five years (12,16). Nonetheless, there seems to be a temporal redistribution of stent thrombosis events with a slight excess of events following bare metal stenting in the first six months and a marginal excess with

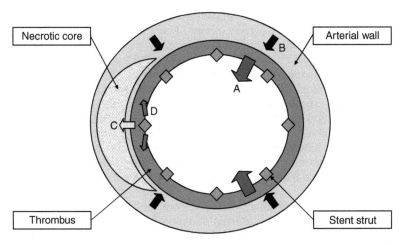

FIGURE 2 Mechanisms of potential late complications following drug-eluting stent implantation in the setting of ST elevation myocardial infarction. Stent implantation is associated with thrombus extrusion (A) that can increase no reflow. Vasoconstriction at the site of plaque rupture (B) increases the risk of stent undersizing. Penetration of the necrotic core by drug-eluting stent struts is a risk factor for delayed healing. Uptake of lipophilic drug is increased in this area (C) resulting in enhanced and prolonged local tissue effects. Thrombus burden further modulates drug release kinetics (D). Dissolution of thrombus jailed behind struts may predispose to late malapposition.

DES after 12 months (16). In addition, pathological and animal studies documented that delayed arterial healing is not an infrequent finding after DES therapy (17,18). Such delayed healing is characterized by persistent fibrin deposition, delayed endothelialization, chronic inflammatory cell infiltration and enhanced platelet responsiveness.

Pathophysiological concerns in relation to stenting of ruptured necrotic-core plaques in the setting of STEMI are illustrated in Figure 2. In point of fact many of these concerns relate just as much to bare metal stent therapy. In addition to the possible effects of thrombus extrusion through the struts in potentiating distal embolization as already mentioned, there is increased potential for late stent malapposition due to dissolution of thrombus jailed behind the stent at the time of intervention. A higher risk of stent undersizing is also possible due to vasoconstriction at the site of the culprit lesion in the setting of myocardial infarction. Furthermore, certain factors may further impair DES-associated delayed vascular healing, namely increased uptake by the necrotic core of the active lipophilic drug (which may lead to prolonged tissue effects), and modulation of release kinetics and drug elution by superimposed thrombus load (19,20).

TYPHOON, PASSION, and HORIZONS-AMI

Bearing in mind these concerns, examination of the outcomes of a number of randomized trials comparing DES with bare metal stenting in the setting of acute myocardial infarction deserves particular scrutiny. The Trial to Assess the Use of the Cypher Stent in Acute Myocardial Infarction Treated with Balloon

Angioplasty (TYPHOON) and the Paclitaxel-Eluting Stent versus Conventional Stent in Myocardial Infarction with ST-Segment Elevation (PASSION) trial were the first large-scale studies addressing this issue and were published simultaneously in 2006 (21,22). The TYPHOON study enrolled 712 patients at 48 international centers with a primary endpoint of target vessel failure at one year (defined as death, myocardial infarction or revascularization pertaining to the target vessel). The rate of this endpoint was significantly lower with the Cypher stent as opposed to its bare metal counterpart (7.3% vs. 14.3%; $P = 0.004$). This reduction was predominantly driven by a decrease in target-vessel revascularization (5.6% vs. 13.4%; $P < 0.001$). There were no significant differences observed with respect to death, myocardial infarction or stent thrombosis; although the high rate of this latter event was a notable feature of the study (3.4% in the Cypher group; 3.6% with BMS).

Somewhat discordant findings emerged from the Paclitaxel-Eluting Stent versus Conventional Stent in Myocardial Infarction with ST-Segment Elevation (PASSION) trial. This was a two-center study from the Netherlands with a marginally smaller sample size ($n = 619$). In terms of the primary outcome measure (composite of death, reinfarction and TLR at 12 months) the trial was negative (8.8% with Taxus vs. 12.8% with bare metal stent; risk ratio 0.63, 95% CI, 0.43–1.10); this finding was accounted for by the lack of statistically significant differences in TLR (5.3% vs. 7.8% respectively; $P = 0.40$). This unexpected negative result may have been due to a combination of less effective neointimal hyperplasia suppression with Taxus (as compared to Cypher), and the enrolment of patients at lower risk for restenosis (though the absence of routine angiographic surveillance may also have attenuated differences in TLR between stent platforms).

The SESAMI and MISSION! Intervention studies were somewhat smaller studies powered primarily for angiographic endpoints (23,24). They demonstrated broadly concordant results in terms of reduced need for TLR and no signal of more frequent safety events in patients randomized to Cypher as compared to bare metal stents, though the MISSION! Intervention study is notable for documenting a significant increase in IVUS-determined late stent malapposition with DES versus bare metal stents (37.5% vs. 12.5% patients; $P < 0.001$).

The STRATEGY trial had earlier investigated a novel hypothesis that in patients undergoing reperfusion for STEMI, a treatment protocol based on Cypher stent implantation in concert with tirofiban bolus administration, would be an attractive alternative to bare metal stent plus abciximab infusion (considered standard of care at that time) (25). The rationale behind the design was that the additional expense associated with DES implantation might be offset by the lower cost of a small molecule glycoprotein inhibitor as compared with abciximab. The composite of death, reinfarction, stroke or target vessel revascularization was significantly reduced by this strategy (18% vs. 32%; risk ratio 0.53; $P = 0.04$). Of course the difficulty with these results lies in the ascription of the observed benefit to differences in stent type alone when it is conceivable that differences between the glycoprotein inhibitors may also have contributed significantly. In this regard the results of the subsequent MULTISTRATEGY trial are somewhat easier to dissect in that a 2 × 2 factorial design was employed in randomizing patients to tirofiban bolus versus abciximab infusion and BMS versus Cypher stent (26). At eight months the composite of death, reinfarction or target vessel revascularization occurred significantly less frequently with the Cypher stent as compared to the BMS (7.8% vs. 14.5%; $P = 0.004$); the observed differences were entirely TLR-driven.

The largest study to date concerning the efficacy of DES in STEMI was published in 2009. In the HORIZONS-AMI study, more than 3000 patients in 11 countries were randomized to either Taxus or bare metal stent implantation in a factorial design that also involved allocation to heparin and routine glycoprotein inhibitor or bivalirudin (a direct thrombin inhibitor) plus bail-out glycoprotein inhibitor (27). The primary endpoint of target lesion revascularization at 12 months was 40% lower following Taxus stent implantation (4.5% vs. 7.5%; odds ratio 0.59; 95% CI, 0.43–0.83). Of note protocol-mandated angiographic follow-up was scheduled at 13 months post index intervention in order that it would take place after primary clinical outcome assessment. While such an approach has the advantage of reducing the influence of surveillance angiography on rates of repeat revascularization, the potential to merely delay the time point at which revascularization is performed should be acknowledged. In terms of safety outcomes the composite of death, reinfarction, stroke and stent thrombosis was very similar in both groups (8.1% with Taxus vs. 8.0% with bare metal stent, risk ratio 1.02; 95% CI, 0.76–1.36), though follow-up is limited to one year.

A full list of the 14 available randomized control trials comparing DES with bare metal stent implantation in STEMI is displayed in Table 1. We recently performed an updated meta-analysis of this data that confirmed both the efficacy and early safety of DES for this indication. Mean follow-up duration was 7 to 24 months. This analysis confirmed that DESs significantly reduce the risk of reintervention in comparison with bare metal stents (risk ratio 0.41; 95% CI, 0.32–0.52) (Fig. 3) without increasing the risk of death (risk ratio 0.90; 95% CI, 0.71–1.15) (Fig. 4) or stent thrombosis (risk ratio 0.84; 95% CI, 0.61–1.17).

Limitations of Data Concerning DES in STEMI

In contrast to the situation in patients with stable coronary disease, the amount of long-term data from randomized trials with DES implantation in the setting of STEMI is relatively limited with few outcome reports beyond 12 months. A number of registry studies have reported two-year follow-up results. However, results have been strikingly divergent. For example, the Global Registry of Acute Coronary Events (GRACE) investigators documented increased late mortality with DES versus bare metal stents (34), while Mauri et al. (35) observed significantly lower adjusted mortality in DES-treated patients. These differences highlight the difficulties with registry reports in which the influence of unmeasured confounding is often inextricable.

In response to the issue of late follow-up, we pooled data from four randomized trials enrolling 658 patients with three to four years of follow-up and detected no evidence of an adverse safety signal between DES and bare metal stents (risk ratio for mortality 0.81; 95% CI, 0.48–1.38; Fig. 5). In fact, the strength of current long-term safety evidence is not dissimilar to that supporting bare metal stenting as compared to balloon angioplasty. Nevertheless, the availability of follow-up results out to four to five years in larger patient numbers remains perhaps the final missing piece of the jigsaw in order that safety concerns might be definitively allayed.

TABLE 1 Randomized Controlled Trials Comparing Drug-eluting and Bare Metal Stent Implantation in Patients Presenting with ST Elevation Myocardial Infarction

Study	Data source	Number of patients	Type of DES	Primary endpoint	Months of clopidogrel	Months of follow-up
BASKET-AMI	(28)	216	PES, SES	MACE	6	18
DEDICATION	(29)	626	PES, SES, ZES	Late luminal loss	12	8
Di Lorenzo	(30)	270	PES, SES	MACE	6	12
Diaz de la Llera	(31)	114	SES	MACE	>1 BMS >9 SES	12
HAAMU-STENT	TCT 2006	164	PES	Late luminal loss	12	17
HORIZONS-AMI	(27)	3006	PES	TLR, Death, MI, stent thrombosis or stroke	6–12	12
MISSION!	(24)	310	SES	Late luminal loss	12	12
MULTISTRATEGY	(26)	745	SES	MACE	≥3	8
PASSION	(21)	619	PES	MACE	6	12
SELECTION	(32)	80	PES	IVUS neointima	9	7
SESAMI	(23)	320	SES	Binary restenosis	12	12
STRATEGY	(25)	175	SES	Death, MI, stroke or binary restenosis	3	24
TITAX AMI	(33)	425	PES	MACE	≥6	12
TYPHOON	(22)	712	SES	MACE	6	12

Abbreviations: AHA, American Heart Association Scientific Sessions; BMS, bare metal stent; DES, drug-eluting stent; ESC, European Society of Cardiology Annual Congress; IVUS, intravascular ultrasound; MACE, major adverse cardiovascular events; MI, myocardial infarction; PES, paclitaxel-eluting stent; SES, sirolimus-eluting stent; TCT, Transcatheter Cardiovascular Therapeutics conference; TLR, target lesion revascularization; ZES, zotarolimus-eluting stent.

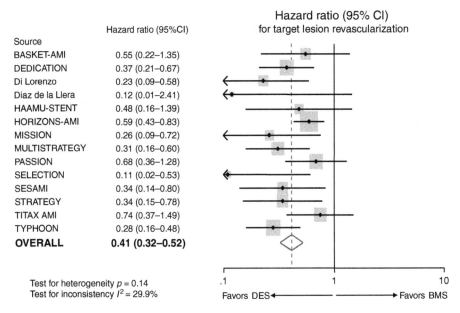

FIGURE 3 Target lesion revascularization with drug-eluting stents versus bare metal stents in acute myocardial infarction. Meta-analysis of randomized clinical trial data. For further details of included studies see Table 1. *Abbreviations*: BMS, bare metal stent; DES, drug-eluting stent.

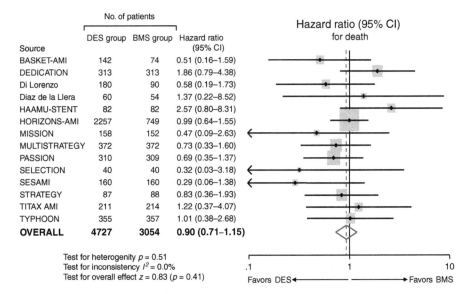

FIGURE 4 Mortality at 7 to 24 months with drug-eluting stents versus bare metal stents in acute myocardial infarction. Meta-analysis of randomized clinical trial data. For further details of included studies see Table 1. *Abbreviations*: BMS, bare metal stent; DES, drug-eluting stent.

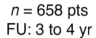

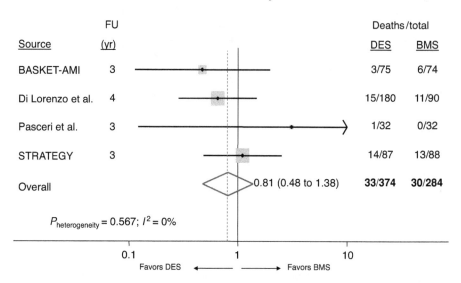

FIGURE 5 Long-term mortality after drug-eluting stent versus bare metal stent implantation following acute myocardial infarction. Meta-analysis of data with long-term follow-up. For further details of included studies see Table 1. BMS, bare metal stent; DES, drug-eluting stent.

The risk: benefit balance of DES and bare metal stents is confounded by one significant issue; namely, the ability to comply with dual antiplatelet therapy for 6 to 12 months postintervention. Current guideline recommendations concerning the optimal duration of dual antiplatelet therapy are limited by a weak evidence base (36). Six months of dual antiplatelet therapy after DES implantation seem to be the minimum duration that can be recommended; patients deemed unlikely or unable to comply with this minimum should be treated with a bare metal stent. Of course the ability to assess broad issues relating to patient compliance with therapy may be difficult to ascertain in the setting of emergency percutaneous intervention and this may impact on choice of stent.

Currently, there is no published data concerning the performance of second or third generation DES in STEMI, though the potential for improved healing with these devices may be of particular relevance in this setting.

CONCLUSION

On the basis of the examined evidence what we can say about the optimal catheter-based revascularization modality in the setting of STEMI is that:

1. In comparison with primary angioplasty, the implantation of a bare metal stent results in a reduction in composite rates of death/myocardial infarction/TLR from approximately 20% to around 10% to 12%. This treatment effect is sizable in absolute terms and is entirely driven by differences in rates of repeat revascularization. There seems to be no reduction in reinfarction

with stenting versus primary angioplasty and no signal of mortality benefit is observed.

2. The implantation of a DES instead of a bare metal stent further reduces the composite of death/myocardial infarction/TLR to in the region of 5% to 8%. The absolute magnitude of this treatment effect is about half that of the effect of bare metal stenting compared to primary angioplasty and is also driven by a reduction in TLR. The absence of mortality benefit in DES is in line with lack of effect on postprocedural TIMI 3 flow and rates of abrupt reocclusion; on the other hand the lack of mortality risk is reassuring in view of safety concerns. Presently available randomized trial data concerning long-term outcomes (≥2 years) in DES-treated STEMI patients is limited but what data are available show no evidence of an adverse safety signal.

In light of the well-proven significant reduction in need for repeat revascularization and the absence of a signal of adverse safety effects, providing that the patient will comply with at least six months of dual antiplatelet therapy, it is our practice to recommend DES implantation in the treatment of culprit lesions in patients presenting with STEMI.

REFERENCES

1. Davies MJ, Woolf N, Robertson WB. Pathology of acute myocardial infarction with particular reference to occlusive coronary thrombi. Br Heart J 1976; 38(7):659–664.
2. Rentrop P, Blanke H, Wiegand V, et al. Recanalization by catheter of the occluded artery after acute myocardial infarction [transluminal recanalization (author's transl.)]. Dtsch Med Wochenschr 1979; 104(40):1401–1405.
3. Zijlstra F, Hoorntje JC, de Boer MJ,et al. Long-term benefit of primary angioplasty as compared with thrombolytic therapy for acute myocardial infarction. N Engl J Med 1999; 341(19):1413–1419.
4. Keeley EC, Boura JA, Grines CL. Primary angioplasty versus intravenous thrombolytic therapy for acute myocardial infarction: a quantitative review of 23 randomised trials. Lancet 2003; 361(9351):13–20.
5. Grines CL, Cox DA, Stone GW, et al. Coronary angioplasty with or without stent implantation for acute myocardial infarction. Stent Primary Angioplasty in Myocardial Infarction Study Group. N Engl J Med 1999; 341(26):1949–1956.
6. Stone GW, Grines CL, Cox DA, et al. Comparison of angioplasty with stenting, with or without abciximab, in acute myocardial infarction. N Engl J Med 2002; 346(13):957–966.
7. Suryapranata H, van 't Hof AW, Hoorntje JC, et al. Randomized comparison of coronary stenting with balloon angioplasty in selected patients with acute myocardial infarction. Circulation 1998; 97(25):2502–2505.
8. Antoniucci D, Santoro GM, Bolognese L, et al. A clinical trial comparing primary stenting of the infarct-related artery with optimal primary angioplasty for acute myocardial infarction: results from the Florence Randomized Elective Stenting in Acute Coronary Occlusions (FRESCO) trial. J Am Coll Cardiol 1998; 31(6):1234–1239.
9. Rodriguez A, Bernardi V, Fernandez M, et al. In-hospital and late results of coronary stents versus conventional balloon angioplasty in acute myocardial infarction (GRAMI trial). Gianturco-Roubin in Acute Myocardial Infarction. Am J Cardiol 1998; 81(11):1286–1291.
10. Suryapranata H, De Luca G, van 't Hof AW, et al. Is routine stenting for acute myocardial infarction superior to balloon angioplasty? A randomised comparison in a large cohort of unselected patients. Heart 2005; 91(5):641–645.

11. De Luca G, Suryapranata H, Stone GW, et al. Coronary stenting versus balloon angioplasty for acute myocardial infarction: a meta-regression analysis of randomized trials. Int J Cardiol 2008; 126(1):37–44.
12. Stettler C, Wandel S, Allemann S, et al. Outcomes associated with drug-eluting and bare-metal stents: a collaborative network meta-analysis. Lancet 2007; 370(9591):937–948.
13. Marroquin OC, Selzer F, Mulukutla SR, et al. A comparison of bare-metal and drug-eluting stents for off-label indications. N Engl J Med 2008; 358(4):342–352.
14. Camenzind E, Steg PG, Wijns W. Stent thrombosis late after implantation of first-generation drug-eluting stents: a cause for concern. Circulation 2007; 115(11):1440–1455; discussion 1455.
15. Byrne RA, Iijima R, Mehilli J, et al. Durability of antirestenotic efficacy in drug-eluting stents with and without permanent polymer. JACC Cardiovasc Interv 2009; 2(4):291–299.
16. Kastrati A, Mehilli J, Pache J, et al. Analysis of 14 trials comparing sirolimus-eluting stents with bare-metal stents. N Engl J Med 2007; 356(10):1030–1039.
17. Joner M, Finn AV, Farb A, et al. Pathology of drug-eluting stents in humans: delayed healing and late thrombotic risk. J Am Coll Cardiol 2006; 48(1):193–202.
18. Joner M, Nakazawa G, Finn AV, et al. Endothelial cell recovery between comparator polymer-based drug-eluting stents. J Am Coll Cardiol 2008; 52(5):333–342.
19. Sianos G, Papafaklis MI, Daemen J, et al. Angiographic stent thrombosis after routine use of drug-eluting stents in ST-segment elevation myocardial infarction: the importance of thrombus burden. J Am Coll Cardiol 2007; 50(7):573–583.
20. Nakazawa G, Finn AV, Joner M, et al. Delayed arterial healing and increased late stent thrombosis at culprit sites after drug-eluting stent placement for acute myocardial infarction patients: an autopsy study. Circulation 2008; 118(11):1138–1145.
21. Spaulding C, Henry P, Teiger E, et al. Sirolimus-eluting versus uncoated stents in acute myocardial infarction. N Engl J Med 2006; 355(11):1093–1104.
22. Laarman GJ, Suttorp MJ, Dirksen MT, et al. Paclitaxel-eluting versus uncoated stents in primary percutaneous coronary intervention. N Engl J Med 2006; 355(11):1105–1113.
23. Menichelli M, Parma A, Pucci E, et al. Randomized trial of Sirolimus-Eluting Stent Versus Bare-Metal Stent in Acute Myocardial Infarction (SESAMI). J Am Coll Cardiol 2007; 49(19):1924–1930.
24. Van Der Hoeven BL, Liem SS, Jukema JW, et al. Sirolimus-eluting stents versus bare-metal stents in patients with ST-segment elevation myocardial infarction: 9-month angiographic and intravascular ultrasound results and 12-month clinical outcome results from the MISSION! Intervention Study. J Am Coll Cardiol 2008; 51(6):618–626.
25. Valgimigli M, Percoco G, Malagutti P, et al. Tirofiban and sirolimus-eluting stent vs abciximab and bare-metal stent for acute myocardial infarction: a randomized trial. JAMA 2005; 293(17):2109–2117.
26. Valgimigli M, Campo G, Percoco G, et al. Comparison of angioplasty with infusion of tirofiban or abciximab and with implantation of sirolimus-eluting or uncoated stents for acute myocardial infarction: the MULTISTRATEGY randomized trial. JAMA 2008; 299(15):1788–1799.
27. Stone GW, Lansky AJ, Pocock SJ, et al. Paclitaxel-eluting stents versus bare-metal stents in acute myocardial infarction. N Engl J Med 2009; 360(19):1946–1959.
28. Pittl U, Kaiser C, Brunner-La Rocca HP. Safety and efficacy of drug-eluting stents versus bare metal stents in primary angioplasty of patients with acute ST-elevation myocardial infarction—a prospective randomized study. Eur Heart J 2006; 27:650 (Abstract Suppl).
29. Tierala I. The Helsinki area acute myocardial infarction treatment reevaluation—should the patient get a drug-eluting or a normal stent (HAAMU-STENT) study, presented at the Annual Scientific Sessions of Transcatheter Cardiovascular Therapeutics 2006.
30. Di Lorenzo E, Varricchio A, Lanzillo T. Paclitaxel and sirolimus stent implantation in patients with acute myocardial infarction. Circulation 2005; 112:II–478 (Abstract Suppl).

31. Diaz de la Llera L, Ballesteros S, Nevado J, et al. Sirolimus-eluting stents compared with standard stents in the treatment of patients with primary angioplasty. Am Heart J 2007; 154:164.e1–6.
32. Chechi T, Vittori G, Biondi Zoccai GG, et al. Single-center randomized evaluation of paclitaxel-eluting versus conventional stent in acute myocardial infarction (SELECTION). J Interv Cardiol 2007; 20:282–291.
33. Karjalainen. TITAX AMI Trial, presented at the Annual Scientific Sessions of Transcatheter Cardiovascular Therapeutics, 2007.
34. Steg PG, Fox KA, Eagle KA, et al. Mortality following placement of drug-eluting and bare-metal stents for ST-segment elevation acute myocardial infarction in the Global Registry of Acute Coronary Events. Eur Heart J 2009; 30(3):321–329.
35. Mauri L, Silbaugh TS, Garg P, et al. Drug-eluting or bare-metal stents for acute myocardial infarction. N Engl J Med 2008; 359(13):1330–1342.
36. Byrne RA, Schulz S, Mehilli J, et al. Rationale and design of a randomized, double-blind, placebo-controlled trial of 6 versus 12 months clopidogrel therapy after implantation of a drug-eluting stent: The Intracoronary Stenting and Antithrombotic Regimen: Safety And EFficacy of 6 Months Dual Antiplatelet Therapy After Drug-Eluting Stenting (ISAR-SAFE) study. Am Heart J 2009; 157(4):620–624.e622.

8 Primary Percutaneous Coronary Intervention: Culprit-Lesion Only versus Multivessel Intervention

Thomas Pilgrim and Stephan Windecker

Department of Cardiology, Bern University Hospital, Bern, Switzerland

INTRODUCTION

Acute myocardial infarction is the leading cause of morbidity and mortality and results from thrombotic occlusion of a major epicardial coronary artery. Primary percutaneous coronary intervention (PCI) is the treatment of choice in patients with acute ST elevation myocardial infarction (STEMI) to improve myocardial salvage by effectively reestablishing coronary perfusion. Randomized clinical trials consistently demonstrated superiority of catheter-based reperfusion of the infarct-related artery (IRA) over fibrinolysis with respect to short- and long-term mortality, nonfatal reinfarction, and hemorrhagic stroke (1). A comprehensive approach with effective integration of potent antithrombotic therapy in combination with timely percutaneous coronary revascularization led to a significant decline in mortality and has prevailed in the contemporary management of acute myocardial infarction.

Multivessel coronary artery disease identified during angiography is encountered in approximately two-thirds of patients undergoing primary PCI (2–4), confers a worse prognosis as compared to single-vessel disease, and is a key predictor of increased in-hospital mortality and long-term morbidity (4,5). Several mechanisms have been suggested to explain the worse outcome in patients with multivessel coronary artery disease. Increased plaque burden, diffuse and more extensive ischemia as well as decreased reperfusion success have been shown to contribute to the adverse prognosis in STEMI patients with multivessel disease undergoing primary PCI (Figs. 1 and 2). Multivessel coronary artery disease in the setting of primary PCI provokes the question whether non-IRA lesions require treatment and if so, at which time.

PATHOPHYSIOLOGICAL CONSIDERATIONS

Multiplicity of Vulnerable Plaques in Patients with Acute Myocardial Infarction

Acute myocardial infarction results from disruption of a vulnerable coronary artery plaque with secondary thrombotic occlusion of the corresponding coronary vessel. As opposed to a stable plaque, a complex or unstable plaque is considered to be present when the surface of the lesion has an ulceration, a fissure or a flap. Several systemic mechanisms such as inflammation, shear stress, platelet

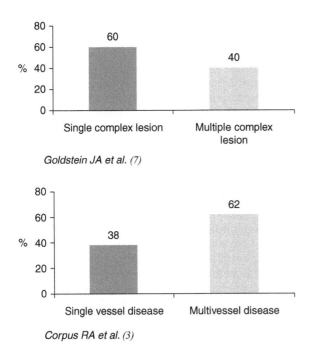

Goldstein JA et al. (7)

Corpus RA et al. (3)

FIGURE 1 Angiographic findings in patients with AMI. *Source*: From Refs. 3,7.

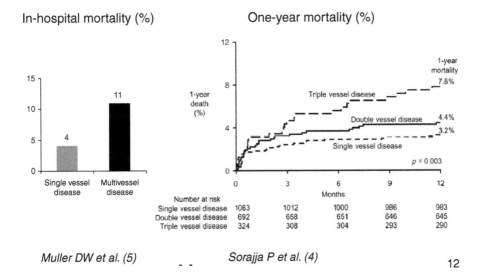

FIGURE 2 Prognosis of patients with multivessel disease in the setting of AMI. *Source*: From Refs. 4,5.

activation, and a generalized procoagulant state are known to contribute to the development of plaque vulnerability and put myocardial infarction in a wider context of a systemic process not confined to a single coronary lesion.

A systemic inflammatory condition in association with an activated coagulation cascade may precipitate plaque instability eventually leading to myocardial infarction. Coronary plaque rupture as evidenced by intravascular ultrasound occurs more often in patients with acute myocardial infarction compared to stable angina patients even in non-IRA vessels (6). As a pathologic correlate, clinical studies evaluating the prevalence of vulnerable plaques in acute coronary syndromes by angiography, angioscopy, and intravascular ultrasound demonstrated more than one unstable coronary plaque in the vast majority of patients. This observation lends support to the concept that development of plaque instability is not limited to the culprit lesion, but rather reflects a pan-coronary process with widespread plaque vulnerability. Coronary angiography in patients with acute myocardial infarction has identified multiple complex lesions in two-fifths of all patients, which was predictive of a poor clinical outcome at one year (7). The presence of multiple complex plaques was independently associated with a higher incidence of recurrent ischemia requiring repeat revascularization and coronary bypass surgery as well as recurrent acute coronary syndromes (7). Investigation of all three coronary arteries by angioscopy in patients with acute myocardial infarction revealed vulnerable plaques in the majority of non-IRA lesions (8). Using intravascular ultrasound imaging in patients with acute coronary syndromes, additional sites of plaque rupture beside the culprit lesion have been observed in 80% of all patients (9).

Blood Flow in Non-IRA Lesions and Regional Wall Motion in Non-Infarct Zone

Perfusion is globally compromised and wall motion abnormalities are observed beyond the territory attributed to the culprit coronary artery in STEMI patients. Assessment of coronary flow in patients with STEMI using corrected TIMI frame counts (CTFC) demonstrates not only the expected decrease in culprit coronary artery flow but also a global flow reduction. Slower global flow measured by CTFC is associated with adverse clinical outcome, including increased in-hospital mortality. Since non-IRA flow in STEMI patients is reduced even after adjustment for hemodynamic abnormalities, it has been speculated that global flow reduction may be the result of vasoconstriction secondary to neurohumoral reflexes or occur as a consequence of more extensive necrosis in the shared microvasculature (10).

Abnormal compared with normal non-IRA flow is more often accompanied by concurrent regional wall motion abnormalities within the distribution of the nonculprit artery, which in turn is associated with a larger infarcted territory and reduced cardiac output. Along this line, it has been shown previously, that the degree of myocardial dysfunction within the noninfarct zone is a predictor of in-hospital mortality (11). Ischemia remote from the IRA may therefore be explained by shared territories of injury or by impaired recruitment of collateral blood flow, thus increasing the hemodynamic significance of a stenosis in the non-IRA vessel.

Multivessel Disease and Reperfusion Success After IRA-Lesion PCI

Multivessel disease is a predictor of decreased reperfusion success and adverse outcome after primary PCI. Reduced myocardial perfusion following restoration of normal epicardial flow (TIMI flow grade 3) by means of PCI correlates with increased mortality and is clinically recognized by persistent ST segment elevation on electrocardiography (12). Thus, the degree of ST segment resolution following primary PCI has been established as a predictor of mortality and reinfarction independent of target vessel patency (13).

In patients undergoing primary PCI for STEMI concomitant coronary artery disease in vessels remote from the IRA has been shown to correlate with reduced myocardial reperfusion success as measured by the degree of ST segment resolution. Furthermore, reduced myocardial perfusion has been reported to result in increased early and late mortality after primary PCI, despite similar rates of final TIMI grade 3 flow in patients with single-, double-, or triple-vessel disease (4). Whether multivessel disease is just a marker of more disseminated atherosclerosis with microcirculatory involvement in the IRA or whether this finding reflects concomitant blood supply of shared territories of injury is currently not clear and needs further investigation. The fact though, that patients who undergo revascularization of the non-IRA coronary artery show improved survival, is evidence in support of the latter.

Progression of Non-IRA Lesions

Apart from the pathophysiologic considerations outlined above, several investigations focusing on prognosis of patients with multivessel disease and multifocal plaque rupture addressed the clinical progression of non-IRA lesions as well as the natural history of myocardium awaiting revascularization. There is mounting evidence to suggest that healing of ruptured plaques results in progression of coronary artery stenosis and that the degree of coronary narrowing increases with repeated plaque rupture at the same site. These observations may explain why patients with acute coronary syndromes and multiple complex lesions on coronary angiography have worse clinical outcome than those with single simple lesions (7). A large cohort of patients treated with culprit vessel PCI and medical therapy for secondary prevention has been examined to determine incidence, presentation, angiographic features, and risk factors associated with clinical plaque progression. Among the 6% of patients that underwent clinically driven repeat PCI of a non-IRA lesion due to plaque progression within one year, two-thirds presented clinically unstable with an acute coronary syndrome. The degree of coronary artery disease at initial PCI, female gender and age below 65 years indicated an increased risk for clinically significant plaque progression in this retrospective analysis (14).

Observations from a postmortem study in patients with sudden cardiac death reported that increased numbers of healed plaque rupture sites correlated with increased coronary luminal narrowing and suggest that repetitive silent plaque disruption results in increased plaque burden and negative remodeling of the coronary vessel (15). The mechanism of luminal narrowing seems to involve repetitive injury, proliferation of smooth muscle cells, and possibly wound contraction (as supported in animal studies) (15).

An angioscopic follow-up study assessing changes in ruptured plaques in non-IRA lesions supports this hypothesis showing that these lesions tend to heal with progression of angiographic stenosis. Analysis by means of QCA showed that diameter stenosis of healed plaques at follow-up angioscopy 13 months after the initial examination significantly increased whereas that of nonhealed plaques remained unchanged. Of note, plaque healing occurred very slowly and several thrombi were still found on the ruptured plaque at one-year follow-up (16).

Ischemic Myocardium Awaiting Revascularization

Ischemic myocardium awaiting revascularization may show contractile deterioration over time that eventually attenuates functional recovery. An observational study of patients awaiting revascularization by coronary artery bypass grafting (CABG) reported a decrease of echocardiographic left ventricular ejection fraction (LVEF) during one year in two-thirds of patients. Overall LVEF decreased from 30.6% ± 11.1% to 27.3% ± 11.5% ($P < 0.001$). This decline went along with a trend toward attenuated improvement in function following revascularization compared to those with stable LVEF (17). The study cohort was small and absolute improvement in function in patients with stable LVEF versus deteriorating LVEF over the preoperative waiting period (delta LVEF) was 10% and 6.3%, respectively. Declining left ventricular function in the setting of delayed revascularization was attributed to worsening hibernation rather than silent infarction since most segments showed at least some improvement postoperatively. However, reduced LVEF is associated with poor prognosis in patients with coronary artery disease (18) and the reported decrease in LVEF over time may eventually translate into increased mortality in patients with delayed complete revascularization.

INTERVENTIONAL STRATEGIES

As outlined above, STEMI patients with multivessel disease pose a challenge to the interventional cardiologists. Three different interventional strategies have been advocated in patients with acute myocardial infarction complicated by multivessel disease, each one carrying its own benefits and risks:

-PCI of the IRA only;
-PCI of the IRA followed by staged treatment of the non-IRA;
-PCI of both the IRA and non-IRA during the initial procedure.

Traditionally, primary PCI was confined to the culprit lesion. Revascularization of non-IRA lesions was considered only following signs of ischemia during noninvasive stress testing with deferred revascularization of significant coronary lesions not related to the infarction.

The completeness of revascularization as important determinant of long-term clinical outcome has been first emphasized in patients undergoing CABG (19). More recently, these findings have been corroborated in PCI populations enrolled into the ARTS I trial (20) and the APPROACH registry (21). Both studies showed a lower need for subsequent revascularization procedures in patients with complete rather than incomplete revascularization. Furthermore, a subgroup analysis from the APPROACH registry restricted to patients with a large area of myocardium at risk suggested improved survival in patients undergoing complete revascularization. A prospective trial that randomized patients to complete versus IRA only revascularization showed a trend toward greater need for repeat revascularization procedures during long-term follow-up in the IRA only group (22). The above-mentioned studies all date to the era prior to the introduction of drug-eluting stents (DES). The latter may impact favorably on the degree of long-term complete revascularization by decreasing the need for repeat interventions owing to restenosis.

While complete percutaneous revascularization has proven beneficial with respect to event-free survival in stable coronary artery disease (20–22), multivessel intervention in the setting of STEMI has been discouraged owing to concerns that periprocedural complications might outweigh the benefit from complete revascularization. Persistent abnormalities of coagulation cascade activation, enhanced inflammatory states, and decreased coronary artery blood flow in patients with acute myocardial infarction provided the rationale for staged procedures rather than immediate complete revascularization. Conversely, pathophysiologic considerations suggest that multivessel interventions might be an asset to the principal objectives of primary PCI by improving plaque stabilization in non-IRA, normalizing blood flow and shear stress, ameliorating overall reperfusion success, and reducing ischemia.

Safety of Multivessel Interventions During Primary PCI

Multivessel disease is a key predictor of in-hospital mortality in patients with acute myocardial infarction, cardiogenic shock being the underlying cause in a majority of cases (4,5). In patients with cardiogenic shock, early revascularization has been shown to portend a survival benefit over a conservative strategy (23) and is recommended according to current guidelines (24). In the SHOCK trial registry, mortality increased from 33% in patients with single-vessel disease to 59% in patients with three-vessel disease. In contrast, there was no significant difference in survival among patients undergoing single-vessel PCI as compared to those undergoing multivessel PCI in the same session (25), supporting the latter approach with the goal of complete revascularization as the preferred strategy in patients with cardiogenic shock.

While complete percutaneous revascularization is associated with a higher event-free survival in patients with stable coronary artery disease (20), multivessel interventions in stable patients with STEMI have been discouraged owing to the potential for additional complications in the past. Although a strategy of complete revascularization may carry the advantage of greater myocardial salvage and prevent recurrent ischemia from non-IRA lesions, concerns have been raised regarding the additional myocardium put at risk, thrombotic complications of non-IRA lesions, and the amount of contrast medium. Clinical data on the safety and efficacy of multivessel interventions during primary PCI is mainly derived from observational studies and remain scarce. With respect to periprocedural mortality, primary multivessel intervention was found to provide similar outcome as culprit-only interventions in most studies (3,26–31). Kalarus et al. (32) reported a survival benefit at 30 days following propensity adjustment in patients with non-IRA intervention and identified incomplete revascularization as an independent risk factor for death in high-risk subgroups with concomitant diabetes, renal failure, and compromised ejection fraction. Likewise, review of the New York State Angioplasty database noted improved in-hospital

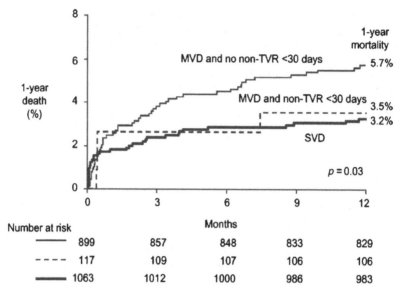

FIGURE 3 Revascularization of noninfarct-related arteries and mortality in the CADILLAC trial (4).

outcome with respect to survival and incidence of major adverse cardiac events in patients undergoing multivessel interventions (33). A mortality benefit was also evident in two large observational studies (4,32). In the CADILLAC trial, that enrolled more than 2000 patients undergoing primary PCI for acute myocardial infarction, patients with multivessel disease who underwent complete revascularization within 30 days had improved one-year survival compared to patients with multivessel disease, who did not undergo non-IRA revascularization and similar survival as patients with single-vessel disease (4) (Fig. 3). A mortality benefit of complete revascularization became evident in another study particularly in diabetic patients and those with decreased left ventricular function or impaired renal function (32) suggesting that patients with acute myocardial infarction and multivessel disease with concomitant risk factors should be treated aggressively to achieve complete revascularization (Fig. 4). Major adverse cardiac events and the need for repeat revascularization procedures during long-term follow-up are also more common among patients with incomplete revascularization (29,32).

While most reports show no difference in the incidence of recurrent myocardial infarction during short-term follow-up (26,27,30,32,34), Corpus et al. (3) documented a higher incidence of nonfatal myocardial infarction within 30 days after primary PCI in patients undergoing multilesion PCI. Similarly, a retrospective case control study reported more recurrent in-hospital myocardial infarctions in patients with multivessel intervention (28). Likewise, data from the large-scale American National Cardiovascular Registry that was confined to patients with non-STEMI showed a somewhat higher rate of periprocedural myocardial infarction. Of note, these observations were not associated with increased mortality (35), and there were no difference in the incidence of renal

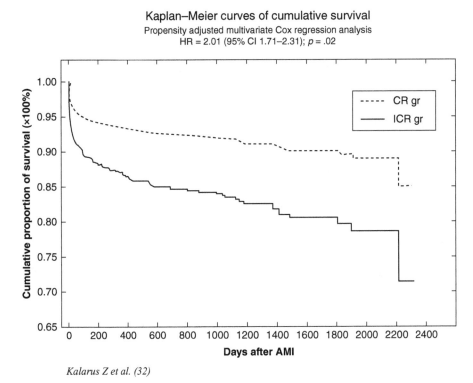

Kaplan–Meier curves of cumulative survival
Propensity adjusted multivariate Cox regression analysis
HR = 2.01 (95% CI 1.71–2.31); *p* = .02

Kalarus Z et al. (32)

FIGURE 4 Complete revascularization (CR) versus culprit vessel only PCI (ICR) in patients with AMI. *Source*: From Ref. 32.

failure (28,35) or bleeding (35). A summary of related articles addressing periprocedural safety is provided in Table 1.

Single-Session Interventions Versus Staged Procedures

Revascularization of non-IRA vessels may be performed in a single session or as a staged procedure. Apart from being safe, single-session interventions reduce hospitalization duration and are cost effective. It has been objected though that this strategy may lead to unnecessary treatment of clinically irrelevant lesions, as lesion severity of non-IRA lesions may be overestimated at the time of primary PCI (36) owing to vasoconstriction.

A small randomized clinical trial comparing the two approaches showed more rapid and substantial improvement of LVEF in patients with single-session complete revascularization, but was underpowered to assess MACE (37). This observation is consistent with observational data from the large-scale American National Cardiovascular Registry that demonstrated a survival benefit in patients with non–ST segment elevation myocardial infarction and multivessel disease treated during a single procedure (35). In contrast, Corpus et al. (3) reported increased in-hospital mortality in patients treated with single-session multivessel intervention as compared to those treated in a staged procedure.

TABLE 1 Primary PCI in AMI: Safety and Efficacy of IRA only versus Non-IRA Intervention

Author	Data	N Pat.	Outcome at 30 days/ in-hospital [a]	IRA-only (%)	Non-IRA (%)	P	Follow-up	Outcome during long-term f/u	IRA-only (%)	Non-IRA (%)	P
Roe et al. (26)	Matched cohort	129	Mortality	11.5	22.1	ns	6 mo	Mortality	16.4	25	ns
			Recurrent MI	0	5.9	ns		Recurrent MI	1.6	8.8	ns
			CABG	0	2.9	ns		CABG	0	4.4	ns
			Repeat PCI	14.8	25	ns		Repeat PCI	11.5	35.3	ns
			Stroke	0	10.3	0.01		Stroke	0	10.3	0.01
Brener et al. (34)	Observational	290 (NST-ACS)	Mortality	1.3	1.5	ns	6 mo	Mortality	2.2	3	ns
			Recurrent MI	4.9	3	ns		Recurrent MI	8	6.1	ns
								Repeat PCI of nonculprit vessel	6.3	1.5	0.04
Corpus et al. (3)	Observational	506	Mortality	6.5	9.9	ns	12 mo	Mortality	12	11	ns
			Recurrent MI	0.6	9.2	<0.001		Recurrent MI	2.8	13	<0.001
			TVR	8.0	5.9	ns		TVR	15	25	0.007
			CABG	8.0	2.6	0.02		CABG	12	6.6	
			MACE	15	22	0.05		MACE	28	40	0.006
Di Mario et al. (27)	RCT	69	Mortality	0	1.9	ns	12 mo	Mortality	0	1.9	ns
			Recurrent MI	0	0	ns		Recurrent MI	5.9	1.9	ns
			PTCA/CABG	0	1.9	ns		PTCA/CABG	35.3	17.3	ns
			MACE	0	3.8	ns		MACE	35.3	21.1	ns
Chen et al. (28)	Case control study	1384	Mortality[a]	2.3	3.8	ns	25 mo	Mortality	9.8	10.9	ns
			Recurrent MI[a]	1.0	2.9	0.015		Composite of death, MI, CABG, TVR	25.7	23.8	ns
			Renal failure	1	0	ns					
			CVA	1	1	ns					
Kong et al. (33)	Observational	1982	Mortality[a]	2.3	1.6	0.02					
			MACE[a]	3.5	0.8	0.018					
			CABG[a]	0.7	0.5	ns					
			Stent thrombosis/acute occlusion[a]	0.7	0.9	ns					
			Stroke[a]	1.0	0.9	ns					
			Renal failure[a]	0.2	0.3	ns					

Study	Design	N	Outcome	Value	Value	p	Follow-up	Outcome	Value	Value	p
Kalarus et al. (32)	Observational	798	Mortality	12.1	3.1	<0.001	29 mo	Mortality	18.5	7.2	<0.001
			Recurrent MI	1.5	0.5	ns		Recurrent MI	9.9	5.7	ns
			Repeat PCI	5.7	3.1	ns		Repeat PCI	15	10.4	ns
			CABG	0.2	0	ns		CABG	9.7	1	<0.001
			MACE	19.5	6.7	<0.001		MACE	53.1	24.3	<0.001
Soraija et al. (4)	Observational	1016					12 mo	Mortality	5.7	3.5	0.03
Qarawani et al. (29)	Observational	120	Mortality[a]	4	4.2	ns		Mortality	8	9.4	ns
								Recurrent MI	16	3.1	0.01
								Repeat PCI	32	7	0.001
								MACE	52	16.7	0.0001
Shishehbor et al. (38)	Propensity-matched	630 (NSTE-ACS)					27 mo	Mortality	14	14	ns
								Composite of Death, MI, repeat PCI	40	30	0.003
Khattab et al. (30)	Observational	73	Mortality	4.5	3.6	ns	12 mo	Repeat PCI	25	17	0.005
			Recurrent MI	4.5	7.1	ns		Mortality	7	8	ns
			TVR	4.5	7.1	ns		Recurrent MI	12	8	ns
			MACE	9.1	10.7	ns		Revascular	28	24	ns
			Stent thrombosis	2.3	7.1	ns		MACE	28	24	ns
			CVA	2.3	7.1	ns					
			Bleeding	4.5	3.6	ns					
Varani et al. (31)	Observational	303	Mortality	6.6	9.9	ns					
Brener et al. (35)	Observational	105366 (NSTE-ACS)	Mortality[a]	1.3	1.2	ns					
			Repeat MI[a]	1.1	1.5	<0.001					
			CABG	0.8	0.3	<0.001					
			Renal failure[a]	1	0.9	ns					
			Bleeding[a]	1.7	1.8	ns					

[a] In hospital outcome.

SUMMARY

Acute myocardial infarction is associated with a widespread vulnerability of atherosclerotic plaques throughout the entire coronary artery tree and is complicated by multivessel coronary artery disease in up to two-thirds of patients. Altered flow in non-IRA and wall motion abnormalities indicating remote ischemia have been observed. Reperfusion success is reduced in patients with multivessel disease, who carry a worse prognosis than patients with single-vessel disease. Multivessel intervention with the goal of complete revascularization appears mandatory in patients with STEMI complicated by cardiogenic shock. In stable STEMI patients, multivessel PCI seems reasonably safe and may portend improved clinical outcome. Careful patient selection and consideration of the appropriate timing of the revascularization (immediate versus staged) procedure are of importance as long as prospective studies establishing the value of multivessel PCI in the setting of acute myocardial infarction are lacking.

REFERENCES

1. Keeley EC, Boura JA, Grines CL. Primary angioplasty versus intravenous thrombolytic therapy for acute myocardial infarction: a quantitative review of 23 randomised trials. Lancet 2003; 361(9351):13–20.
2. Cannon CP, Weintraub WS, Demopoulos LA, et al. Comparison of early invasive and conservative strategies in patients with unstable coronary syndromes treated with the glycoprotein IIb/IIIa inhibitor tirofiban. N Engl J Med 2001; 344(25):1879–1887.
3. Corpus RA, House JA, Marso SP, et al. Multivessel percutaneous coronary intervention in patients with multivessel disease and acute myocardial infarction. Am Heart J 2004; 148(3): 493–500.
4. Sorajja P, Gersh BJ, Cox DA, et al. Impact of multivessel disease on reperfusion success and clinical outcomes in patients undergoing primary percutaneous coronary intervention for acute myocardial infarction. Eur Heart J 2007; 28(14):1709–1716.
5. Muller DW, Topol EJ, Ellis SG, et al. Multivessel coronary artery disease: a key predictor of short-term prognosis after reperfusion therapy for acute myocardial infarction. Thrombolysis and Angioplasty in Myocardial Infarction (TAMI) Study Group. Am Heart J 1991; 121 (4, pt 1):1042–1049.
6. Hong MK, Mintz GS, Lee CW, et al. Comparison of coronary plaque rupture between stable angina and acute myocardial infarction: a three-vessel intravascular ultrasound study in 235 patients. Circulation 2004; 110(8):928–933.
7. Goldstein JA, Demetriou D, Grines CL, et al. Multiple complex coronary plaques in patients with acute myocardial infarction. N Engl J Med 2000; 343(13):915–922.
8. Asakura M, Ueda Y, Yamaguchi O, et al. Extensive development of vulnerable plaques as a pan-coronary process in patients with myocardial infarction: an angioscopic study. J Am Coll Cardiol 2001; 37(5):1284–1288.
9. Rioufol G, Finet G, Ginon I, et al. Multiple atherosclerotic plaque rupture in acute coronary syndrome: a three-vessel intravascular ultrasound study. Circulation 2002; 106(7):804–808.
10. Gibson CM, Ryan KA, Murphy SA, et al. Impaired coronary blood flow in nonculprit arteries in the setting of acute myocardial infarction. The TIMI Study Group. Thrombolysis in myocardial infarction. J Am Coll Cardiol 1999; 34(4):974–982.
11. Grines CL, Topol EJ, Califf RM, et al. Prognostic implications and predictors of enhanced regional wall motion of the noninfarct zone after thrombolysis and angioplasty therapy of acute myocardial infarction. The TAMI Study Groups. Circulation 1989; 80(2):245–253.
12. Schröder R, Wegscheider K, Schröder K, et al. Extent of early ST segment elevation resolution: a strong predictor of outcome in patients with acute myocardial infarction and a sensitive measure to compare thrombolytic regimens: a substudy of the

International Joint Efficacy Comparison of Thrombolytics (INJECT) trial. J Am Coll Cardiol 1995; 26(7):1657–1664.

13. McLaughlin MG, Stone GW, Aymong E, et al. Prognostic utility of comparative methods for assessment of ST-segment resolution after primary angioplasty for acute myocardial infarction: the controlled abciximab and device investigation to lower late angioplasty complications (CADILLAC) trial. J Am Coll Cardiol 2004; 44(6):1215–1223.

14. Glaser R, Selzer F, Faxon DP, et al. Clinical progression of incidental, asymptomatic lesions discovered during culprit vessel coronary intervention. Circulation 2005; 111(2):143–149.

15. Burke AP, Kolodgie FD, Farb A, et al. Healed plaque ruptures and sudden coronary death: evidence that subclinical rupture has a role in plaque progression. Circulation 2001; 103(7):934–940.

16. Takano M, Inami S, Ishibashi F, et al. Angioscopic follow-up study of coronary ruptured plaques in nonculprit lesions. J Am Coll Cardiol 2005; 45(5):652–658.

17. Pitt M, Dutka D, Pagano D, et al. The natural history of myocardium awaiting revascularisation in patients with impaired left ventricular function. Eur Heart J 2004; 25(6):500–507.

18. Mock MB, Ringqvist I, Fisher LD, et al. Survival of medically treated patients in the coronary artery surgery study (CASS) registry. Circulation 1982; 66(3):562–568.

19. Bell MR, Gersh BJ, Schaff HV, et al. Effect of completeness of revascularization on long-term outcome of patients with three-vessel disease undergoing coronary artery bypass surgery. A report from the Coronary Artery Surgery Study (CASS) Registry. Circulation 1992; 86(2):446–457.

20. van den Brand MJ, Rensing BJ, Morel MA, et al. The effect of completeness of revascularization on event-free survival at one year in the ARTS trial. J Am Coll Cardiol 2002; 39(4):559–564.

21. McLellan CS, Ghali WA, Labinaz M, et al. Association between completeness of percutaneous coronary revascularization and postprocedure outcomes. Am Heart J 2005; 150(4):800–806.

22. Ijsselmuiden AJ, Ezechiels J, Westendorp IC, et al. Complete versus culprit vessel percutaneous coronary intervention in multivessel disease: a randomized comparison. Am Heart J 2004; 148(3):467–474.

23. Hochman JS, Sleeper LA, White HD, et al. One-year survival following early revascularization for cardiogenic shock. JAMA 2001; 285(2):190–192.

24. Smith SC, Feldman TE, Hirshfeld JW, et al. ACC/AHA/SCAI Practice Guidelines Update for Percutaneous Coronary Intervention. A Report of the American College of Cardiology/American Heart Association Task Force on Practice Guidelines (ACC/AHA/SCAI Writing Committee to Update the 2001 Guidelines for Percutaneous Coronary Intervention). Circulation, 2006; 113(7):e166–286.

25. Webb JG, Sanborn TA, Sleeper LA, et al. Percutaneous coronary intervention for cardiogenic shock in the SHOCK Trial Registry. Am Heart J 2001; 141(6):964–970.

26. Roe MT, Cura FA, Joski PS, et al. Initial experience with multivessel percutaneous coronary intervention during mechanical reperfusion for acute myocardial infarction. Am J Cardiol 2001; 88(2):170–173, A6.

27. Di Mario C, Mara S, Flavio A, et al. Single vs multivessel treatment during primary angioplasty: results of the multicentre randomised HEpacoat for cuLPrit or multivessel stenting for Acute Myocardial Infarction (HELP AMI) Study. Int J Cardiovasc Intervent 2004; 6 (3–4):128–133.

28. Chen LY, Lennon RJ, Grantham JA, et al. In-hospital and long-term outcomes of multivessel percutaneous coronary revascularization after acute myocardial infarction. Am J Cardiol 2005; 95(3):349–354.

29. Qarawani D, Nahir M, Abboud M, et al. Culprit only versus complete coronary revascularization during primary PCI. Int J Cardiol 2008; 123(3):288–292.

30. Khattab AA, Abdel-Wahab M, Hazanov Y, et al. Multi-vessel stenting during primary percutaneous coronary intervention for acute myocardial infarction. A single-center experience. Clin Res Cardiol 2008; 97(1):32–38.

31. Varani Balducelli M, Aquilina M, et al. Single or multivessel percutaneous coronary intervention in ST-elevation myocardial infarction patients. Catheter Cardiovasc Interv 2008; 72(7):934–936.
32. Kalarus Z, Lenarczyk R, Kowalczyk J, et al. Importance of complete revascularization in patients with acute myocardial infarction treated with percutaneous coronary intervention. Am Heart J 2007; 153(2):304–312.
33. Kong JA, Chou ET, Minutello RM, et al. Safety of single versus multi-vessel angioplasty for patients with acute myocardial infarction and multi-vessel coronary artery disease: report from the New York State Angioplasty Registry. Coron Artery Dis 2006; 17(1):71–75.
34. Brener SJ, Murphy SA, Gibson CM, et al. Efficacy and safety of multivessel percutaneous revascularization and tirofiban therapy in patients with acute coronary syndromes. Am J Cardiol 2002; 90(6):631–633.
35. Brener SJ, Milford-Beland S, Roe MT, et al. Culprit-only or multivessel revascularization in patients with acute coronary syndromes: an American College of Cardiology National Cardiovascular Database Registry report. Am Heart J 2008; 155(1):140–146.
36. Hanratty CG, Koyama Y, Rasmussen HH, et al. Exaggeration of nonculprit stenosis severity during acute myocardial infarction: implications for immediate multivessel revascularization. J Am Coll Cardiol 2002; 40(5):911–916.
37. Ochala A, Smolka GA, Wojakowski W, et al. The function of the left ventricle after complete multivessel one-stage percutaneous coronary intervention in patients with acute myocardial infarction. J Invasive Cardiol 2004; 16(12):699–702.
38. Shishehbor MH, Lauer MS, Singh IM, et al. In unstable angina or non-ST-segment acute coronary syndrome, should patients with multivessel coronary artery disease undergo multivessel or culprit-only stenting? J Am Coll Cardiol 2007; 49(8):849–854.

9 Management of Mechanical Complications of Myocardial Infarction: Ventricular Septal Defect, Mitral Regurgitation, Free-Wall Rupture

Imran Saeed and Marjan Jahangiri

Department of Cardiothoracic Surgery, St. George's Hospital, University of London, London, U.K.

INTRODUCTION

Mechanical complications account for 15% to 20% of deaths following myocardial infarction (MI) (1). These complications include acute ventricular septal defect (VSD), acute ischemic regurgitation (IMR), and free ventricular wall rupture.

VENTRICULAR SEPTAL DEFECT

Definition and Epidemiology

A postinfarction VSD is a perforation of the muscular ventricular septum that occurs through a necrotic area of myocardium following a transmural infarct (1,2).

Postinfarct VSDs have historically complicated 1% to 3% of all infarcts, however, data from the postthrombolysis era report an incidence of 0.2%. Data in the current era of primary angioplasty are limited but suggest an incidence of a similar order (3,4).

The time between infarction the development of a VSD has also decreased. Earlier studies reported average times from infarction to perforation of two to four days whilst more recent data report average times nearer to one day. This time frame can, however, range quite widely from a few hours to several weeks (3,4).

Men are affected marginally more often than women and the mean age of presentation is 63 years (2).

Pathophysiology

Postinfarction VSD almost exclusively occurs following full thickness infarction. This typically follows complete occlusion of a coronary artery in patients with poorly collateralized infarct territories following first-time infarcts. Whilst patients are classically thought to have single-vessel disease, double or triple vessel lesions are present in just over 50% of patients (3).

Postinfarction VSDs can be classified according to their acuity of onset, their anatomical location or based on their morphology. All three aspects are

TABLE 1 Classification of Postinfarction Ventricular Septal Defect (VSD)

Acuity	Acute	• Occurs within 4–6 weeks of infarction
	Chronic	• Occurs 4–6 weeks after infarction
Anatomical location	Anterior	• Occur in anteroapical septum
		• Follow anteroseptal MI from LAD occlusion
		• Comprise 60% of ischemic VSD
	Posterior	• Occur in posterior septum
		• Follow inferoseptal MI from RCA or dominant circumflex occlusion
		• Comprise 30–40% of ischemic VSD
Morphology	Simple	• Direct through and through defects
		• Usually associated with anterior VSD
	Complex	• Serpiginous dissection tract remote from primary tear
		• Usually associated with inferior VSD

Abbreviations: LAD, left anterior descending artery; RCA, right coronary artery.

complimentary and are important to consider when managing patients. These elements are summarized in Table 1. Average defect size is 1.7 cm (1).

The magnitude of the left to right shunt and infarct size are key determinants for the development of cardiac failure, cardiogenic shock, and hence mortality. Preoperative shock and inferior infarction have consistently been shown to be associated with poorer outcomes (5).

Clinical Presentation and Diagnosis

Patients typically present with congestive cardiac failure and the development of a pansystolic murmur following MI. The clinical presentation can, however, vary from the development of an asymptomatic murmur to the development of cardiogenic shock. Data from the SHOCK trial registry showed that postinfarct VSD accounted for almost 4% of patients where shock complicated MI (6).

The commonest differential diagnosis is with acute mitral valve regurgitation secondary to papillary muscle rupture. The distinction between the two conditions can be made on clinical examination and based on ECG findings. Distinguishing features of the two conditions are shown in Table 2.

Two-dimensional transthoracic echocardiography (TTE) with color flow Doppler is the imaging modality of choice. As well as characterizing the location and size of the VSD and shunt, it discriminates between a VSD and papillary muscle rupture. If echocardiography is not diagnostic, right heart catheterization can be used to confirm the diagnosis if a step up in oxygen saturation between the right atrium and pulmonary artery is shown (5).

TABLE 2 Common Distinguishing Features of Postinfarction VSD and Acute Ischemic MR

Postinfarction VSD	Acute Ischemic MR
CCF – predominantly right-sided failure	Pulmonary edema
Pansystolic murmur – left sternal edge	Pansystolic murmur – LV apex
Left parasternal thrill (50%)	No thrill
ECG: right axis deviation and RBBB	ECG: inferior infarction most common, conduction abnormalities unusual

Abbreviations: CCF, congestive cardiac failure; RBBB, right bundle branch block.

Natural History

The GUSTO-1 trial reports that medically treated VSD has a one-month mortality of 94% in comparison to 47% for surgically managed patients (3).

Management

Based on these data, emergent surgery is currently accepted as the treatment option of choice and should ideally proceed before shock ensues.

This approach differs from earlier years where surgery was often deferred for a number of weeks in the hope of providing more favorable (fibrosed) tissues to hold surgical sutures. The dire prognosis of this condition, however, means that the majority of patients will die whilst awaiting surgery and deferral of surgery should probably be reserved for the few patients who are completely stable (5).

On acceptance for surgery patients are aggressively managed to minimize the shunt and to maximize cardiac output. This is usually done using a combination of diuretics, vasodilators, inotropes, and intra-aortic balloon counterpulsation.

The value of concomitant coronary revascularization is not clearly proven and hence there is currently no consensus about the need for preoperative coronary angiography. Advocates of concomitant revascularization, as well as reporting improved results, highlight that there appears to be no additional harm to adding bypass surgery (7).

Given the potential to ease weaning from cardiopulmonary bypass (CPB) and longer-term benefits of revascularizing areas of ischemic myocardium, we advocate coronary angiography.

There are currently only very limited data about the impact of primary angioplasty on the outcome of patients with subsequent or preceding VSD repairs. Yip et al. report that two out of three patients who developed a postinfarct VSD after primary PCI had surgery and survived. This was in comparison to 9 out of 15 patients who underwent VSD repair following elective PCI due to late presentation following MI (4).

OPERATIVE SURGERY, TRANSCATHETER INTERVENTIONS, AND OUTCOMES

There are several well-described surgical techniques that are used to repair postinfarct VSDs. These include the following:

- Apical amputation (Daggett Procedure) – for apical septal defects.
- Infarctectomy – for anterior and posterior defects.
- Infarct exclusion – for anterior and posterior defects.

There are a number of common surgical principles that are applicable to these techniques. These include the following:

- Hypothermic CPB with rigorous myocardial protection.
- A transinfarct approach to the VSD.
- Trimming infarct margins back to viable muscle to prevent delayed rupture.
- Tension-free closure of the VSD – normally using a patch repair.
- Tension-free closure of the infarctectomy with epicardial placement of the patch to the VSD and buttressing of suture lines with prosthetic material.

The infarct exclusion technique does not require resection of myocardium and is thought to maintain better ventricular geometry and may improve ventricular function (2).

Postoperative problems commonly include low cardiac output and bleeding. These are managed with inotropes, continuing intra-aortic balloon counterpulsation, and the use of blood products. In some cases of low cardiac output, the use of ventricular assist devices is sometimes considered.

The largest published series is of 179 patients from Southampton in the United Kingdom. The authors of this study report an in-hospital mortality of 31%, and 1-, 5-, and 10-year survival of 60%, 49%, and 31% respectively (8). A multicenter study from the United Kingdom has also reported a risk-adjusted hazard improvement of 0.17 (0.04–0.784) for midterm survival with concomitant coronary artery bypass surgery (7). Overall, studies report an operative mortality that varies from 30% to 50% (2,5,8).

Transcatheter devices have also been used to close postinfarction VSDs. Thiele et al. have recently reported data on 29 consecutive patients who underwent primary transcatheter closure of postinfarct VSDs using amplatzer ASD and VSD devices. The procedural success rate was 86% whilst the procedural complication rate (including major residual shunting, left ventricular rupture, and device embolization) was close to 40%. Overall 30-day mortality was 35% and was 88% in the patients with cardiogenic shock (9).

Holzer et al. have reported a 30-day mortality of 28% in 18 patients using the Amplatzer postinfarct muscular VSD device (10). Refinement of this technology and further data are needed to assess the long-term efficacy of these devices.

ACUTE ISCHAEMIC MITRAL REGURGITATION

Definition and Epidemiology
Ischemic mitral regurgitation (IMR) is mitral incompetence that occurs as a result of MI or ischemia. The leaflets of the mitral valve are by definition normal (11).

IMR results in a spectrum of clinical presentations from an asymptomatic chronic condition identified only on echocardiography to an acute condition with a precipitous decline to cardiogenic shock.

IMR occurs in 8% to 50% of patients following MI depending on the modality used to detect mitral insufficiency (12). Acute severe MR was the etiology of shock in 7% of patients in the SHOCK trial registry (13).

Pathophysiology
IMR following MI is most commonly associated with transmural posteroinferior infarcts. This can result in papillary muscle rupture or more commonly in the remodelling of a dysfunctional left ventricular wall that results in a relative failure of leaflet coaptation.

Papillary muscle rupture is the cause of death in 1% to 5% of patients following MI. Papillary muscle rupture may be partial (two-thirds of patients) or complete. Acute complete rupture results in massive MR with flailing of both anterior and posterior leaflets and cardiovascular collapse. Partial rupture usually results in lesser degrees of regurgitation (14). Though single-vessel disease is common in patients with acute IMR, three-vessel disease is present in approximately 50% of these patients (11).

The posteromedial papillary muscle is affected in two-thirds of cases because of single dominant RCA supply. The anteromedial papillary muscle is better protected by its dual blood supply from the LAD and circumflex arteries (11).

Acute IMR in the absence of papillary muscle rupture is associated with geometric changes in the left ventricle. These include annular dilatation (primarily in the anteroposterior diameter) and more subtle changes in subvalvar geometry.

The Carpentier classification is used to understand the mechanism of MR and guide operative strategy (15):

- Type I: normal leaflet motion, MR results from annular dilatation.
- Type II: leaflet prolapse or excessive leaflet motion.
- Type IIIa: restricted leaflet motion in diastole.
- Type IIIb: restricted leaflet motion in systole.

IMR is associated with type I, II (papillary muscle rupture), and IIIb lesions.

Clinical Presentation and Diagnosis

Papillary muscle rupture presents with a sudden onset of pulmonary edema, cardiovascular collapse, and cardiogenic shock. The median time to presentation is 22 hours following MI (13). Patients with acute MR in the absence of papillary muscle rupture with moderate to severe regurgitation may also present with heart failure and cardiogenic shock.

Patients usually have a pansystolic murmur over the region of the apex though this may not be present because of early equalization of pressures between a nondilated left atrium and the left ventricle. ECG shows evidence of infarction in 40% of patients (13). The presentation is similar to postinfarct VSD. Distinguishing features are listed in Table 2.

Transthoracic echocardiogram (TTE) is the diagnostic modality of choice quantifies the severity and mechanism of MR, evaluates left ventricular function, and may demonstrate a mobile papillary muscle head. Transesophageal echocardiography (TOE) is useful in patients who are mechanically ventilated and in whom TTE images are inadequate.

Natural History

Papillary muscle rupture is a catastrophic complication that carries a 75% and 30% mortality at 24 hours for complete and partial rupture, respectively (14).

There are some small case series that suggest that PCI may positively impact the degree of IMR acutely (16,17).

Even with successful percutaneous revascularization, however, moderate-to-severe MR appears to persist and continues to carry a high mortality. Pastorius et al. report long-term outcomes in 711 patients. Patients at the time of PCI with moderate-to-severe MR had a five-year survival of 57% compared with 97% for those with no MR (18). Whilst there is still debate about whether surgery can alter the natural history of IMR, there are some data that suggest surgical revascularization may give rise to better outcomes (19).

Management

Emergent surgery is the only effective treatment for patients with severe MR secondary to papillary muscle rupture. In addition, there may be four additional groups of patients who may need surgery for acute MR following MI (12):

• Patients with surgical coronary disease – left main stem or three-vessel.
• Patients with acute postinfarction angina.
• Patients with acute postinfarction angina and mild–moderate MR.
• Patients with acute severe MR with heart failure and shock.

Mitral valve surgery is probably indicated in the first three groups if there is persistent moderate regurgitation on intraoperative TOE following revascularization. The indications for surgery in the last group of patients vary between centers but include pulmonary edema and failure of nonsurgical revascularization to diminish MR.

Patients with severe MR with severely impaired left ventricular function in whom there is concern that the mechanism of MR is secondary to left ventricular failure should be managed medically in the first instance.

Prior to surgery, patients require aggressive medical management to reduce regurgitant flow and volume overload, and to increase cardiac output. This is usually achieved using vasodilators, inotropes, and intra-aortic balloon counterpulsation. Patients should have coronary angiography unless precluded by their clinical condition.

Operative Surgery and Outcomes

Surgery entails mitral valve repair or replacement with or without concomitant coronary surgery.

Although MV repair yields improved outcomes for most patients with IMR, MV repair and replacement yield similar outcomes for patients in higher risk groups (20).

Hence, elderly patients, patients in extremis, and patients in whom there is doubt about the feasibility or durability of repair should receive chord sparing mitral valve replacement. As many chordal attachments to the annulus should be preserved or resuspended with the goal of preserving left ventricular geometry. The choice of valve (bioprosthetic or mechanical) is based upon an estimation of life expectancy and patient comorbidities.

The most commonly used repair technique is MV annuloplasty. Freedom from recurrent MR is probably best achieved by using downsized complete annuloplasty rings (as opposed to incomplete bands) (19). Factors favoring repair include simple, central regurgitant jets, and minimally tethered leaflets. Techniques to reimplant ruptured papillary muscles and the use of artificial chordae are described but are used infrequently in the acute setting because of the caveats already described.

Thirty-day mortality following surgery for acute MR secondary to MI is of the order of 20% (21). Once shock ensues this rises to 40%. This, nevertheless, compares well with the 71% mortality in patients who receive medical management (13).

Five-year survival is of the order of 50% to 65% reflecting the impact of infarct size and progressive left ventricular failure on survival (20,21).

VENTRICULAR FREE-WALL RUPTURE

Definition and Epidemiology
Rupture of the free wall of the left ventricle accounts for approximately 20% to 30% of deaths following acute MI and is the second commonest cause of death after pump failure (22).

The incidence has decreased progressively with the introduction of thrombolysis and percutaneous interventions. Figueras et al. (23) have reported an incidence of 3.2% in the current era, almost half of the incidence seen in their series 30 years earlier.

Moreno et al. suggest further improvements with primary angioplasty with 1.8% of patients developing free-wall rupture in comparison with 3.3% of their patients who had thrombolysis. They also report that primary angioplasty reduces the risk of developing this condition [odds ratio 0.46 (95% CI, 0.22–0.96)] (24).

Female sex, older age (>70 years), first time infarcts, hypertension and anteriorly located ruptures are amongst the risk factors reported for cardiac rupture (2).

Prior to the era of thrombolysis free-wall rupture occurred with a peak incidence at five days following infarction. This appears to occur earlier in the post-thrombolysis era (25).

Pathophysiology
Left ventricular free-wall rupture occurs as a result of infarct expansion after full-thickness infarction in poorly collateralized myocardium. Rupture occurs most frequently on the anterior and lateral free walls at midventricular level at the junction between viable and necrotic myocardium (2,22).

Like postinfarction VSD, free-wall ruptures can be simple or complex. There are three clinicopathological categories (2):

- Acute
- Subacute
- Chronic (with false aneurysm formation).

Clinical Presentation and Diagnosis
Acute rupture results in death within minutes as a result of hemorrhage into the pericardial cavity. It presents with pulseless electrical activity and shock. It is not generally amenable to medical or surgical therapy.

Subacute rupture accounts for approximately 20% to 40% of the cases of free-wall rupture (1,26). It begins as a small endocardial tear that becomes temporarily sealed off by clot and fibrinous adhesions. It presents with symptoms and signs of cardiac tamponade that may progress to shock. Clinical predictors of impending rupture include pericarditis, repetitive vomiting, restlessness, and agitation. Transient bradycardia associated with hypotension occurs in approximately 21% of patients who proceed to rupture. Patients with subacute rupture are also likely to have persistent or recurrent ST elevation on ECG (61%) (27).

Echocardiography is the diagnostic modality of choice and may demonstrate a pericardial effusion with clots as well as demonstrating the site of rupture. For patients who present for primary angioplasty, rounded areas of persistent contrast accumulation (at angiography) have been associated with sites of future free-wall rupture (28).

Chronic rupture is rare and is associated with pseudoaneurysm formation that develops as a result of a contained leakage of blood. Pseudoaneurysms tend to form posteriorly and have narrow necks. Their walls are comprised of pericardium and adhesions.

Chronic ruptures present with symptoms of congestive heart failure, chest pain, or dyspnoea, but >10% of patients will be asymptomatic. More than two-thirds of patients will have a murmur and more than 95% will have CXR or ECG abnormalities. Coronary angiography shows an abnormality in most cases and provides a diagnosis in 87% of patients (29).

The use of Doppler color flow and increasingly MRI can be used to distinguish true and false aneurysms (false aneurysms demonstrating marked delayed pericardial enhancement on MRI) (30).

Natural History

Survival following subacute rupture varies from minutes to weeks. Pollack et al. report a median survival of 8 hours with a range from 45 minutes to 6.5 weeks (31).

The relative rarity of chronic rupture means that the true natural history is difficult to establish. It has traditionally been thought to carry a high risk of rupture (30% to 45%) when untreated (22). However, there are some data that demonstrate a considerably more benign course with a one-year survival approaching 90% (albeit with a significantly high stroke risk) in conservatively managed patients (29,32).

Management

Patients with subacute rupture are usually managed with a view to undergoing urgent surgery. This involves fluid resuscitation, the use of blood products, and blood pressure control as needed prior to rapid transfer to the operating theatre. Pericardiocentesis can be used to treat tamponade in the interim if needed (12).

There are some case reports that describe the use of percutaneously directed fibrin glues at the time of pericardiocentesis that have been used to treat acute and subacute ruptures successfully (33).

Though the natural history of chronic ruptures is not well-known, it has been suggested that the timing and need for surgery is dependent on the time interval between infarction and diagnosis (34). Patients who are within a few months of infarction are still considered to be at high risk of rupture and should undergo urgent cardiac catheterization followed by surgical repair. Indications for surgery after this time point include the following:

- Symptomatic disease;
- Asymptomatic patients with pseudoaneurysm size >3 cm;
- Increasing size;
- Concomitant coronary artery disease or mitral valve regurgitation.

Operative Surgery and Outcomes

Operations are performed through a standard median sternotomy. The location of the tear, hemodynamic status of the patient, the presence of concomitant cardiac lesions, and the choice of repair determine the need for CPB.

Four surgical techniques have been described to repair subacute free-wall ruptures (2):

- Primary suture using a buttressed horizontal mattress sutures.
- Infarct excision and buttressed or patch closure of the defect.
- Limited infarctectomy, buttressed or patch closure with additional coverage of tear site with Teflon onlay patch to the epicardium.
- Epicardial patch applied using biocompatible glue only (sutureless technique).

The need for concomitant coronary artery bypass grafting is a subject of debate. The majority of patients will have multivessel disease but the urgency of presentation will mean that the majority will not have a coronary angiogram. Some surgeons recommend bypassing all vessels regardless whilst others cite that most long-term survivors have not undergone bypass procedures. Other surgeons will bypass clinically palpable disease only (12).

Operative mortality for subacute rupture appears to be of the order of 24% with medium-term survival just under 50% (35,36). Padro et al. have reported 100% five-year survival for 13 patients using the sutureless technique (37).

Chronic anterior ruptures can usually be repaired by direct closure, posterior defects require patch repair. Both procedures should be performed using CPB and crossclamping to prevent systemic embolization of thrombotic debris from within the pseudoaneurysm (1).

Operative mortality following surgery for chronic rupture is approximately 25%. This compares to a mortality of 48% for those managed conservatively. As mentioned earlier, however, there is a small subset of patients who survive to medium and long-term with medical management alone (29).

REFERENCES

1. Berry MF, Gardner TJ. Surgery for complications of myocardial infarction. In: Kaiser LR KI, Spray TL, eds. Mastery of Cardiothoracic Surgery. 2nd ed. Philadelphia, PA: Lippincott Williams & Wilkins, 2007:510–526.
2. Agnihotri AK, Madsen JC, Daggett WM. Surgical treatment of complications of myocardial infarction: postinfarction ventricular septal defect and free wall rupture. In: LH C, ed. Cardiac Surgery in the Adult. 3rd ed. New York: McGraw-Hill, 2008:753–784.
3. Crenshaw BS, Granger CB, Birnbaum Y, et al. Risk factors, angiographic patterns, and outcomes in patients with ventricular septal defect complicating acute myocardial infarction. GUSTO-I (Global Utilization of Streptokinase and TPA for Occluded Coronary Arteries) Trial Investigators. Circulation 2000; 101:27–32.
4. Yip HK, Fang CY, Tsai KT, et al. The potential impact of primary percutaneous coronary intervention on ventricular septal rupture complicating acute myocardial infarction. Chest 2004; 125:1622–1628.
5. Murday A. Optimal management of acute ventricular septal rupture. Heart 2003; 89:1462–1466.
6. Menon V, Webb JG, Hillis LD, et al. Outcome and profile of ventricular septal rupture with cardiogenic shock after myocardial infarction: a report from the SHOCK Trial

Registry. SHould we emergently revascularize Occluded Coronaries in cardiogenic shocK? J Am Coll Cardiol 2000; 36(3 suppl A):1110–1106.

7. Barker TA, Ramnarine IR, Woo EB, et al. Repair of post-infarct ventricular septal defect with or without coronary artery bypass grafting in the northwest of England: a 5-year multi-institutional experience. Eur J Cardiothorac Surg 2003; 24:940–946.

8. Dalrymple-Hay MJ, Monro JL, Livesey SA, et al. Postinfarction ventricular septal rupture: the Wessex experience. Semin Thorac Cardiovasc Surg 1998; 10:111–116.

9. Thiele H, Kaulfersch C, Daehnert I, et al. Immediate primary transcatheter closure of postinfarction ventricular septal defects. Eur Heart J 2009; 30:81–88.

10. Holzer R, Balzer D, Amin Z, et al. Transcatheter closure of postinfarction ventricular septal defects using the new Amplatzer muscular VSD occluder: results of a U.S. Registry. Catheter Cardiovasc Interv 2004; 61:196–201.

11. Szeto WY, Gorman RC, Joseph H, et al. Ischemic mitral regurgitation. In: LH C, ed. Cardiac Surgery in the Adult. 3rd ed. New York: McGraw-Hill, 2008:785–802.

12. Davies RR, Coady M. Mechanical complications of myocardial infarction. In: Yuh DD, Vricella LA, Baumgartner WA, eds. Johns Hopkins Manual of Cardiothoracic Surgery. 1st ed. New York: McGraw-Hill, 2007:489–560.

13. Thompson CR, Buller CE, Sleeper LA, et al. Cardiogenic shock due to acute severe mitral regurgitation complicating acute myocardial infarction: a report from the SHOCK Trial Registry. SHould we use emergently revascularize Occluded Coronaries in cardiogenic shocK? J Am Coll Cardiol 2000; 36(3 suppl A):1104–1109.

14. Kouchoukos NT, Blackstone EH, Doty DB, et al. Mitral regurgitation from ischemic heart disease. In: Kouchoukos NT, Blackstone EH, Doty DB, et al., eds. Kirklin/Barrat-Boyes Cardiac Surgery. 3rd ed. Philadelphia, PA: Churchill Livingstone, 2003:472–482.

15. Carpentier A. Cardiac valve surgery – the "French correction". J Thorac Cardiovasc Surg 1983; 86:323–337.

16. Le Feuvre C, Metzger JP, Lachurie ML, et al. Treatment of severe mitral regurgitation caused by ischemic papillary muscle dysfunction:indications for coronary angioplasty. Am Heart J 1992; 123(4, pt 1):860–865.

17. Shawl FA, Forman MB, Punja S, et al. Emergent coronary angioplasty in the treatment of acute ischemic mitral regurgitation: long-term results in five cases. J Am Coll Cardiol 1989; 14:986–991.

18. Pastorius CA, Henry TD, Harris KM. Long-term outcomes of patients with mitral regurgitation undergoing percutaneous coronary intervention. Am J Cardiol 2007; 100:1218–1223.

19. Anyanwu AC, Adams DH. Ischemic mitral regurgitation: recent advances. Curr Treat Options Cardiovasc Med 2008; 10:529–537.

20. Gillinov AM, Wierup PN, Blackstone EH, et al. Is repair preferable to replacement for ischemic mitral regurgitation? J Thorac Cardiovasc Surg 2001; 122:1125–1141.

21. Tavakoli R, Weber A, Vogt P, et al. Surgical management of acute mitral valve regurgitation due to post-infarction papillary muscle rupture. J Heart Valve Dis 2002; 11: 20–25.

22. Kouchoukos NT, Blackstone EH, Doty DB, et al. Left ventricular aneurysm. In: Kouchoukos NT, Blackstone EH, Doty DB, Hanley FL, Karp RB, eds. Kirklin/Barratt-Boyes Cardiac Surgery. 3rd ed. Philadelphia, PA: Churchill Livingstone, 2003:437–455.

23. Figueras J, Alcalde O, Barrabes JA, et al. Changes in hospital mortality rates in 425 patients with acute ST-elevation myocardial infarction and cardiac rupture over a 30-year period. Circulation 2008; 118:2783–2789.

24. Moreno R, Lopez-Sendon J, Garcia E, et al. Primary angioplasty reduces the risk of left ventricular free wall rupture compared with thrombolysis in patients with acute myocardial infarction. J Am Coll Cardiol 2002; 39:598–603.

25. Becker RC, Charlesworth A, Wilcox RG, et al. Cardiac rupture associated with thrombolytic therapy: impact of time to treatment in the Late Assessment of Thrombolytic Efficacy (LATE) study. J Am Coll Cardiol 1995; 25:1063–1068.

26. Dellborg M, Held P, Swedberg K, et al. Rupture of the myocardium. Occurrence and risk factors. Br Heart J 1985; 54:11–16.

27. Oliva PB, Hammill SC, Edwards WD. Cardiac rupture, a clinically predictable complication of acute myocardial infarction: report of 70 cases with clinicopathologic correlations. J Am Coll Cardiol 1993; 22:720–726.
28. Rigatelli G, Cardaioli P, Dell'Avvocata F, et al. Peculiar angiographic predictors of impending left ventricular rupture after primary coronary angioplasty. Cardiovasc Revasc Med 2008; 9:235–237.
29. Frances C, Romero A, Grady D. Left ventricular pseudoaneurysm. J Am Coll Cardiol 1998; 32:557–561.
30. Konen E, Merchant N, Gutierrez C, et al. True versus false left ventricular aneurysm: differentiation with MR imaging – initial experience. Radiology 2005; 236:65–70.
31. Pollak H, Diez W, Spiel R, et al. Early diagnosis of subacute free wall rupture complicating acute myocardial infarction. Eur Heart J 1993; 14:640–648.
32. Moreno R, Gordillo E, Zamorano J, et al. Long term outcome of patients with postinfarction left ventricular pseudoaneurysm. Heart 2003; 89:1144–1146.
33. Murata H, Masuo M, Yoshimoto H, et al. Oozing type cardiac rupture repaired with percutaneous injection of fibrin-glue into the pericardial space: case report. Jpn Circ J 2000; 64:312–315.
34. Pretre R, Linka A, Jenni R, et al. Surgical treatment of acquired left ventricular pseudoaneurysms. Ann Thorac Surg 2000; 70:553–557.
35. Canovas SJ, Lim E, Dalmau MJ, et al. Midterm clinical and echocardiographic results with patch glue repair of left ventricular free wall rupture. Circulation 2003; 108(suppl 1):II237–II240.
36. Lopez-Sendon J, Gonzalez A, Lopez de Sa E,et al. Diagnosis of subacute ventricular wall rupture after acute myocardial infarction: sensitivity and specificity of clinical, hemodynamic and echocardiographic criteria. J Am Coll Cardiol 1992; 19:1145–1153.
37. Padro JM, Mesa JM, Silvestre J, et al. Subacute cardiac rupture: repair with a sutureless technique. Ann Thorac Surg 1993 55:20–23.

10 Primary Coronary Angioplasty: The Role of Mechanical Circulatory Support

Luiz Alberto Mattos

Instituto Dante Pazzanese de Cardiologia, Santa Casa de Marília, Marília, São Paulo, Brazil

Pedro Beraldo de Andrade

Santa Casa de Marília, Marília, São Paulo, Brazil

INTRODUCTION

Cardiogenic shock is a major cause of death among patients hospitalized for acute myocardial infarction (AMI) with a mortality rate of nearly 50% (1). Although the incidence of cardiogenic shock at admission has remained stable ranging from 5% to 10%, over the last 25 years, it has decreased during hospitalization. Mortality rates have been reduced related to the progressive increase in primary percutaneous coronary intervention (PCI) as the preferred reperfusion strategy (2–6).

The mortality rates remain elevated despite early percutaneous or surgical revascularization interventions mainly in patients in whom hemodynamic instability is maintained despite the procedure having been done (7,8). The performance of revascularization procedures in the first 18 hours of the onset of the cardiogenic shock has led to an absolute mortality rate reduction of 13% in one year (9) and the beneficial result has lasted up to six years (10).

The vast majority of cardiogenic shock, up to 85%, was related to left ventricular failure and the minority, an average of 15%, is due to mechanical complications of AMI (11). The use of mechanical circulatory support might be an important adjunctive therapy to treat these patients. A few days were required for the functional recovery of the myocardium after the revascularization procedure, and mechanical circulatory support devices might work synergistically, promoting hemodynamic stability and additional mortality decrease (12).

We are going to review the major evidence in the literature regarding the different mechanical circulatory support devices used in combination with primary PCI for the treatment of AMI with cardiogenic shock.

INTRA-AORTIC BALLOON PUMP

The intra-aortic balloon pump (IABP) is the device most commonly applied for patients that develop cardiogenic shock and the one that has the most evidence from clinical experience, in randomized controlled trials or national registries. The mechanism of action is related to increasing coronary perfusion pressure during diastole, reduction in afterload, and in the impedance on left ventricular ejection and consequently reduction of myocardial energy expenditure. The IABP promotes temporary support to circulatory failure observed in cardiogenic shock patients, balancing oxygen supply and consumption and therefore preserving and restoring cardiac function after AMI (13,14). Its physiological effects also probably reduce infarct area, as shown in an experimental model (15).

This device has been established for many years, being used for up to 40 years since it was first reported by Kantrowitz et al. (16). IABP is used in nearly 20% to 39% of patients that developed cardiogenic shock after AMI (2,4,5), despite being a class I–C recommendation according to European and North American clinical guidelines (17,18). The lack of randomized clinical trials assessing the efficacy of IABP in this high-risk mortality clinical scenario, constraints in the reimbursement policies, and technical difficulties might explain this finding.

Two recent meta-analyses tried to clarify the role of the IABP in reducing mortality of patients with AMI (19). The first one included seven randomized controlled trials gathering a total of 1009 patients with high-risk AMI (20–26) (Table 1). The high-risk inclusion criteria were: PCI failure, lack of ST segment resolution, fibrinolytic failure, Killip class >1 or large myocardial area at risk. The use of IABP was not associated with mortality decrease after 30 days (risk difference 1%; 95% CI: −3% to 4%; $P = 0.75$), nor it was associated with left ventricular ejection fraction improvement (mean difference −0.1%; 95% CI: −2.2% to 2.0%; $P = 0.93$). On the other hand, it was associated with a 2% increase in the rate of stroke (95% CI: 0–4%; $P = 0.03$) and a 6% increase in the bleeding rate (95% CI: 1–11%; $P = 0.02$).

The second meta-analysis evaluated the result of nine observational registries (14,27–35), involving 10,529 patients with cardiogenic shock diagnosed after AMI (Table 2). In these registries the primary reperfusion strategy was fibrinolytic administration, and the usage of IABP was associated with an absolute mortality reduction of 18% at 30 days (95% CI: 16–20%; $P < 0.0001$). Those patients who received the IABP support were younger (66 vs. 73 years), greater proportion of men (63% vs. 53%), and had a higher revascularization rate (39% vs. 9%, relative risk 4.0, 95% CI: 3.6–4.5; $P < 0.001$). These factors might have had a favorable impact on the occurrence of major adverse events for those that used this device.

In the series whose reperfusion strategy was primary PCI, the use of IABP was associated with an absolute increase of 6% in the 30-day mortality rate (95% CI: 3–10%; $P = 0.0008$). The possible explanations for these unexpected results, since these are registries without a strict methodology, were probably related to the selection of IABP usage in more severely ill patients and in ones transferred to regional centers to carry out primary PCI, with consequent increment in ischemia time. Nevertheless, the influence of the negative results observed in the large nationwide NRMI-2 registry (33) might had been associated with the high mortality rates among patients undergoing primary PCI with IABP support.

In summary, the use of IABP does not appear to provide clinical benefit for patients with AMI without cardiogenic shock even in the high-risk ones, as demonstrated by the PAMI-II trial (25). On the other hand, its usage in patients with cardiogenic shock is not properly supported by robust scientific evidence, raising doubts about the current guidelines.

However, the objective physiological benefits and its intuitive advantages still support its use in these patients. The performance of randomized studies with defined clinical endpoints and adequate statistical power are needed in order to obtain conclusive answers.

TABLE 1 Characteristics of Randomized Controlled Trials with Intra-aortic Balloon Pump Usage in Patients with Cardiogenic Shock After Acute Myocardial Infarction

Study	Period	Setting	No. of patients	Reperfusion therapy	CS excluded	Primary outcome	Mean age (yr) IABP	Mean age (yr) Control
O'Rourke et al. (20)	1976–1979	Multicenter	30	No	No	Hospital/long-term mortality/infarct size	60	54
Flaherty et al. (21)	NR	Single center	20	No	Yes	14-day mortality/infarct size	52	53
Kono et al. (22)	1992–1995	Single center	45	Thrombolysis	Yes	Patency of IRA at 3-week FUP	54	60
Ohman et al. (23) (TACTICS)	1996–1999	Multicenter	57	Thrombolysis	No	All cause mortality at 6 mo	68	67
Ohman et al. (24)	1989–1992	Multicenter	182	Primary PCI	Yes	Reocclusion of IRA during hospitalization	56	55
Stone et al. (25)	1993–1995	Multicenter	437	Primary PCI	Yes	Composite of death, re-MI, stroke, hypotension/CHF	65	64
van 't Hof et al. (26)	1993–1996	Single center	238	Primary PCI	No	Composite of death, re-MI, stroke, LVEF <30% at 6-mo FUP	59	56

Abbreviations: CS, cardiogenic shock; IABP, intra-aortic balloon pump; NR, not reported; IRA, infarct related artery; FUP, follow-up; MI, myocardial infarction; CHF, cardiac heart failure; LVEF, left ventricular ejection fraction.
Source: Modified from Ref. 19.

TABLE 2 Characteristics of the Cohort of Patients Receiving Intra-aortic Balloon Pump Assisted Support for Acute Myocardial Infarction Complicated by Cardiogenic Shock

Study	Period	Clinical enrolment	No. of patients	Reperfusion therapy	Mean age (yr)		Male gender (%)	
					IABP	Control	IABP	Control
Mouloopoulos et al. (27)	1985	Single center	49	No	60	61	85	87
Stomel et al. (28)	1985–1991	Single center	64	Thrombolysis/rescue PCI	66	66	45[a]	62[a]
Kovack et al. (29)	1985–1995	Multicenter	46	Thrombolysis/rescue PCI	62	64	59	63
Bengtson et al. (30)	1987–1988	Single center	200	Thrombolysis/rescue PCI	64	67	NR	NR
Waksman et al. (31)	1989	Single center	41	Thrombolysis/rescue PCI	66	68	70	71
GUSTO-I (32)	1990–1993	Multicenter	310	Thrombolysis/rescue PCI	64	68	68	62
NRMI-2 (33)	1994–1998	Multicenter	8671	Thrombolysis/rescue PCI	67[a]	74[a]	61[a]	51[a]
SHOCK registry (14)	1995–2000	Multicenter	856	Thrombolysis/rescue PCI or primary PCI	65[a]	72[a]	67[a]	60[a]
AMC CS cohort (34,35)	1997–2005	Single center	292	Primary PCI	65	62	68	66

[a] $P < 0.05$.

Abbreviations: IAPB, intra-aortic balloon pump; PCI, percutaneous coronary intervention; NR, not reported.
Source: From Ref. 19.

TABLE 3 Technical Features of Currently Available Percutaneous Left Ventricular Assisted Devices

Device	Tandem Heart™	Impella Recover® LP 5.0	Impella Recover® LP 2.5
Catheter size (French)	–	9	9
Cannula size (French)	21 (venous)–17 (arterial)	21	12
Flow (L/min)	Max. 4.0	Max. 5.0	Max. 2.0
Pump speed (r.p.m.)	Max. 7.500	Max. 33.000	Max. 33.000
Insertion/placement	Peripheral (transseptal puncture + femoral artery)	Peripheral surgical cutdown (femoral artery)	Percutaneous (femoral artery)
Anticoagulation	+	+	+
Maximal duration of usage	14 days	7 days	5 days

Source: From Ref. 12.

PERCUTANEOUS LEFT VENTRICULAR ASSIST DEVICES

IABP is the first-line device prescription for cardiogenic shock patients. However, it has limitations including lack of active cardiac support in face of large amount of jeopardized myocardium, the need of synchronization with the cardiac cycle, and this in the presence of poor residual left ventricular function. In patients with severe left ventricular dysfunction, hemodynamic support provided by IABP is often insufficient to revert the shock status (11). In this regard, the use of left ventricular assist devices (LVAD), with active circulatory support is an attractive option for patients who have not responded to the initial standard therapy and works as a bridge to functional recovery or referral to surgical repair (12). Currently, different active circulatory assist devices and modalities are available (Table 3).

PERCUTANEOUS CARDIOPULMONARY BYPASS

This is a system involving 16 to 18 French cannulas inserted through the femoral artery and vein. Blood is removed from the right atrium by a pump, goes through an oxygenating membrane, and returns to systemic circulation by the femoral artery. There are few reports of its use in AMI (36), and its major limitations are the use of large caliber cannulas, with potential risk of ischemic lower limb complications, need for the assistance of skilled perfusionists, lack of direct left ventricle emptying, augmentation of afterload, and limited support time exposure.

AXIAL FLOW PUMPS

These devices are retrogradely inserted through the aortic valve, aspiring left ventricular blood and pumping it to the ascending aorta by an external pump. The early models were associated with high complication rates, especially at the puncture site, or required surgical techniques for implantation (37). The more recent models have been introduced in the clinical practice. The Impella Recover® (Abiomed Europe GmbH, Aachen, Germany) is a microaxial flow pump capable of generating a continuous flow of 5 L/min or 2.5 L/min. It is percutaneously inserted through a 13 French introducer and is equipped with a pigtail catheter to ensure stable positioning in the left ventricle (Fig. 1).

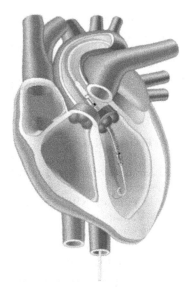

FIGURE 1 Impella Recover® 2.5 L/min positioned across the aortic valve into the left ventricle. *Source:* From Ref. 12.

Compared to IABP in a randomized controlled study that enrolled 26 patients with cardiogenic shock after AMI, it proved to be safe, feasible, and provided better hemodynamic support and greater increase of the cardiac index 30 minutes after implant and was associated with greater reduction of serum lactate dosage, promoting similar 30-day mortality rates (46%) (38).

LEFT ATRIAL-TO-FEMORAL ARTERIAL DEVICE
This device is inserted by a transseptal puncture with introduction of a venous cannula in the left atrium. The oxygenated blood is removed by a centrifugal pump and returned to the abdominal aorta by means of a 17-French arterial cannula also inserted in the femoral artery, enabling flow of up to 4 L/min (Fig. 2).

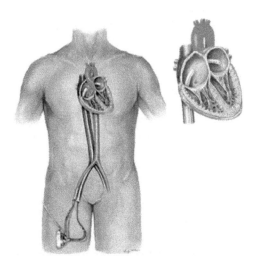

FIGURE 2 TandemHeart™ centrifugal pump. *Right upper corner*: Close-up of the transseptal catheter with large end hole and 14 side holes in the left atrium. *Source:* From Ref. 12.

The commercially available model, TandemHeart™ (Cardiac Assist Technologies, Inc., Pittsburgh, PA, USA), was compared to IABP in a randomized study that gathered 41 patients with cardiogenic shock after AMI (39). A significant improvement was observed in hemodynamic and metabolic parameters favoring this device, but at the expense of a larger number of complications, such as severe bleeding, lower limb ischemia, and fever, without differences in mortality after 30 days (42% vs. 45%; $P = 0.86$).

INTRA-AORTIC BALLOON PUMP VERSUS LEFT VENTRICULAR ASSISTED DEVICE

A contemporary meta-analysis had the objective to compare differences in the hemodynamic performances parameters between these two devices, assessing the 30-day mortality and the major adverse events in patients with AMI and cardiogenic shock treated with IABP assistance or LVAD implant (40). Because of a lack of previous controlled clinical research with these devices, the analysis included three series, two of them using the TandemHeart® device™ (39,41) and one using the Impella® device (38) in comparison to IABP, involving a total of 100 patients.

The hemodynamic assessments were performed two hours after installation of the circulatory support showing that the use of LVAD was associated with a higher cardiac index (MD 0.35 L/min/m², 95% CI: 0.09–0.61), greater mean arterial blood pressure (MD 12.8 mm Hg; 95% CI: 3.6–22.0), and lower pulmonary artery pressure (MD 25.3 mm Hg; 95% CI: 29.4 to 21.2), when compared to IABP (Fig. 3).

However, the improvement in hemodynamic parameters was not translated into clinical benefit and mortality rates at 30 days were similar (RR 1.06; 95% CI: 0.68–1.66; Fig. 4). There was no difference between the devices for the occurrence of lower limb ischemia (RR 2.59; 95% CI: 0.75–8.97). However, the use of TandemHeart™ was associated with greater bleeding rates (RR 2.35; 95% CI: 1.40–3.93) when compared to IABP usage.

Although the primary objective was to determine the most effective and safest mechanical circulatory assist device for the treatment of cardiogenic shock, limitations were evident, such as the small number of patients, a comparison between different LVADs, and the short clinical follow-up period.

CONCLUSIONS AND RECOMMENDATIONS

The mortality rates related to cardiogenic shock remain unacceptably high, despite the advances in reperfusion strategies, despite primary PCI and modern adjunctive pharmacotherapy. Mechanical circulatory support, although based on physiological backgrounds, has not proven to be effective in reducing mortality in randomized controlled clinical trials.

However, AMI patients with cardiogenic shock represent an extremely high-risk group and the trials have been complicated by biased selection criteria and high cross over rates.

IABP is a mature technology and it is the first-line choice assisted device for offering hemodynamic support in the treatment of AMI patients with cardiogenic shock. It is relatively easy to use and widely available. It requires a lower level of expertise for insertion than other devices (Table 4).

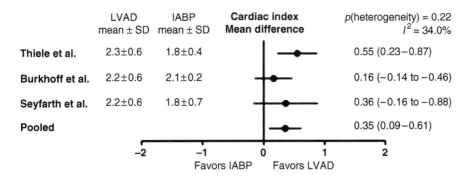

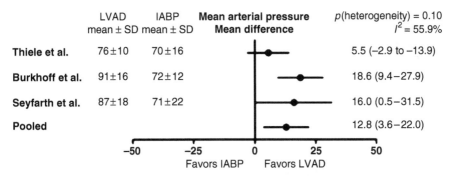

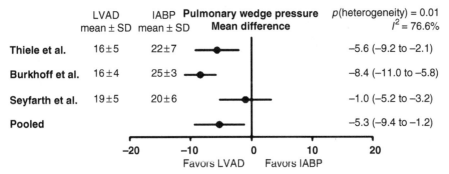

FIGURE 3 Comparative analysis in the hemodynamic parameters after the use of percutaneous left ventricular assist devices. *Source:* From Ref. 40.

Second-line treatments involve LVADs that can provide additional and active cardiac support in critically ill patients and require a higher level of skill, a team of health professionals to support the device, and there is a learning curve for successful use (Table 4).

The most recent European Guidelines recommended these devices as class "IIa" with "C" level of evidence (17). However, there are few comparative series with these different devices assessing major endpoints other than crude mortality. There is clearly a need for multicenter randomized controlled trials to properly assess the use of these devices, so that clear and robust guidelines can be developed.

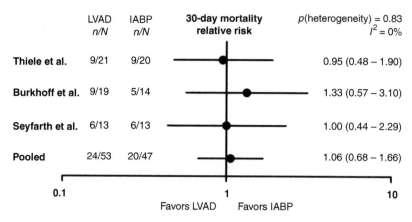

FIGURE 4 Thirty-day mortality with use of percutaneous left ventricular assist devices. *Source:* Modified from Ref. 40.

TABLE 4 Comparative Performance Analysis Between Intra-aortic Balloon Pump and Left Ventricular Assisted Devices

Device	Cumulative clinical experience and favorable evidences	Health professionals capable for insertion	Percutaneous insertion	Console usage and monitoring	Magnitude of hemodynamic support	Longevity of support permanence (>48 hr)
Intra-aortic balloon pump	Higher	ER/CCU physicians, interventional cardiologists and cardiac surgeons	Always	More easier	Lower	Similar (progressively higher complication rate >48 hr of insertion)
Left ventricular assisted devices	Lower	Interventional cardiologists with/out cardiac surgeons	Not always	Less easier	Higher	Similar (progressively higher complication rate >48 hr of insertion)

REFERENCES

1. Becker RC, Gore JM, Lambrew C, et al. A composite view of cardiac rupture in the United States National Registry of Myocardial Infarction. J Am Coll Cardiol 1996; 27:1321–1326.
2. Babaev A, Frederick PD, Pasta DJ, et al; NRMI Investigators. Trends in management and outcomes of patients with acute myocardial infarction complicated by cardiogenic shock. JAMA 2005; 294:448–454.
3. Goldberg RJ, Gore JM, Alpert JS, et al. Cardiogenic shock after acute myocardial infarction: incidence and mortality from a community-wide perspective, 1975–1988. N Engl J Med 1991; 325:1117–1122.
4. Goldberg RJ, Samad NA, Yarzebski J, et al. Temporal trends in cardiogenic shock complicating acute myocardial infarction. N Engl J Med 1999; 340:1162–1168.
5. Zeymer U, Vogt A, Zahn R, et al. Predictors of in-hospital mortality in 1333 patients

with acute myocardial infarction complicated by cardiogenic shock treated with primary percutaneous coronary intervention (PCI). Eur Heart J 2004; 25:322–328.

6. Jeger RV, Radovanovic D, Hunziker PR, et al. Ten-year incidence and treatment of cardiogenic shock. Ann Intern Med 2008; 149:618–626.

7. Hochman JS, Sleeper LA, Webb JG, et al. Early revascularization in acute myocardial infarction complicated by cardiogenic shock. N Engl J Med 1999; 341:625–634.

8. The TRIUMPH Investigators. Effect of tilarginine acetate in patients with acute myocardial infarction and cardiogenic shock. The TRIUMPH Randomized Controlled Trial. JAMA 2007; 297:1657–1666.

9. Hochman JS, Sleeper LA, White HD, et al; SHOCK Investigators. One-year survival following early revascularization for cardiogenic shock. JAMA 2001; 285:190–192.

10. Hochman JS, Sleeper LA, Webb JG, et al. Early revascularization and long-term survival in cardiogenic shock complicating acute myocardial infarction. JAMA 2006; 295:2511–2515.

11. Hochman JS, Buller CE, Sleeper LA, et al. Cardiogenic shock complicating acute myocardial infarction—etiologies, management and outcomes: a report from the SHOCK trial registry. J Am Coll Cardiol 2000; 36:1063–1070.

12. Thiele H, Smalling RW, Schuler G. Percutaneous left ventricular assist devices in cardiogenic shock. Eur Heart J 2007; 28:2057–2063.

13. Kern MJ, Aguirre F, Bach R, et al. Augmentation of coronary blood flow by intra-aortic balloon pumping in patients after coronary angioplasty. Circulation 1993; 87: 500–511.

14. Sanborn TA, Sleeper LA, Bates ER, et al. Impact of thrombolysis, intra-aortic balloon pump counterpulsation, and their combination in cardiogenic shock complicating acute myocardial infarction: a report from the SHOCK Trial Registry. SHould we emergently revascularize Occluded Coronaries for cardiogenic shocK? J Am Coll Cardiol 2000; 36:1123–1129.

15. Smalling RW, Cassidy DB, Barrett R, et al. Improved regional myocardial blood flow, left ventricular unloading, and infarct salvage using an axial-flow, transvalvular left ventricular assist device. A comparison with intra-aortic balloon counterpulsation and reperfusion alone in a canine infarction model. Circulation 1992; 85:1152–1159.

16. Kantrowitz A, Tjonneland S, Freed PS, et al. Initial clinical experience with intraaortic balloon pumping in cardiogenic shock. JAMA 1968; 203:113–118.

17. Van de Werf F, Bax J, Betriu A, et al. Management of acute myocardial infarction in patients presenting with persistent ST-segment elevation: the Task Force on the management of ST-segment elevation acute myocardial infarction of the European Society of Cardiology. Eur Heart J 2008; 29:2909–2945.

18. Antman EM, Anbe DT, Armstrong PW, et al. 2007 Focused Update of the ACC/AHA 2004 Guidelines for the Management of Patients With ST-Elevation Myocardial Infarction. A Report of the American College of Cardiology/American Heart Association Task Force on Practice Guidelines. J Am Coll Cardiol 2008; 51:210–247.

19. Sjauw KD, Engström AE, Vis MM, et al. A systematic review and meta-analysis of intra-aortic balloon pump therapy in ST-elevation myocardial infarction: should we change the guidelines? Eur Heart J 2009; 30:459–468.

20. O'Rourke MF, Norris RM, Campbell TJ, et al. Randomized controlled trial of intraaortic balloon counterpulsation in early myocardial infarction with acute heart failure. Am J Cardiol 1981; 47:815–820.

21. Flaherty JT, Becker LC, Weiss JL, et al. Results of a randomized prospective trial of intraaortic balloon counterpulsation and intravenous nitroglycerin in patients with acute myocardial infarction. J Am Coll Cardiol 1985; 6:434–446.

22. Kono T, Morita H, Nishina T, et al. Aortic counterpulsation may improve late patency of the occluded coronary artery in patients with early failure of thrombolytic therapy. J Am Coll Cardiol 1996; 28:876–881.

23. Ohman EM, Nanas J, Stomel RJ, et al. Thrombolysis and counterpulsation to improve survival in myocardial infarction complicated by hypotension and suspected

cardiogenic shock or heart failure: results of the TACTICS Trial. J Thromb Thrombolysis 2005; 19:33–39.

24. Ohman EM, George BS, White CJ, et al. Use of aortic counterpulsation to improve sustained coronary artery patency during acute myocardial infarction. Results of a randomized trial. The Randomized IABP Study Group. Circulation 1994; 90:792–799.

25. Stone GW, Marsalese D, Brodie BR, et al. A prospective, randomized evaluation of prophylactic intraaortic balloon counterpulsation in high risk patients with acute myocardial infarction treated with primary angioplasty. Second Primary Angioplasty in Myocardial Infarction (PAMI-II) Trial Investigators. J Am Coll Cardiol 1997; 29:1459–1467.

26. van 't Hof AW, Liem AL, de Boer MJ, et al. A randomized comparison of intra-aortic balloon pumping after primary coronary angioplasty in high risk patients with acute myocardial infarction. Eur Heart J 1999; 20:659–665.

27. Moulopoulos S, Stamatelopoulos S, Petrou P. Intraaortic balloon assistance in intractable cardiogenic shock. Eur Heart J 1986; 7:396–403.

28. Stomel RJ, Rasak M, Bates ER. Treatment strategies for acute myocardial infarction complicated by cardiogenic shock in a community hospital. Chest 1994; 105:997–1002.

29. Kovack PJ, Rasak MA, Bates ER, et al. Thrombolysis plus aortic counterpulsation: improved survival in patients who present to community hospitals with cardiogenic shock. J Am Coll Cardiol 1997; 29:1454–1458.

30. Bengtson JR, Kaplan AJ, Pieper KS, et al. Prognosis in cardiogenic shock after acute myocardial infarction in the interventional era. J Am Coll Cardiol 1992; 20:1482–1489.

31. Waksman R, Weiss AT, Gotsman MS, et al. Intra-aortic balloon counterpulsation improves survival in cardiogenic shock complicating acute myocardial infarction. Eur Heart J 1993; 14:71–74.

32. Anderson RD, Ohman EM, Holmes DR Jr, et al. Use of intraaortic balloon counterpulsation in patients presenting with cardiogenic shock: observations from the GUSTO-I Study. Global Utilization of Streptokinase and TPA for Occluded Coronary Arteries. J Am Coll Cardiol 1997; 30:708–715.

33. Barron HV, Every NR, Parsons LS, et al. The use of intra-aortic balloon counterpulsation in patients with cardiogenic shock complicating acute myocardial infarction: data from the National Registry of Myocardial Infarction 2. Am Heart J 2001; 141:933–939.

34. Vis MM, Sjauw KD, van der Schaaf RJ, et al. In patients with ST-segment elevation myocardial infarction with cardiogenic shock treated with percutaneous coronary intervention, admission glucose level is a strong independent predictor for 1-year mortality in patients without a prior diagnosis of diabetes. Am Heart J 2007; 154:1184–1190.

35. Vis MM, Sjauw KD, Van Der Schaaf RJ, et al. Prognostic value of admission hemoglobin levels in ST-segment elevation myocardial infarction patients presenting with cardiogenic shock. Am J Cardiol 2007; 99:1201–1202.

36. Shawl FA, Domanski MJ, Hernandez TJ, et al. Emergency percutaneous cardiopulmonary bypass support in cardiogenic shock from acute myocardial infarction. Am J Cardiol 1989; 64:967–970.

37. Baughman KL, Jarcho JA. Bridge to life—cardiac mechanical support. N Engl J Med 2007; 357:846–849.

38. Seyfarth M, Sibbing D, Bauer I, et al. A randomized clinical trial to evaluate the safety and efficacy of a percutaneous left ventricular assist device versus intra-aortic balloon pumping for treatment of cardiogenic shock caused by myocardial infarction. J Am Coll Cardiol 2008; 52:1584–1588.

39. Thiele H, Sick P, Boudriot E, et al. Randomized comparison of intra-aortic balloon support with a percutaneous left ventricular assist device in patients with revascularized acute myocardial infarction complicated by cardiogenic shock. Eur Heart J 2005; 26:1276–1283.

40. Cheng JM, den Uil CA, Hoeks SE, et al. Percutaneous left ventricular assist devices vs. intra-aortic balloon pump counterpulsation for treatment of cardiogenic shock: a meta-analysis of controlled trials. Eur Heart J 2009; 30(17):2102–2108.
41. Burkhoff D, Cohen H, Brunckhorst C, et al. A randomized multicenter clinical study to evaluate the safety and efficacy of the TandemHeart percutaneous ventricular assist device versus conventional therapy with intraaortic balloon pumping for treatment of cardiogenic shock. Am Heart J 2006; 152:469.e461–e468.

Primary Angioplasty: Methods of Reducing Infarct Size and Reperfusion Injury

Michael Gick and Jan Minners

Herz-Zentrum Bad Krozingen, Bad Krozingen, Germany

Franz-Josef Neumann

Herz-Zentrum Bad Krozingen, Bad Krozingen, and University of Freiburg, Freiburg, Germany

INTRODUCTION

In acute myocardial infarction, effective and sustained reperfusion can salvage myocardium and improve survival and convalescence. Although there is no alternative to reperfusion when pursuing these treatment goals, some aspects of reperfusion may cause additional injury and, thus, constitute potential therapeutic targets. Reperfusion arrhythmia, myocardial stunning, reperfusion-induced microvascular damage, and reperfusion-induced myocardial necrosis are generally considered as the principle manifestations of reperfusion injury. There is, however, debate whether microvascular damage and expansion of the necrotic zone truly represent reperfusion injury or rather extension of the consequences of the ischemic insult into the reperfusion period.

Animal experiments performed in a variety of species have demonstrated that the burst of oxygen free radical formation, which occurs upon reperfusion, plays a key role in the pathophysiology of each of the manifestations of reperfusion injury. In addition, it has been shown both in experimental animals and in patients that myocardial salvage during reperfusion critically depends on adequate recovery of the coronary microcirculation. Apart from inadequate patency of the infarct-related artery (which will be discussed in other chapters of this book), distal embolization of thrombus and plaque material as well as inflammatory interactions of blood cells with the microvasculature limit the quality of reperfusion in acute myocardial infarction. In the current chapter, we will discuss therapeutic options to interfere with these two mechanisms. In addition, we will address measures of interfering with the metabolic conditions that lead to the extension of myocardial necrosis during reperfusion.

PREVENTION OF DISTAL EMBOLIZATION

Studies in percutaneous coronary intervention (PCI) of saphenous vein grafts established the potential of mechanical embolic protection devices. The SAFER trial on saphenous vein graft intervention demonstrated a substantial, statistically significant reduction in the incidence of peri-interventional myocardial infarction with a first generation mechanical protection device as compared to standard care (1). The FIRE trial confirmed that similar results could be obtained with a much simpler second generation filter device (2,3).

In acute myocardial infarction, distal embolization of plaque and thrombus material is considered a major cause of insufficient reperfusion despite a fully patent infarct-related artery. Angiographic evidence of distal embolization is found in 9% to 15% of the patients after primary PCI for acute myocardial infarction, but the true incidence of distal embolization may be considerably higher, as suggested by autopsy studies (4). In a recent study, angiographic evidence of distal embolization was associated with an eightfold increase in 5-year mortality (5). Therefore, it was hypothesized that distal protection devices with primary PCI may improve clinical outcome of primary PCI substantially.

Devices

Technical solutions for reduction of embolization include distal or proximal protection devices minimizing the dislocation of thrombotic material into the distal segments of the coronary vasculature, thromboaspiration devices reducing the thrombotic burden of the affected artery, and finally a combination of the two. The first pure distal protection device was the prototypical FilterWire® (3) tested in saphenous vein graft intervention. A filter system is unfolded distally to the culprit lesion retaining all particles larger than 50 μm. Another distal protection device is the Percusurge® system (1). Here, a small balloon inflated distally to the culprit lesion stops blood flow during intervention and thereby prevents distal embolization. Before balloon deflation and reestablishment of blood flow accumulated thrombus material and debris have to be removed with an aspiration catheter. This device therefore represents a combination of embolic protection and thrombaspiration device. Proximal protection is achieved using the Proxis® system (6), also first applied in saphenous vein graft interventions. A sealing balloon is inflated proximally to the lesion, temporarily suspending antegrade blood flow and thus protecting all downstream vessels, including collateral branches and bifurcations. Again, before restoring blood flow aspiration of thrombi and debris is performed with an evacuation syringe.

A number of dedicated thrombaspiration/thrombectomy devices have been developed. Either by hand or with a motorized suction pump, thrombotic material is removed as far as it fits into the catheter. The suction catheter area is about one square millimeter and the catheter is guided by a wire through the lesion into the vessel. There are different designs for the tip to ease the passage into the lesion and remove material from the surrounding area. A special aspiration catheter, the X-SIZER® (ev3, Inc.) (7), houses an atraumatic helical cutter on its tip. The Archimedes screw is designed to grab thrombus on contact, drawing it in shearing and removing it with a vacuum effect. Another aspiration strategy has been named "rheolytic thrombectomy." Thrombectomy is accomplished with the introduction of a pressurized saline jet stream through the directed orifices on the distal tip of the catheter tip. The jet generates a localized low pressure zone via the Bernoulli effect and thus entrains and macerates thrombus. The saline and clot particles are then sucked back into the exhaust lumen of the catheter based on the Venturi principle (AngioJet®) (8).

Clinical Trials of Embolic Protection in Primary PCI

In the setting of primary PCI for acute myocardial infarction, embolic protection devices are employed with the intent to reduce infarct size and to improve long-term outcome. Measurement of infarct size in clinical trials can be performed using sestamibi SPECT calculating the difference between the area at risk and the final infarct size determined at 30 days postinfarction. Alternatively, estimation of infarct size is feasible by magnetic resonance imaging (MRI). However, most of the pertinent clinical trials did not investigate hard clinical endpoints due to the low incidence of clinical events. Instead, surrogate parameters including visible distal embolizations, TIMI flow grade, "corrected TIMI flow grade," flow velocity, "myocardial blush grade" or ST segment resolution were used. Although these parameters of epicardial and microcirculatory perfusion have been shown repeatedly to correlate with long time outcome, the use of a variety of surrogate parameters complicates the comparison of the different trials and devices.

Regarding distal protection devices, a number of trials have shown a reduction of visible distal embolization with a meta-analysis by de Luca reporting on six trials demonstrating a significant reduction of this surrogate parameter. Flow characteristics of the affected epicardial vessel were very heterogeneous with no significant improvement in the pooled analysis (9). Similarly the effect of distal protection on myocardial blush grade is controversial, although the pooled data showed a significant improvement in the device group. Coronary flow velocity representing a sensitive parameter of the functional integrity of the microvasculature was investigated extensively in the PROMISE trial (10). This randomized study involving 200 patients failed to demonstrate an improvement of maximal adenosine-induced coronary flow in the device group. Also, there was no improvement in ST segment resolution in the EMERALD, ASPARAGUS, or DEDICATION trial (11–13). In the PROMISE trial, neither infarct size nor ejection fraction as measured by MRI was different between the study groups (10). Similar results were obtained in the EMERALD trial (11). Only few trials investigating distal protection devices report on hard clinical endpoints. With a lack of benefit regarding infarct size an improved outcome is unlikely. Consistently, two recent meta-analyses did not reveal any significant difference in mortality between the distal protection and usual care (9,14). In summary, so far, none of the clinical trials has demonstrated an improvement in infarct size or mortality with the use of distal protection devices.

Clinical Trials of Thrombaspiration in Primary PCI

An alternative approach to myocardial protection consists of aspiration of thrombotic material during primary PCI in an attempt to reduce thrombotic burden and improve epicardial and microvascular flow. Of the surrogate endpoints discussed above, thrombaspiration has repeatedly been shown to reduce visible distal embolizations. Effects on flow characteristics of the epicardial vessels are inconsistent; large trials like the EXPORT Study (15) showed no improvement of the rate of TIMI III flow grade by thrombaspiration. ST segment resolution was significantly improved in the small EXPORT trial (15) and in the X-Amine ST Trial (16). A meta-analysis published in 2007 demonstrated a trend for improvement in some of the surrogate endpoints (9). However, thrombaspiration devices have been undergoing a renaissance since the publication of the TAPAS trial in 2008 (17) that showed an improvement in myocardial blush grade and ST segment resolution in patients treated with a thrombaspiration device. Even more convincingly, rates of cardiac death or nonfatal reinfarction were significantly reduced after one year (5.6 vs. 9.9%; $P < 0.01$) (Fig. 1) (18). Consequently, an updated meta-analysis reporting on eight trials including TAPAS demonstrated a significant improvement in mortality with thrombaspiration (19).

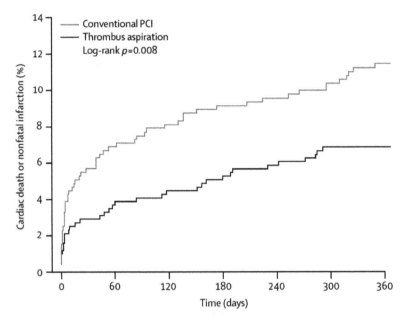

FIGURE 1 Thrombaspiration significantly decreases the combined endpoint of cardiac death or nonfatal reinfarction after one-year of follow-up in the TAPAS trial. *Source*: From Ref. 18.

A differentiation between manual (e.g., Export or Pronto catheter) and mechanical (e.g., Angiojet or X-sizer) aspiration devices showed improved survival for the manual and increased mortality for the mechanical approach (14). In this review, increased mortality was driven by excess deaths in the AiMI trial, however, investigators were unable to identify a specific device-related reason for these findings.

In summary, results from a multitude of clinical trials regarding mechanical embolic protection and thrombaspiration/thrombectomy are inconsistent. Whereas surrogate endpoints are repeatedly improved, a clinical benefit for these devices has only been suggested by the TAPAS trial, so far.

INHIBITION OF INFLAMMATORY AND THROMBOTIC RESPONSES

Apart from oxygen free radicals that are immediately formed upon reperfusion, inflammatory interactions of leucocytes and platelets with endothelial cells and myocytes play a central role in the pathophysiology of reperfusion. Although these inflammatory mechanisms are essential to the removal of necrotic tissue and formation of a stable scar, they may also cause further damage both to the microvasculature and to viable myocytes. As early as the 1970s, clinicians attempted to limit inflammatory damage in acute myocardial infarction by the administration of corticosteroids. This, however, increased the risk of aneurysm formation and ventricular rupture (20). Since then, a number of pharmacological approaches to limit inflammatory responses during reperfusion have been developed in experimental animals. Many of these pharmacological strategies, although very effective under experimental conditions, yielded disappointing results in initial clinical studies. Specifically, among the more promising pharmacological strategies both the application of radical scavengers (21) and the inhibition of Mac-1, a key leucocyte adhesion molecule (22), were unable to demonstrate any clinical benefit and were thus abandoned at an early stage of clinical development. Among the many promising therapeutic principles derived from animal experiments, only three found their way into large-scale clinical trials: adenosine, complement inhibition, and inhibition of the glycoprotein (GP) IIb/IIIa, a β_3 integrin on platelets. These approaches will be discussed below.

Adenosine

In experimental animals, adenosine inhibits oxygen free radical formation as well as neutrophil activity and accumulation and improves microvascular function. In addition, adenosine participates in ischemic preconditioning (see below). Thus, in animal models of reperfusion injury, adenosine has consistently reduced infarct size.

Based on these findings, the concept of adenosine for reperfusion in acute myocardial infarction was tested in the AMISTAD (Acute Myocardial Infarction Study of Adenosine) trial in the setting of thrombolytic therapy (23). The study randomly assigned 362 patients within six hours after onset of ST elevation myocardial infarction to either adenosine infusion or placebo. Although the primary endpoint, reduction of infarct size, was missed in the entire cohort, there was an impressive reduction in infarct size in patients with anterior myocardial infarction, from 44.5% in 38 patients of the placebo group to 15% in 39 patients of the adenosine group ($P = 0.014$). Based on these findings the concept that adenosine infusion improves outcome in patients with entire myocardial infarction was tested in the AMISTAD-2 trial (24). In this trial, patients with anterior ST elevation myocardial infarction were randomly assigned to placebo ($n = 703$) or adenosine infusion at a rate of 50 µg/kg/min ($n = 701$) or 70 µg/kg/min ($n = 713$). The primary endpoint, the composite six-month incidence of death, new congestive heart failure or rehospitalization for a heart failure, did not show any significant benefit of the adenosine infusions as compared with placebo (16.3% vs. 17.9%; $P = 0.043$). Likewise, in the entire adenosine group infarct size was not significantly lower than in the placebo group. Based on these findings, adenosine did not find its way into routine clinical practice for patients with acute myocardial infarction.

Complement Inhibition

The canine model of myocardial infarction revealed neutrophil activation and complement C5a activity and complement depletion by cobra venom treatment reduced the infarct size (25–27). Based on these findings the antibody pexelizumab was developed for complement inhibition and tested in various clinical settings including myocardial infarction. In the COMMA (COMplement inhibition in Myocardial infarction treated with Angioplasty) trial comprising 960 patients (28) pexelizumab missed the primary endpoint of the reduction in infarct size. Nevertheless, a significant reduction in 90-day mortality was observed with bolus and infusion of pexelizumab. Based on these findings, pexelizumab was tested in the large APEX-AMI (Assessment of Pexelizumab in Acute Myocardial Infarction) trial (29). This trial was stopped prematurely for presumed futility. At this time, 5745 patients had been randomly assigned to pexelizumab or placebo. Mortality in the pexelizumab group was 4.1% versus 3.9% in the placebo group (hazard ratio 1.10; 95% confidence interval: 0.86–1.39;

$P = 0.45$). Similarly the combined incidence of death, cardiogenic shock, or congestive heart failure was almost identical in the two treatment arms (hazard ratio 1.01; 95% confidence interval: 0.89–1.19; $P = 0.91$). Thus, although very promising from a theoretical point of view, pexelizumab did not yield any clinical benefit during reperfusion in acute myocardial infarction.

GPIIb/IIIa Receptor Blockade and Other Antithrombotic Therapies

Experimental models of myocardial infarction document the preeminent role of platelets in limiting blood flow during reperfusion in acute myocardial infarction (30). By occlusive thrombus formation, distal embolization of small aggregates, and release of vasoconstrictive mediators, platelets interfere with both large vessel patency and microvascular flow. Activated platelets can also adhere to the endothelial cells in the reperfused region. Binding of platelet GP IIb/IIIa to the endothelial vitronectin receptor plays a key role in this interaction (31). Due to the platelet's proinflammatory cytokine activity, adhesion of platelets to endothelial cells becomes an important mechanism for procoagulant, vasoconstrictor, and inflammatory responses, including leukocyte attachment. Platelets are, thus, important players in the inflammatory cell interactions that limit the benefit from reperfusion.

The ISAR-2 trial (Intracoronary Stenting and Antithrombotic Regimen) demonstrated improved recovery of perfusion and improved recovery of wall motion in the infarct area in patients receiving abciximab as an adjunct to primary PCI in acute myocardial infarction as compared with patients receiving only heparin (32). This was taken as a proof-of-principle that the inhibition of the GPIIb/IIIa receptor improved recovery of microvascular and myocardial function in reperfused myocardial infarction. De Luca et al. (33) analyzed the available evidence of the effect of abciximab in clinical outcome in patients undergoing PCI for acute myocardial infarction. This meta-analysis comprised six studies that included 3912 patients with primary PCI. They found a 28% relative reduction in 6- to 12-month mortality by abciximab as compared with the control group (4.4% vs. 6.2%; $P = 0.01$). The BRAVE-3 (Bavarian Reperfusion Alternatives Evaluation) trial investigated the effect of abciximab versus placebo in patients preloaded with the thienopyridine clopidogrel. The primary endpoint infarct size was not significantly different in the 401 patients assigned to abciximab as compared with the 399 patients assigned to placebo (34). In addition, there was no significant difference in the incidence of mortality (3.2% in the abciximab group vs. 2.5% in the placebo group; $P = 0.53$) (34). The HORIZONS-AMI study (35) randomly assigned 1802 patients to unfractionated heparin plus anti-GPIIb/IIIa and 1800 patients to bivalirudin. In the bivalirudin group, provisional administration of GPIIb/IIIa inhibitors was allowed for high-risk settings, such as large thrombus burden or poor flow. Accordingly 8.2% of the patients of the bivalirudin group received GPIIb/IIIa inhibitors. HORIZONS-AMI showed no significant benefit of GPIIb/IIIa inhibitors with respect to ischemic complications, but a significant reduction in major bleeding by bivalirudin from 8.3% to 4.9% ($P \leq 0.001$). Thus the net clinical outcome was superior in the bivalirudin group as compared with the unfractionated heparin plus anti-GPIIb/IIIa group (12.1% vs. 9.2%; $P = 0.06$). Although, mortality was not a primary endpoint, it is noteworthy that there was a significant reduction in mortality from 4.8% in the heparin plus GPIIb/IIIa group to 3.4% in the bivalirudin group ($P = 0.029$).

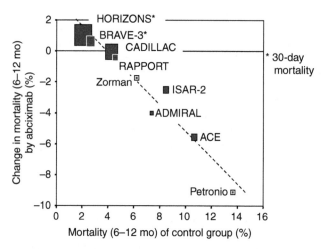

FIGURE 2 Mortality reduction by abciximab as a function of the mortality of the control group.

When comparing the various randomized trials that addressed GPIIb/IIIa receptor blockade as compared with control treatments it is noteworthy that there is a large variability in the mortality of the control arm (Fig. 2). The benefit of GPIIb/IIIa receptor blockade was the larger the higher the mortality of the control group. Hence, effective GPIIb/IIIa receptor blockade may still be needed in high-risk patients.

On the other hand, it has to be considered that mortality of the control group in BRAVE-3 and HORIZONS-AMI might have been low because of the effective antithrombotic treatment regimen that was instituted in the control arm. BRAVE-3 was the first study in which patients with acute myocardial infarction had been systematically pretreated with a thienopyridine prior to PCI. It is known that blockade of the $P2Y_{12}$-receptor by thienopyridines inhibits the activation of the GPIIb/IIIa receptor upon stimulation with ADP and by this mechanism also inhibits platelet leucocyte interactions and other inflammatory responses. Effective $P2Y_{12}$-receptor blockade may thus obviate the need for additional GPIIb/IIIa receptor blockade. This interpretation is corroborated by recent findings from the TRITON-TIMI 38 trial (36). In this trial, the third generation thienopyridine prasugrel that induces a more rapid consistent and potent platelet inhibition reduced a 30-day mortality in patients undergoing PCI for acute myocardial infarction as compared with the less potent thienopyridine clopidogrel (37). As far as HORIZONS-AMI is concerned, it has to be considered that by acting as a direct thrombin inhibitor bivalirudin interferes with the one of the most powerful stimulants for platelets, capable of inducing increased surface expression and activation of the GPIIb/IIIa receptors. On the contrary, heparin by itself that was used in the control arm directly activates platelets. Hence, reduction of platelet activation by bivalirudin as compared with heparin might have contributed to the beneficial results in HORIZONS-AMI.

In summary, among the many pharmacological attempts to improve microvascular reperfusion only optimization of antithrombotic therapy proved to be successful in improving reperfusion and clinical outcome.

MEASURES TO IMPROVE METABOLIC CONDITIONS

Pre- and Postconditioning

Our growing understanding of the mechanisms leading to myocardial cell death in ischemia/reperfusion has lead to a number of interesting concepts regarding myocardial protection going beyond the swift reestablishment of coronary blood flow. For instance, cardiac preconditioning first described in 1986 (38) represents the most powerful method for the reduction of infarct size known today. Preconditioning describes a phenomenon whereby a set of short cycles of ischemia/reperfusion renders the heart more resistant to a subsequent prolonged ischemia/reperfusion insult with a reduction in infarct size up to 75% depending on cell type and protocol (39). Unraveling the cellular pathways resulting in the profound protection seen lead to the discovery of a number of agents (amongst others adenosine, bradykinine, nicorandil) able to mimic the cardioprotective effects of ischemic preconditioning at least in vitro. Clinically, results were disappointing (24). Moreover, in the clinical setting patients presenting with myocardial infarction already suffer from the prolonged ischemia/reperfusion insult and the application of a preconditioning stimulus – be it ischemia or a preconditioning mimetic drug – is therefore no longer feasible.

The cellular protection achieved by preconditioning is also obtained when the short cycles of ischemia/reperfusion are applied after the index ischemia (40). This phenomenon was consequently termed postconditioning and has recently been tested in a small pilot study in the setting of primary angioplasty. Four one-minute cycles of balloon inflation and deflation after successful opening of the culprit vessel resulted in a significant reduction in infarct size (41). That cardioprotection at reperfusion can also be achieved using a pharmacological agent has been suggested by a number of trial involving adenosine (see section "Inhibition of Inflammatory and Thrombotic Responses" above) and nicorandil. When the latter was tested in a multicenter study (545 patients) no reduction in infarct size or improvement in left ventricular ejection fraction during follow-up was noted (42). Cyclosporine A represents another preconditioning mimetic (43) shown to be cardioprotective when administered at reperfusion (44). In a pilot study randomizing 58 patients presenting with acute myocardial infarction to either IV cyclosporine or placebo, Piot et al. recently demonstrated that cyclosporine A reduces infarct size as indicated by creatine kinase release and MRI (Fig. 3) (45).

Cooling

A number of experimental studies strongly suggest that mild hypothermia induces myocardial protection during ischemia/reperfusion by decreasing metabolic demand (46). In patients with STEMI undergoing primary PCI mild hypothermia has been induced using both an invasive (47) as well as a non-invasive approach (48) demonstrating the feasibility and safety of this method. Unfortunately, data from a randomized trial (COOL-MI, published as an abstract only) including 357 patients showed no benefit (49). On the other hand, induction of mild hypothermia has been integrated into the recommendations for the treatment of successfully resuscitated patients (50). Since the majority of these patients can be expected to have underlying myocardial infarction it is tempting to speculate that mild hypothermia may be beneficial in this setting. A recent observational study (51) including resuscitated patients presenting with STEMI

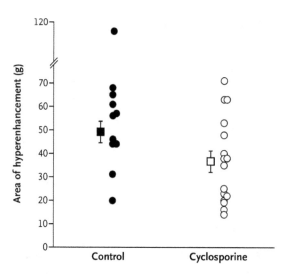

FIGURE 3 Mean infarct size as assessed by MRI is decreased by administration of cyclosporine prior to PCI ($P < 0.04$). *Source*: From Ref. 45.

undergoing primary PCI supports this notion. However, no data from randomized trials are available.

Glucose–Insulin Infusion
In the setting of ischemia, reperfusion glucose will reduce oxygen demand compared to fatty acids. Application of this concept in the clinical setting with the infusion of glucose, insulin, and potassium (GIK) in 20,201 patients with acute myocardial infarction, however, has shown no benefit (52).

Other Pharmacological Approaches
Calcium overload represents an important step in the cascade ultimately leading to cellular death. Conceptually, inhibition of cellular calcium accumulation using cariporide – a selective inhibitor of the sodium/hydrogen exchanger – therefore held much value. However, a study in patients presenting with myocardial infarction undergoing primary angioplasty failed to demonstrate a benefit for the inhibition of the sodium/hydrogen exchanger (53).

In summary, of the multitude of approaches to improve metabolic conditions in patients with acute myocardial infarction, postconditioning and cyclosporine A currently show potential clinical benefit and warrant further testing in large-scale clinical trials. Until results of such trials become available, speedy reestablishment of coronary blood flow preferably by primary angioplasty remains the main stay of contemporary treatment of acute myocardial infarction.

REFERENCES
1. Baim DS, Wahr D, George B, et al. Randomized trial of a distal embolic protection device during percutaneous intervention of saphenous vein aorto-coronary bypass grafts. Circulation 2002; 105:1285–1290.

2. Halkin A, Masud AZ, Rogers C, et al. Six-month outcomes after percutaneous intervention for lesions in aortocoronary saphenous vein grafts using distal protection devices: results from the FIRE trial. Am Heart J 2006; 151:915. e1–e7.
3. Stone GW, Rogers C, Hermiller J, et al. Randomized comparison of distal protection with a filter-based catheter and a balloon occlusion and aspiration system during percutaneous intervention of diseased saphenous vein aorto-coronary bypass grafts. Circulation 2003; 108:548–553.
4. Saber RS, Edwards WD, Bailey KR, et al. Coronary embolization after balloon angioplasty or thrombolytic therapy: an autopsy study of 32 cases. J Am Coll Cardiol 1993; 22:1283–1288.
5. Henriques JP, Zijlstra F, Ottervanger JP, et al. Incidence and clinical significance of distal embolization during primary angioplasty for acute myocardial infarction. Eur Heart J 2002; 23:1112–1127.
6. Mauri L, Cox D, Hermiller J, et al. The PROXIMAL trial: proximal protection during saphenous vein graft intervention using the Proxis Embolic Protection System: a randomized, prospective, multicenter clinical trial. J Am Coll Cardiol 2007; 50:1442–1449.
7. Beran G, Lang I, Schreiber W, et al. Intracoronary thrombectomy with the X-sizer catheter system improves epicardial flow and accelerates ST-segment resolution in patients with acute coronary syndrome: a prospective, randomized, controlled study. Circulation 2002; 105:2355–2360.
8. Ali A, Cox D, Dib N, et al. Rheolytic thrombectomy with percutaneous coronary intervention for infarct size reduction in acute myocardial infarction: 30-day results from a multicenter randomized study. J Am Coll Cardiol 2006; 48:244–252.
9. De Luca G, Suryapranata H, Stone GW, et al. Adjunctive mechanical devices to prevent distal embolization in patients undergoing mechanical revascularization for acute myocardial infarction: a meta-analysis of randomized trials. Am Heart J 2007; 153:343–553.
10. Gick M, Jander N, Bestehorn HP, et al. Randomized evaluation of the effects of filter-based distal protection on myocardial perfusion and infarct size after primary percutaneous catheter intervention in myocardial infarction with and without ST-segment elevation. Circulation 2005; 112:1462–1469.
11. Stone GW, Webb J, Cox DA, et al. Distal microcirculatory protection during percutaneous coronary intervention in acute ST-segment elevation myocardial infarction: a randomized controlled trial. JAMA 2005; 293:1063–1072.
12. Muramatsu T, Kozuma K, Tsukahara R, et al. Comparison of myocardial perfusion by distal protection before and after primary stenting for acute myocardial infarction: angiographic and clinical results of a randomized controlled trial. Catheter Cardiovasc Interv 2007; 70:677–682.
13. Kelbaek H, Terkelsen CJ, Helqvist S, et al. Randomized comparison of distal protection versus conventional treatment in primary percutaneous coronary intervention: the drug elution and distal protection in ST-elevation myocardial infarction (DEDICATION) trial. J Am Coll Cardiol 2008; 51:899–905.
14. Bavry AA, Kumbhani DJ, Bhatt DL. Role of adjunctive thrombectomy and embolic protection devices in acute myocardial infarction: a comprehensive meta-analysis of randomized trials. Eur Heart J 2008; 29:2989–3001.
15. Chevalier B, Gilard M, Lang I, et al. Systematic primary aspiration in acute myocardial percutaneous intervention: a multicentre randomised controlled trial of the export aspiration catheter. EuroIntervention 2008; 4:222–228.
16. Lefevre T, Garcia E, Reimers B, et al. X-sizer for thrombectomy in acute myocardial infarction improves ST-segment resolution: results of the X-sizer in AMI for negligible embolization and optimal ST resolution (X AMINE ST) trial. J Am Coll Cardiol 2005; 46:246–252.
17. Svilaas T, Vlaar PJ, van der Horst IC, et al. Thrombus aspiration during primary percutaneous coronary intervention. N Engl J Med 2008; 358:557–567.
18. Vlaar PJ, Svilaas T, van der Horst IC, et al. Cardiac death and reinfarction after 1 year in the Thrombus Aspiration during Percutaneous coronary intervention in

Acute myocardial infarction Study (TAPAS): a 1-year follow-up study. Lancet 2008; 371:1915–1920.

19. De Luca G, Dudek D, Sardella G, et al. Adjunctive manual thrombectomy improves myocardial perfusion and mortality in patients undergoing primary percutaneous coronary intervention for ST-elevation myocardial infarction: a meta-analysis of randomized trials. Eur Heart J 2008; 29:3002–3010.

20. Bulkley BH, Roberts WC. Steroid therapy during acute myocardial infarction. A cause of delayed healing and of ventricular aneurysm. Am J Med 1974; 56:244–250.

21. Flaherty JT, Pitt B, Gruber JW, et al. Recombinant human superoxide dismutase (h-SOD) fails to improve recovery of ventricular function in patients undergoing coronary angioplasty for acute myocardial infarction. Circulation 1994; 89:1982–1991.

22. Faxon DP, Gibbons RJ, Chronos NA, et al. The effect of blockade of the CD11/CD18 integrin receptor on infarct size in patients with acute myocardial infarction treated with direct angioplasty: the results of the HALT-MI study. J Am Coll Cardiol 2002; 40:1199–1204.

23. Mahaffey KW, Puma JA, Barbagelata NA, et al. Adenosine as an adjunct to thrombolytic therapy for acute myocardial infarction: results of a multicenter, randomized, placebo-controlled trial: the Acute Myocardial Infarction STudy of ADenosine (AMISTAD) trial. J Am Coll Cardiol 1999; 34:1711–1720.

24. Ross AM, Gibbons RJ, Stone GW, et al. A randomized, double-blinded, placebo-controlled multicenter trial of adenosine as an adjunct to reperfusion in the treatment of acute myocardial infarction (AMISTAD-II). J Am Coll Cardiol 2005; 45:1775–1780.

25. Dreyer WJ, Smith CW, Michael LH, et al. Canine neutrophil activation by cardiac lymph obtained during reperfusion of ischemic myocardium. Circ Res 1989; 65:1751–1762.

26. Birdsall HH, Green DM, Trial J, et al. Complement C5a, TGF-beta 1, and MCP-1, in sequence, induce migration of monocytes into ischemic canine myocardium within the first one to five hours after reperfusion. Circulation 1997; 95:684–692.

27. Griselli M, Herbert J, Hutchinson WL, et al. C-reactive protein and complement are important mediators of tissue damage in acute myocardial infarction. J Exp Med 1999; 190:1733–1740.

28. Granger CB, Mahaffey KW, Weaver WD, et al. Pexelizumab, an anti-C5 complement antibody, as adjunctive therapy to primary percutaneous coronary intervention in acute myocardial infarction: the COMplement inhibition in Myocardial infarction treated with Angioplasty (COMMA) trial. Circulation 2003; 108:1184–1190.

29. Armstrong PW, Granger CB, Adams PX, et al. Pexelizumab for acute ST-elevation myocardial infarction in patients undergoing primary percutaneous coronary intervention: a randomized controlled trial. JAMA 2007; 297:43–51.

30. Topol EJ. Toward a new frontier in myocardial reperfusion therapy: emerging platelet preeminence. Circulation 1998; 97:211–218.

31. Gawaz M, Neumann FJ, Schomig A. Evaluation of platelet membrane glycoproteins in coronary artery disease: consequences for diagnosis and therapy. Circulation 1999; 99:E1–E11.

32. Neumann FJ, Blasini R, Schmitt C, et al. Effect of glycoprotein IIb/IIIa receptor blockade on recovery of coronary flow and left ventricular function after the placement of coronary-artery stents in acute myocardial infarction. Circulation 1998; 98:2695–2701.

33. De Luca G, Suryapranata H, Stone GW, et al. Abciximab as adjunctive therapy to reperfusion in acute ST-segment elevation myocardial infarction: a meta-analysis of randomized trials. JAMA 2005; 293:1759–1765.

34. Mehilli J, Kastrati A, Schulz S, et al. Abciximab in patients with acute ST-segment-elevation myocardial infarction undergoing primary percutaneous coronary intervention after clopidogrel loading: a randomized double-blind trial. Circulation 2009; 119:1933–1940.

35. Stone GW, Witzenbichler B, Guagliumi G, et al. Bivalirudin during primary PCI in acute myocardial infarction. N Engl J Med 2008; 358:2218–2230.

36. Wiviott SD, Braunwald E, McCabe CH, et al. Prasugrel versus clopidogrel in patients with acute coronary syndromes. N Engl J Med 2007; 357:2001–2015.

37. Montalescot G, Wiviott SD, Braunwald E, et al. Prasugrel compared with clopidogrel in patients undergoing percutaneous coronary intervention for ST-elevation myocardial infarction (TRITON-TIMI 38): double-blind, randomised controlled trial. Lancet 2009; 373:723–731.
38. Murry CE, Jennings RB, Reimer KA. Preconditioning with ischemia: a delay of lethal cell injury in ischemic myocardium. Circulation 1986; 74:1124–1136.
39. Yellon DM, Downey JM. Preconditioning the myocardium: from cellular physiology to clinical cardiology. Physiol Rev 2003; 83:1113–1151.
40. Zhao ZQ, Corvera JS, Halkos ME, et al. Inhibition of myocardial injury by ischemic postconditioning during reperfusion: comparison with ischemic preconditioning. Am J Physiol Heart Circ Physiol 2003; 285:H579–H588.
41. Thibault H, Piot C, Staat P, et al. Long-term benefit of postconditioning. Circulation 2008; 117:1037–1044.
42. Kitakaze M, Asakura M, Kim J, et al. Human atrial natriuretic peptide and nicorandil as adjuncts to reperfusion treatment for acute myocardial infarction (J-WIND): two randomised trials. Lancet 2007; 370:1483–1493.
43. Minners J, van den Bos EJ, Yellon DM, et al. Dinitrophenol, cyclosporin A, and trimetazidine modulate preconditioning in the isolated rat heart: support for a mitochondrial role in cardioprotection. Cardiovasc Res 2000; 47:68–73.
44. Weinbrenner C, Liu GS, Downey JM, et al. Cyclosporine A limits myocardial infarct size even when administered after onset of ischemia. Cardiovasc Res 1998; 38:678–684.
45. Piot C, Croisille P, Staat P, et al. Effect of cyclosporine on reperfusion injury in acute myocardial infarction. N Engl J Med 2008; 359:473–481.
46. Hale SL, Kloner RA. Myocardial temperature in acute myocardial infarction: protection with mild regional hypothermia. Am J Physiol 1997; 273:H220–H227.
47. Dixon SR, Whitbourn RJ, Dae MW, et al. Induction of mild systemic hypothermia with endovascular cooling during primary percutaneous coronary intervention for acute myocardial infarction. J Am Coll Cardiol 2002; 40:1928–1934.
48. Ly HQ, Denault A, Dupuis J, et al. A pilot study: the Noninvasive Surface Cooling Thermoregulatory System for Mild Hypothermia Induction in Acute Myocardial Infarction (the NICAMI Study). Am Heart J 2005; 150:933.
49. O'Neill. COOL-MI. A prospective, randomized trial of mild systemic hypothermia during PCI treatment of ST elevation MI. Paper presented at: Transcatheter Cardiovascular Therapeutics (TCT) Meeting; 2003; Washington DC.
50. Nolan JP, Morley PT, Hoek TL, et al. Therapeutic hypothermia after cardiac arrest. An advisory statement by the Advancement Life Support Task Force of the International Liaison Committee on Resuscitation. Resuscitation 2003; 57:231–235.
51. Wolfrum S, Pierau C, Radke PW, et al. Mild therapeutic hypothermia in patients after out-of-hospital cardiac arrest due to acute ST-segment elevation myocardial infarction undergoing immediate percutaneous coronary intervention. Crit Care Med 2008; 36.1780–1786.
52. Mehta SR, Yusuf S, Diaz R, et al. Effect of glucose-insulin-potassium infusion on mortality in patients with acute ST-segment elevation myocardial infarction: the CREATE-ECLA randomized controlled trial. JAMA 2005; 293:437–446.
53. Theroux P, Chaitman BR, Danchin N, et al. Inhibition of the sodium-hydrogen exchanger with cariporide to prevent myocardial infarction in high-risk ischemic situations. Main results of the GUARDIAN trial. Guard during ischemia against necrosis (GUARDIAN) Investigators. Circulation 2000; 102:3032–3038.

12 Primary Angioplasty: The Importance of Time to Reperfusion, Door to Balloon Times, and How to Reduce Them

Atman P. Shah

Department of Medicine, Division of Cardiology, The University of Chicago, Chicago, Illinois, U.S.A.

William J. French

Department of Medicine, Division of Cardiology, Harbor-UCLA Medical Center, Torrance, California, U.S.A.

Acute ST segment myocardial infarction (STEMI) is a growing, international health concern with at least 500,000 events annually in the United States (1). The pathophysiology of STEMI involves complete occlusion of a coronary artery with a thrombus arising from the site of a ruptured plaque. Cessation of blood flow to the area of affected myocardium would lead to myocardial necrosis and subsequent loss of function. "Time is muscle" (2) became the guiding practice and opening up the occluded artery became standard of care. Mortality from STEMI increases by 7.5% for every 30 minutes revascularization is delayed (3,4). Prompt revascularization can increase survival for patients. Initially the fastest way to revascularize STEMI patients was with fibrinolytic therapy. Currently, percutaneous coronary intervention offers better clinical outcomes than treatment with fibrinolytics and has become the revascularization method of choice (5). Hospitals and public health officials can influence (6) outcomes by developing systems and processes that minimize the intervals between onset of patient systems and revascularization.

While fibrinolytics can be administered in ambulances, the ability to perform primary percutaneous coronary interventions (PCIs) requires a skilled cardiac catheterization laboratory, defined by the American College of Cardiology and the American Heart Association as a laboratory that performs over 200 PCIs annually, of which 36 are for STEMI and is staffed by physicians who perform at least 75 PCIs a year (1). Therefore, there is currently a strong desire to transport STEMI patients to centers that are primary PCI "ready."

Early and complete revascularization after STEMI has been associated consistently with lower mortality. Gibson et al. have reported data from the NRMI database that mortality from STEMI dropped from 8.6% in 1994 to 3.1% in patients undergoing primary PCI. This drop in mortality was commensurate with a decrease in the door-to-balloon time of 111 minutes in 1994 to 79 minutes in 2006 (7). These contemporary findings were echoed by results published from the Global Registry of Acute Coronary Events (GRACE) investigators that reported a decrease in mortality from 6.9% to 5.4% from 1999 to 2006 correlating with a decrease in time to reperfusion (8). However, this same study also reported that up to 40% of patients with STEMI do not receive timely reperfusion and 33% of the patients in the study, despite having presented with a STEMI, do not receive any reperfusion therapy at all.

Timely reperfusion of the infarct artery requires coordination between a variety of healthcare providers. However, initiation of the system of care begins with the patient, but the average patient with a STEMI does not seek medical care for approximately two hours after symptom onset (9). Furthermore, there was an increased delay in seeking care on behalf of non-Hispanic blacks, the elderly, and publicly supported recipients compared to Medicare recipients (10). Part of the reason for the delay in seeking care has to deal with confusion about their symptoms (not having the symptoms classically seen on TV and in the movies) as well as being embarrassed for calling a "false alarm" (11).

While emergency medical services (EMS) are available to almost 95% of the American population, just 53% of patient with a STEMI were transported to the hospital by an ambulance (12), a statistic that is sobering given that approximately 1 in 300 patients who are having chest pain being transported to the hospital by a non-EMS vehicle go into cardiac arrest while en route (13), underlining the importance that patients contact EMS so that they are transported safely.

Public health programs that have stressed the need for early self-recognitions of the signs and symptoms of a possible STEMI and the need to notify EMS have been reported to increase EMS use by 20% to 40% (14). Therefore, despite all the efforts that can be put toward improving public EMS and hospital systems, improving public education and access to EMS will provide an important first step in reducing DTB times.

Once the patient has contacted EMS, there are a number of strategies that can be employed that will reduce the time necessary to open the occluded artery. A door-to-balloon time of less than 90 minutes is the goal. However, a recent study of 365 U.S. hospitals found that the median DTB time was 100 minutes and only 14% of the studied hospitals had a DTB <90 minutes (15). A large part of the problem is that almost 35% of all Americans presenting with STEMI present to hospitals that do not have the capacity to perform primary PCI therefore necessitating the use of fibrinolytics and/or a transfer to a PCI-capable hospital and incorporating a delay (16). Implementation of systems designed to quickly transport and reperfuse patients has proven to be successful with either a "spoke and hub" model whereby all patients with STEMI are transported to a PCI-ready hospital (17) or a model where non–PCI capable hospitals adopt strategies to treat patients with lytics prior to transport; (18) the fact that a system exists reduces DTB times.

Recently, many municipalities have recognized the benefit of having suspected STEMI patients transferred directly from the field to a PCI-capable hospital. This triage point has been facilitated by the early adoption by many municipalities of 12-lead ECG systems that are placed in the ambulance. Rapid interpretation of 12-lead ECGs of suspected STEMI patients by trained paramedics could lead to a reduction in DTB times by correct and early triage of patients (19,20). Le May et al. (21) reported a nearly 50% reduction in DTB times in STEMI patients who were triaged to PCI-capable hospitals based on 12-lead ECGs obtained by paramedics in the field compared to STEMI patients taken to the nearest hospital and then to a PCI-capable hospital. Recently, Rokos et al. (22) have reported that the implementation of prehospital ECGs in 10 communities

(Royal Oak MI, Atlanta GA, Charlotte NC, Minneapolis-St. Paul MN, Medford OR, Marin County CA, Ventura County CA, Los Angeles County CA, Orange County CA, and San Diego County CA) has led to 86% of STEMI patients having a DTB of less than 90 minutes.

Obtaining a prehospital ECG allows not only preferential transfer to those hospitals best equipped to handle STEMIs, but it also allows early notification of the Cardiac Catheterization Laboratory Team that allows quicker mobilization. Bradley et al. (15) reported that direct activation of the CCL team from the field is associated with a 15-minute reduction in DTB times. However, activation of the CCL team by paramedics or ED physicians can be associated with a false-positive activation rate of almost 30% (23). False activations of the CCL team carry a human and economic cost; so a number of studies have investigated methods to reduce the number of false-positive activations. These methods include direct transmission of the ECG from the ambulance to either the emergency department physician or the cardiologist or simply by taking a picture of the ECG with a handheld device and transmitting the image to the cardiologist (24).

Simplifying the process for activating the CCL team will lead to a reduction in DTB times. For example, many hospitals have employed a system whereby the emergency department physician will consult a cardiologist in order to activate the CCL team for a STEMI patient. Simply allowing direct activation of the CCL team by the emergency department physician can lead to improved DTB times without a crippling number of false-positive activations (25). In addition, utilization of a single page operator to activate the CCL team instead of multiple pages can also lead to significant reductions in DTB times.

The CCL team comprises physicians, nurses, and technologists. Most primary PCI-capable institutions require that team members live within 30 minutes of the hospital. Recently, a number of centers have created an on-call CCL team that stays in the hospital thereby reducing DTB times by eliminating commuting times by the team. Bradley et al. report that creation of an on-call team can be expected to reduce DTB times by at least 14 minutes (Table 1).

Having an experienced CCL is also very important in the treatment of STEMI patients. Physicians and nurses who are skilled and experienced can not only achieve rapid reperfusion, but can also make astute clinical decisions that lead to better clinical outcomes. Therefore, very important strategies that can be implemented are the aforementioned AHA/ACC requirements for primary PCI cath labs.

Treatment of a STEMI patient requires close coordination between EMS, the emergency department, the CCL, and the hospital administration. In order

TABLE 1   Adjusted Associations between Hospital Strategies and Door-to-Balloon Times

Strategy	Door-to-balloon time (95%CI) minutes
ED activation of CCL team	-8.2 (-14.3 to -2.0)
Single call to page operator	-13.8 (-21.2 to -6.4)
Activation of CCL team while the patient is en route to the hospital	-15.4 (-24.2 to -6.6)
In-house MD	-14.6 (-25.7 to -3.6)
Real time feedback to ED from CCL	-8.8 (-13.6 to -3.6)

Source: Adapted from Ref. 15.

to improve DTB times and outcomes, there needs to be close coordination of policies and clear channels of communication and to tailor particular strategies to each individual community (26).

In conclusion, there have been considerable advances in reducing DTB times in patients with STEMI with corresponding decreases in mortality. Implementation of STEMI systems of care with prehospital ECGs, dedicated PCI hospitals, and close collaboration between interventional cardiologists, ED physicians, EMS, and hospital administrations are necessary for further reductions in DTB.

REFERENCES

1. Antman EM, Anbe DT, Armstrong PW, et al. ACC/AHA guidelines for the management of patients with ST-elevation myocardial infarction: a report of the ACC/AHA Task Force on Practice Guidelines. J Am Coll Cardiol 2004; 44:E1–E211.
2. Reimer KA, Jennings RB. The "wavefront phenomenon" of myocardial ischemic cell death. II. Transmural progression of necrosis within the framework of ischemic bed size (myocardium at risk) and collateral flow. Lab Invest 1979; 40:633–644.
3. De Luca G, Suryapranata H, Ottervanger JP, et al. Time delay to treatment and mortality in primary angioplasty for acute myocardial infarction: every minute of delay counts. Circulation 2004; 109:1223–1225.
4. McNamara RL, Wang Y, Herrin J, et al. Effect of door-to-balloon time on mortality in patients with ST-segment elevation myocardial infarction. J Am Coll Cardiol 2006; 47:2180–2186.
5. Keeley EC, Boura JA, Grines CL. Primary angioplasty versus intravenous thrombolytic therapy for acute myocardial infarction: a quantitative review of 23 randomised trials. Lancet. 2003; 361(9351):13–20.
6. Cannon CP, Gibson CM, Lambrew CT, et al. Relationship of symptom onset-to-balloon time and door-to-balloon time with mortality in patients undergoing angioplasty for acute myocardial infarction. JAMA 2000; 283:2941–2947.
7. Gibson CM, Pride YB, Frederick PD, et al. Trends in reperfusion strategies, door-to-needle and door-to-balloon times, and in-hospital mortality among patients with ST-segment elevation myocardial infarction enrolled in the National Registry of Myocardial Infarction from 1990–2006. Am Heart J 2008; 156:1035–1044.
8. Eagle KA, Nallamothu BK, Mehta RH, et al. Trends in acute reperfusion therapy for ST-segment elevation myocardial infarction from 1999 to 2006: we are getting better but we have got a long way to go. Euro Heart J 2008; 29:607–617.
9. Welsh RC, Ornato J, Armstrong PW. Prehospital management of acute ST-elevation myocardial infarction: a time for reappraisal in North America. Am Heart J 2003; 145:1–8.
10. Goff DC, Feldman H, McGovern PG, et al.; for the Rapid Early Action for Coronary Treatment (REACT) Study Group. Prehospital delay in patients hospitalized with heart attach symptoms int he United States. Am Heart J 1999; 138:1046–1057.
11. McKinley S, Moser DK, Dracup K. Treatment-seeking behavior for acute myocardial infarction symptoms in North America and Australia. Heart Lung 2000; 29:237–247.
12. Canto JG, Zalenski RJ, Ornato JP, et al.; for the National Registry of Myocardial Infarction 2 Investigators. Use of emergency medical services in acute myocardial infarction and subsequent quality of care. Circulation 2002; 106:3018–3023.
13. Becker L, Larsen MP, Eisenberg MS. Incidence of cardiac arrest during self-transport for chest pain. Ann Emerg Med 1996; 28:612–616.
14. Wright RS, Kopecky SL, Timm M, et al.; for the Wabasha Heart ATtack Team. Impact of community-based education on health care evaluation in patients with acute chest pain syndromes: the Wabasha Heart Attack Team (WHAT) project. Fam Pract 2001; 18:537–539.

15. Bradley EH, Herrin J, Wang Y, et al. Strategies for reducing the door-to-balloon time in acute myocardial infarction. N Engl J Med 2006; 355:2308–2320.

16. Boersma E. Does time matter? A pooled analysis of randomized clinical trials comparing primary percutaneous coronary intervention and in-hospital fibrinolysis in acute myocardial infarction patients. Eur Heart J 2006; 27:779–788.

17. Ting HH, Rihal CS, Gersh BJ, et al. Regional systems of care to optimize timeliness or reperfusion therapy for ST-elevation myocardial infarction: The Mayo clinic STEMI protocol. Circulation 2007; 116:729–736.

18. Jollis JG, Roettig ML, Aluko AO, et al. Implementation of a statewide system for coronary reperfusion for ST-segment elevation myocardial infarction. JAMA 2007; 298(20):2371–2380.

19. Canto JG, Rogers WJ, Bowlby LJ, et al. The prehospital electrocardiogram in acute myocardial infarction: is its full potential being realized? J Am Coll Cardiol 1997; 29:498–505.

20. Brown JP, Mahmud E, Dunford JV, et al. Effect of prehospital 12-lead electrocardiogram on activation of the cardiac catheterization laboratory and door-to-balloon time in ST-segment elevation acute myocardial infarction. Am J Cardiol 2008; 101(2):158–161.

21. Le May MR, So DY, Dionne R, et al. A city-wide protocol for primary PCI in ST segment elevation myocardial infarction. N Engl J Med 2008; 358:231–240.

22. Rokos IC, French WJ, Koenig WJ, et al. Integration of Pre-hospital electrocardiograms and ST-elevation myocardial infarction receiving center (SRC) networks impact on door-to-balloon times across 10 independent regions. JACC Cardiovasc Interv 2009; 2:339–346.

23. Youngquist ST, Shah AP, Niemann JT, et al. A comparison of door-to-balloon times and false-positive activations between emergency department and out-of-hospital activation of the coronary catheterization team. Acad Emerg Med 2008; 15(8):784–787.

24. Clemmensen P, Sejersten M, Sillesen M, et al. Diversion of ST-elevation myocardial infarction patients for primary angioplasty based on wireless prehospital 12-lead electrocardiographic transmission directly to the cardiologist's handheld computer: a progress report. J Electrocardiol 2005; 38(suppl 4):194–198.

25. Khot UN, Johnson ML, Ramsey C, et al. Emergency department physician activation of the catheterization laboratory and immediate transfer to an immediately available catheterization laboratory reduce door-to-balloon time in ST elevation myocardial infarction. Circulation 2007; 116:67–76.

26. Rokos IC, Larson DM, Henry TD, et al. Rationale for establishing regional ST-elevation myocardial infarction receiving center (SRC) networks. Am Heart J 2006; 152(4):661–667.

13 Systems of Care for Primary Percutaneous Coronary Intervention

Abhiram Prasad

Cardiac Catheterization Laboratory, Mayo Clinic, Rochester, Minnesota, U.S.A.

Tremendous progress has been made over the past decade in the field of primary percutaneous coronary intervention (PPCI). It is estimated from data derived from clinical trials that compared to fibrinolytics, mechanical reperfusion with PPCI reduces mortality by 25%, as well markedly decreasing the rate of recurrent infarction, intracranial hemorrhage, and stroke (1). The superior outcomes are to a large extent attributable to the advances in adjunctive interventional techniques and pharmacological therapy that have made it possible to achieve normal epicardial flow in as many as 90% to 95% of patients with ST elevation myocardial infarction (STEMI) as compared to 40% to 60% after fibrinolytics (2). These benefits have resulted in PPCI becoming the preferred strategy for reperfusion in the United States and many countries in Europe (3). Despite these advances, a significant proportion of patients still experience adverse outcomes highlighting the need for further improvements in treatment strategies (1). An important step in this direction is to maximize the delivery of evidence-based practice to as many, if not all patients with STEMI, recognizing that approximately one-third of patients around the world do not receive any form of reperfusion therapy (4,5). Second, there remains the need to develop novel adjunctive cardioprotective treatment in order to improve myocardial salvage (6). Third, it is essential to reduce treatment delays by adhering to the national guidelines that in the United States recommend a first medical contact-to-balloon time of ≤90 minutes (3), and in Europe a first medical contact-to-balloon time of ≤120 minutes (7). It is recognized that the benefits of PPCI over fibrinolytics are lost if there is excessive incremental delay in getting a patient to a cardiac catheterization laboratory compared to the time when fibrinolytics could have been administered. A widely quoted estimate for this incremental delay is >60 minutes (8), however, another analysis reported that the mortality benefit of PPCI may persist with incremental delays of up to 120 minutes (9). Given the importance of time to treatment and the shift toward PPCI as the preferred reperfusion strategy, it has become important for health care organizations to restructure with the goal of developing integrated systems of care for STEMI that provide greater access to timely, high-quality catheter-based reperfusion and other evidence-based therapy (10).

CHALLENGES TO INCREASING DELIVERY OF PPCI
The majority of patients with STEMI do not present to PCI centers, but rather to local emergency services or directly to community hospitals. Thus, a major challenge even in well-resourced countries is the limitation in the number of

cardiac catheterization laboratories at the institution where there is an initial contact with the patient. To take the example of the United States, only 1200 (~25%) out of the approximate 5000 acute care hospitals have the capability to perform PPCI. There are two strategies to increase the availability of PPCI. The first is to develop mechanical reperfusion capability at hospitals with catheterization laboratories that do not have on-site cardiac surgery and the second is to transfer patients directly or via noninterventional hospitals to tertiary facilities that act as regional "heart attack" centers.

PPCI WITHOUT ON-SITE CARDIAC SURGERY

The appeal of this strategy for PPCI is that it avoids the delay and cost associated with transportation of patients to a "heart attack" center. The major concern regarding the strategy is that PPCI has generally been performed at tertiary centers and the majority of the published literature is derived from such institutions and therefore, there is limited data regarding the safety and efficacy. The Cardiovascular Patient Outcomes Research Team (C-PORT) trial is the only randomized study on this subject. It was underpowered to assess mortality as an endpoint having enrolled 451 patients with STEMI who presented within 12 hours of symptom onset at 11 community hospitals with cardiac catheterization laboratories that did not perform angioplasty and did not have on-site cardiac surgery (11). After conducting appropriate training of the staff, patients were randomized to either PPCI or fibrinolysis at the community hospitals. Treatment with PPCI resulted in a reduction in the duration of hospitalization and the composite endpoint of the incidence of death, recurrent myocardial infarction, and stroke at six weeks (10.7% vs. 17.7%; $p = 0.03$) and six months (12.4% vs. 19.9%; $p = 0.03$) predominantly as a result of significant reductions in reinfarction with trends toward lower mortality and stroke. Of note, none of the patients required emergency CABG. Additional data regarding PPCI without on-site cardiac surgery is available from several observational studies that report in-hospital mortality rates ranging from 2.0% to 11.3% with exceedingly low rates of emergency coronary bypass surgery (CABG) being needed for failed PPCI (12–18). The largest of these is from 52,532 Medicare patients treated with PPCI. Of these, 1795 (3.4%) were performed at centers without on-site surgery. There was no difference in the in-hospital mortality between those treated at hospitals with or without on-site cardiac surgery (11.3% vs. 12.2% respectively, $p = 0.34$). An estimate of the frequency of CABG for failed PCI from the randomized clinical trials of PPCI is 0.3% (17).

Thus the apparent feasibility, efficacy, and safety have led to the gradual adoption of this strategy at many institutions. The European STEMI guidelines do not include recommendations on the role of PPCI at centers without on-site surgery (7). The American College of Cardiology/American Heart Association (ACC/AHA) guidelines have established criteria, though the recommendation is given a class IIb indication reflecting the lack of consensus over its appropriateness (Tables 1 and 2) (19). The consensus statement from the Society of Cardiovascular Angiography and Interventions endorses the ACC/AHA recommendations and emphasizes the importance of strict quality control (20). The debate over the appropriateness of PPCI without on-site surgery is likely to continue and for the moment this strategy must be individualized to each community with the primary goal of providing optimal care. There is clearly a potential for unnecessary or inappropriate development of multiple, potentially low-volume

TABLE 1 ACC/AHA Criteria for Performance of Primary PCI at Hospitals Without Onsite Cardiac Surgery

- The operators must be experienced interventionalists who regularly perform elective PCI at a surgical center (at least 75 cases/yr)
- The catheterization laboratory must perform a minimum of 36 primary PCI procedures per year
- The nursing and technical catheterization laboratory staff must be experienced in handling acutely ill patients and must be comfortable with interventional equipment. They must have acquired experience in dedicated interventional laboratories at a surgical center
- They participate in a 24-hr, 365-day call schedule
- The catheterization laboratory itself must be well equipped, with optimal imaging systems, resuscitative equipment, and IABP support, and must be well stocked with a broad array of interventional equipment
- The cardiac care unit nurses must be adept in hemodynamic monitoring and IABP management
- The hospital administration must fully support the program and enable the fulfillment of the above institutional requirements
- There must be formalized written protocols in place for immediate and efficient transfer of patients to the nearest cardiac surgical facility that are reviewed/tested on a regular (quarterly) basis
- Primary PCI must be performed routinely as the treatment of choice around the clock for a large proportion of patients with STEMI, ensure streamlined care paths and increased case volumes
- Case selection for the performance of primary PCI must be rigorous (Table 2)
- There must be an ongoing program of outcomes analysis and formalized periodic case review
- Institutions should participate in a 3- to 6-month period of implementation during which time development of a formalized primary PCI program is instituted that includes establishment of standards, training of staff, detailed logistic development, and creation of a quality assessment and error management system

Source: From Ref. 19.

PPCI programs in a given geographic region that must be strongly discouraged. Cardiologists and institutions must not succumb to incentives related to financial gain, market share, prestige as a primary motivation for establishing a PPCI program. However, the establishment of a high-quality PPCI program at selected hospitals where a clear need exists is likely to lead to improved outcomes.

TABLE 2 Patient Selection for PPCI and Emergency Aortocoronary Bypass at Hospitals Without Onsite Cardiac Surgery

Avoid intervention in hemodynamically stable patients with
- Significant (greater than or equal to 60%) stenosis of an unprotected left main coronary artery upstream from an acute occlusion in the left coronary system that might be disrupted by the angioplasty catheter
- Extremely long or angulated infarct-related lesions with TIMI grade 3 flow
- Infarct-related lesions with TIMI grade 3 flow in stable patients with 3-vessel disease
- Infarct-related lesions of small or secondary vessels
- Hemodynamically significant lesions in other than the infarct artery

Transfer for emergency aortocoronary bypass surgery patients
- After primary PCI of occluded vessels if high-grade residual left main or multivessel coronary disease with clinical or hemodynamic instability present. Preferably with IABP support

Abbreviations: TIMI, thrombolysis in myocardial infarction; IABP, intra-aortic balloon pump.
Source: From Ref. 19.

REGIONAL "HEART ATTACK" CENTERS

An alternative model for increasing the availability of timely and a high-quality PPCI service is the development of regional "heart attack" centers that receive patients from noninterventional hospitals. However, the logistics of maintaining consistently low transfer times require the establishment of systems care that involve multiple stake holders and vary depending on geographical location. It has been estimated that in the United States 79% of the population lives within 60 minutes of a hospital with PPCI capability (21). The estimates include the time for activation of the emergency services, initial assessment by the paramedical crew, and the transportation time to the hospital. Among patients whose nearest hospital was a noninterventional facility, in 74% of case the additional time to reach a PPCI center was estimated to add less than 30 minutes. These data suggest that a transfer strategy in the United States would be feasible at a national level. The feasibility of the strategy in Europe has been demonstrated in Denmark, Czech Republic, and Sweden.

Several randomized trials have reported improved outcomes with transfer for PPCI compared to the administration of fibrinolytics at community hospitals (22–25). The two largest trials are the DANAMI-2 and PRAGUE-2 in which the majority of patients initially presented to hospitals without interventional facilities. In DANAMI-2, 1572 patients were randomized to either front-loaded alteplase at the presenting hospital or PPCI with transfer if necessary to a PCI center. PPCI was associated with a marked reduction (8.0% vs. 13.7%) in the primary composite endpoint of mortality, reinfarction, or stroke at 30 days driven largely by a reduction in the rate of reinfarction (1.6% vs. 6.3%; $P < 0.001$). There was no significant reduction mortality or stroke. Ninety-six percent of patients were transferred from referral hospitals to a PPCI center within two hours. The benefits persisted at three years (22). In the PRAGUE-2 trial, 850 patients were randomized to either streptokinase at the presenting community hospital or transfer to a PPCI center (23). PPCI was associated with a trend toward lower mortality at 30 days (6.8% vs. 10.0%). Data from a meta-analysis of the six published trials indicate a clear benefit with a 42% reduction in the composite endpoint of death, recurrent myocardial infarction, or stroke (Fig. 1); as well as the individual endpoints of recurrent myocardial infarction (68%) and stroke (56%), and a clear trend for mortality reduction (19%) though this did not reach statistical significance (25).

Despite the favorable outcomes and the relatively short transport times (70 to 103 minutes) documented in clinical trials, experience in everyday practice suggests that transport times for PPCI are longer. For example, in the NRMI registry for the period 1999 to 2002, the median first-door-to-second-door time was 120 minutes, and the first-door-to-balloon time was 180 minutes. The times have decreased in the more recent cohorts with the median first-door-to-balloon time in the NRMI registry in 2006 decreasing to 139 minutes that has been accompanied by a reduction in mortality such that the mortality in transfer and nontransfer patients was similar (26). The improvement in performance measures reflect increasing awareness of the importance of treatment delay, establishment of quality measures for individual hospitals, and the impact of national campaigns by the ACC (D2B: An Alliance for Quality that focuses on reducing door-to-balloon time in the interventional hospital) (27), and the AHA (Mission Lifeline that aims to establish a framework for integrative strategies for developing systems of care) (10).

Death/reinfarction/stroke

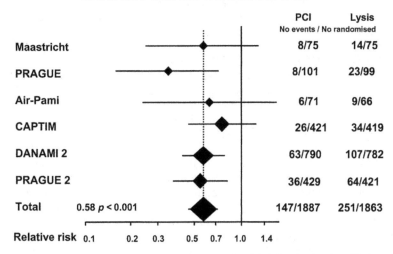

FIGURE 1 Relative risks for the composite of death/reinfarction/stroke with thrombolysis and transfer for primary PCI in individual trials and the combined analysis. *Source*: From Ref. 25.

In general, there are two models of systems of care for "heart attack" centers. The first is the *bypass* model, in which patients with STEMI are transported by the emergency services to a "heart attack" center bypassing noninterventional hospitals that may be closer. A prerequisite of this system is the capacity to perform prehospital electrocardiograms (ECG) (28). The Boston EMS Bypass STEMI Triage Plan and Treatment Registry is an example of such as system in which a consortium of tertiary hospitals has agreed upon uniform standards and established oversight for the monitoring quality (29). The second model is the *transfer* ("hub and spoke") model in which STEMI patients who present at a noninterventional hospital, either self-transported or via the emergency services, are immediately transferred to a PPCI facility. Several publications from around the world in rural and urban settings have reported the feasibility and efficacy of this model (30–34). Our experience at the Mayo Clinic from an initial cohort of 597 patients with STEMI presenting to Saint Marys Hospital ("heart attack center") and 28 regional hospitals up to 150 miles away has demonstrated a median door-to-balloon time of 71 minutes for those presenting at the PCI center and 116 minutes for those transferred by a helicopter from community hospitals (30). Notably, the establishment of the integrated system resulted in an immediate reduction in the door-to-balloon times at the PCI center when compared to historical controls, and this has further decreased with the introduction of prehospital ECG. Similarly, at the Minneapolis Heart Institute, STEMI patients are rapidly transferred by air ambulance for PPCI to the hub hospital from community hospitals within a 210-mile radius. Median door-to-balloon times of 95 minutes for hospitals within a 60-mile radius, and 120 minutes for hospitals between 61 and 210-mile radius have been achieved in an all comers population (31). There were no deaths during transportation in the Mayo Clinic study. At the Minneapolis Heart Institute, endotracheal intubation was required during transportation in 0.7% patients, and a cardiopulmonary arrest occurred 2.0% of patients, with all but one being successfully resuscitated. The two studies were the first to establish the feasibility and safety of the transfer model in daily practice. Studies reporting the efficacy of the transfer/bypass systems of care have since also been published from Canada (32) and Europe (33,34).

ESTABLISHING INTEGRATED SYSTEMS OF CARE

Due to the diversity in health care systems, geography, population density, and financial resources, a single integrated care model is unlikely to be applicable to all, though certain general principles are critically important. These include the acceptance by physicians, allied health care workers, and hospital administrators involved in the care of STEMI patients that PPCI is the preferred reperfusion strategy (fibrinolysis being available as the back-up for situations where mechanical reperfusion may not be deliverable in a timely fashion) when performed at high-volume experienced "heart attack" centers. With this in mind, the initiation of a STEMI system of care requires reorganization and integration of prehospital pathways, community emergency rooms, and services at the "heart attack" center.

Fundamental issues that must be overcome with regards to prehospital care are regulatory reform of laws that in some parts of the world require patients with STEMI to be transported to the nearest hospital with a coronary care unit regardless of whether or not it has a PPCI capability. Furthermore, financial and political incentives must be addressed, especially from the perspective of small community hospitals that may see the diversion of patients to "heart attack" centers as a loss of revenue. Integration of prehospital services by streamlining emergency transportation systems that have historical links to specific hospitals often owned by competing health care organizations is essential. If required, emergency services must be restructured so that patients requiring transfer from a noninterventional hospital to a PCI facility are given top priority. Currently, in many systems stable patients with STEMI requiring inter-hospital are given lower priority than a primary transfer of an emergency case from the field to a hospital. Standardized treatment protocols for evidence-based therapies such as antiplatelet, anti-ischemic, and anticoagulant agents must be formulated to deliver uniform and prompt care in the setting of an emergency. This can be achieved by using locally designed standing orders, tool kits, and transfer forms. Examples of tools developed by the ACC D2B initiative are available at: http://interventions.onlinejacc.org/cgi/content/full/1/1/97/DC1.

Bradley et al. have identified core qualitative characteristics of institutions that have successfully reorganized their systems of care (35). The starting point is an explicit shared organizational goal of reducing door-to-balloon time and improving other quality metrics that is generally driven by internal and external pressures. This effort must be championed by a core group of individuals that provides strong leadership and works with interdepartmental and interdisciplinary collaborative teams. The support of senior management who are active participants is critical for overcoming issues related to staffing, space limitations, or resistance among individuals to implementing the process changes. Specific techniques such as root-causes analyses, flowcharting, and brainstorming need to be instituted to identify limitations of existing systems and develop and refine protocols. Developing innovative protocols often involves breaking the process of door-to-balloon time into smaller segments such as door-to-ECG,

ECG-to-decision, decision-to-laboratory, and laboratory-to-balloon times and tackling them individually. Once a local system is established, real-time patient specific data feedback, though resource intensive, is integral to identify areas for ongoing improvement, motivate changes, reinforce adherence to protocols, make successes visible, and sustain new processes over the longer term. However, the data need to be valid, formatted in a readily understandable way, presented by a credible clinician, and reviewed in a nonblaming fashion in order to influence changes in clinical processes. A "nonblaming" approach to identifying problems needs to be developed so that systems failures can be discussed in open forums and lessons learned from mistakes. All this must be conducted in an organizational culture that fosters resilience to challenges or setbacks.

In a larger analysis, Bradley et al. identified specific processes that lead to shorter door-to balloon times at PCI centers (36). Based on this and other work, the ACC D2B initiative has formulated seven key strategies for reducing door-to-balloon times (Table 3) (27). A key paradigm shift in these recommendations is for cardiologists to relinquish the control of catheterization laboratory activation to emergency room physicians that appears to be feasible, even in complex systems, though false activation rates of at least 10% are likely (37). Thus, the financial and other consequences of false-positive catheterization laboratory activation must be considered in such systems that can be minimized by the immediate notification of the cardiology services that must review the ECG and clinical information and abort the activation if deemed to be inappropriate. An inherent consequence of maintaining short door-to-balloon times is that patients will arrive in the catheterization laboratory without being subjected to the conventional admission process of a sequential history, physical examination, and laboratory tests. This must be replaced with parallel processes that are performed simultaneously involving the emergency, coronary care unit, and interventional cardiology services. Information technology solutions to facilitate a reliable single-call system for activating the entire catheterization laboratory staff and the transmission of medical information (e.g., ECG) to the on-call staff are not always simple and often require innovative solutions. Finally, appropriate staffing, facilities, and financial remuneration are required to maintain a cardiac catheterization team that is available within 20 to 30 minutes at all times.

In conclusion, STEMI systems of care are evidence-based process-of-care initiatives. It is very likely that improving access to rapid PPCI at high-volume

TABLE 3 Key Strategies for Reducing Door-to-Balloon Times

- Activation of the catheterization laboratory by emergency medicine physicians
- Establishment of a single-call system for activating the catheterization laboratory
- Expectation that the catheterization team be available within 20 to 30 min of being paged
- Use of data monitoring and prompt data feedback to emergency department and catheterization laboratory staff
- Senior management support and organizational environment that fosters and sustains organizational change directed at improving door-to-balloon time
- Team-based approach from ambulance to balloon, within a culture of continuous quality improvement

Optional strategy
- Use of prehospital ECG to activate the catheterization laboratory

Source: From Ref. 27.

centers will improve outcomes and quality of care. Although the challenges to establishing such systems are significant, the experience from around the world demonstrates that is feasible.

TREATMENT OF NON–ST ELEVATION ACUTE CORONARY SYNDROME IN A "HEART ATTACK" CENTER

There is considerable evidence that an invasive strategy improves outcomes in high-risk non–ST elevation acute coronary syndromes (NSTACS) (38,39) (Fig. 2). Early risk stratification is essential to direct care in these patients and may be readily performed using clinical, ECG, and serum biomarker indices (Fig. 3). Unlike STEMI, an early invasive strategy does not reduce mortality, but appears to decrease recurrent myocardial infarction and refractory ischemia. There is considerable variability in the management of NSTACS depending on local practices that are often determined by the availability of a cardiac catheterization laboratory. The recently presented TIMACS (TIMing of Intervention in patient with Acute Coronary Syndromes) trial demonstrated that coronary angiography, and revascularization if needed, within 24 hours versus more than 36 hours after presentation resulted in a marked reduction in refractory ischemia [hazard ratio: 0.30 (0.17–0.53), $P < 0.00001$]. The study was underpowered to show a reduction in the primary composite endpoint of death, myocardial infarction, or stroke, nevertheless, there was a significant reduction in this endpoint in high-risk patients treated within 24 hours. Based on this data and experience at our institution, it is reasonable to conclude that coronary angiography within 24 hours is desirable for high-risk NSTACS because it improves outcomes and almost certainly will decrease the duration of hospitalization. The establishment of "heart attack" centers for STEMI offers an opportunity to provide expeditious care for these patients and thereby expand the utilization of the PCI facility. This approach will require weekend operation of catheterization laboratories with implications for staffing and financial resources. However, the strategy is likely to

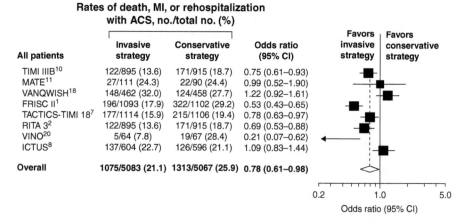

Rates of death, MI, or rehospitalization with ACS, no./total no. (%)

All patients	Invasive strategy	Conservative strategy	Odds ratio (95% CI)
TIMI IIIB[10]	122/895 (13.6)	171/915 (18.7)	0.75 (0.61–0.93)
MATE[11]	27/111 (24.3)	22/90 (24.4)	0.99 (0.52–1.90)
VANQWISH[18]	148/462 (32.0)	124/458 (27.7)	1.22 (0.92–1.61)
FRISC II[1]	196/1093 (17.9)	322/1102 (29.2)	0.53 (0.43–0.65)
TACTICS-TIMI 18[7]	177/1114 (15.9)	215/1106 (19.4)	0.78 (0.63–0.97)
RITA 3[2]	122/895 (13.6)	171/915 (18.7)	0.69 (0.53–0.88)
VINO[20]	5/64 (7.8)	19/67 (28.4)	0.21 (0.07–0.62)
ICTUS[8]	137/604 (22.7)	126/596 (21.1)	1.09 (0.83–1.44)
Overall	1075/5083 (21.1)	1313/5067 (25.9)	0.78 (0.61–0.98)

Favors invasive strategy | Favors conservative strategy

0.2   1.0   5.0
Odds ratio (95% CI)

FIGURE 2 A meta-analysis of the rates of death, myocardial infarction, or rehospitalization from randomized trials of an invasive versus a conservative treatment strategy for a non–ST elevation acute coronary syndrome. *Source*: From Ref. 38.

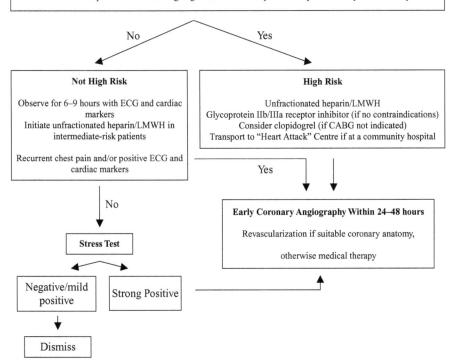

FIGURE 3 Early risk stratification-based management strategy for non–ST segment elevation acute coronary syndromes. *Abbreviations*: CABG, coronary artery bypass graft; ECG, electrocardiogram; LMWH, low-molecular-weight heparin; TIMI, thrombolysis in myocardial infarction. *Source*: From Ref. 39.

be feasible in the context of large hub "heart attack" centers. High-risk NSTACS patients admitted to community hospitals within a STEMI network should be transferred to the "heart attack" center to follow this treatment pathway. Specific standardized order sets and tool kits for NSTACS that can be used at the community hospitals must be developed in order to optimize risk stratification, decision making, and pharmacological therapy.

REFERENCES

1. Keeley EC, Boura JA, Grines CL. Primary angioplasty versus intravenous thrombolytic therapy for acute myocardial infarction: a quantitative review of 23 randomised trials. Lancet 2003; 361:13–20.

2. Prasad A, Stone GW, Aymong E, et al. Impact of ST-segment resolution following primary angioplasty on outcomes after myocardial infarction in the elderly: an analysis from the CADILLAC trial. Am Heart J 2004; 147:669–675.
3. Antman EM, Hand M, Armstrong PW, et al. 2007 Focused Update of the ACC/AHA 2004 Guidelines for the Management of Patients with ST-Elevation Myocardial Infarction: a report of the American College of Cardiology/American Heart Association Task Force on Practice Guidelines. Circulation 2008; 117:296–329.
4. Bates ER, Nallamothu BK. The role of percutaneous coronary intervention in ST-segment–elevation myocardial infarction. Circulation 2008; 118:567–573.
5. Eagle KA, Goodman SG, Avezum A, et al. Practice variation and missed opportunities for reperfusion in ST-segment-elevation myocardial infarction. Lancet 2002; 359:373–377.
6. Hausenloy DJ, Yellon DM. Myocardial protection: is primary PCI enough? Nat Clin Pract Cardiovasc Med 2009; 6:12–13.
7. Van de Werf F, Bax J, Betriu A, et al. Management of acute myocardial infarction in patients presenting with persistent ST-segment elevation: the Task Force on the Management of ST-Segment Elevation Acute Myocardial Infarction of the European Society of Cardiology. Eur Heart J 2008; 29:2909–2945.
8. Nallamothu BK, Antman EM, Bates ER. Primary percutaneous coronary intervention versus fibrinolytic therapy in acute myocardial infarction: does the choice of fibrinolytic agent impact on the importance of time-to-treatment? Am J Cardiol 2004; 94:772–774.
9. Boersma E; for the Primary Coronary Angioplasty vs. Thrombolysis Group. Does time matter? A pooled analysis of randomized clinical trials comparing primary percutaneous coronary intervention and in-hospital fibrinolysis in acute myocardial infarction patients. Eur Heart J 2006; 27:779–788.
10. Jacobs AK, Antman Em, Faxon DP, et al. Development of systems of care for ST-elevation myocardial infarction patients: executive summary. Circulation 2007; 116:217–230.
11. Aversano T, Aversano LT, Passamani E, et al. Thrombolytic therapy vs primary percutaneous coronary intervention for myocardial infarction in patients presenting to hospitals without on-site cardiac surgery: a randomized controlled trial. JAMA 2002; 287:1943–1951.
12. Wharton TP Jr, McNamara NS, Fedele FA, et al. Primary angioplasty for the treatment of acute myocardial infarction: experience at two community hospitals without cardiac surgery. J Am Coll Cardiol 1999; 33:1257–1265.
13. Weaver WD, Litwin PE, Martin JS. Use of direct angioplasty for treatment of patients with acute myocardial infarction in hospitals with and without on-site cardiac surgery: the Myocardial Infarction, Triage, and Intervention Project investigators. Circulation 1993; 88:2067–2075.
14. Smyth DW, Richards AM, Elliott JM. Direct angioplasty for myocardial infarction: one-year experience in a center with surgical back-up 220 miles away. J Invasive Cardiol 1997; 9:324–332.
15. Iannone LA, Anderson SM, Phillips SJ. Coronary angioplasty for acute myocardial infarction in a hospital without cardiac surgery. Tex Heart Inst J 1993; 20:99–104.
16. Brush JE Jr, Thompson S, Ciuffo AA, et al. Retrospective comparison of a strategy of primary coronary angioplasty versus intravenous thrombolytic therapy for acute myocardial infarction in a community hospital without cardiac surgical backup. J Invasive Cardiol 1996; 8:91–98.
17. Singh M, Ting HH, Gersh BJ, et al. Percutaneous coronary intervention for ST-segment and non-ST-segment elevation myocardial infarction at hospitals with and without on-site cardiac surgical capability. Mayo Clin Proc 2004; 79:738–744.
18. Wennberg DE, Lucas FL, Siewers AE, et al. Outcomes of percutaneous coronary interventions performed at centers without and with onsite coronary artery bypass graft surgery. JAMA 2004; 292:1961–1968.

19. Antman EM, Anbe DT, Armstrong PW, et al. ACC/AHA guidelines for the manage-ment of patients with ST-elevation myocardial infarction: a report of the American College of Cardiology/American Heart Association Task Force on Practice Guide-lines (Committee to Revise the 1999 Guidelines for the Management of Patients with Acute Myocardial Infarction). J Am Coll Cardiol 2004; 44:e1–e211.
20. Dehmer GJ, Blankenship J, Wharton TP Jr, et al. The current status and future direc-tion of percutaneous coronary intervention without on-site surgical backup: an expert consensus document from the Society for Cardiovascular Angiography and Interven-tions. Catheter Cardiovasc Interv 2007; 69:471–478.
21. Nallamothu BK, Bates ER, Wang Y, et al. Driving times and distances to hospitals with percutaneous coronary intervention in the United States: implications for prehospital triage of patients with ST-elevation myocardial infarction. Circulation 2006; 113:1189–1195.
22. Busk M, Maeng M, Rasmussen K, et al. The Danish multicentre randomized study of fibrinolytic therapy vs. primary angioplasty in acute myocardial infarction (the DANAMI-2 trial): outcome after 3 years follow-up. Eur Heart J 2008; 29:1259.
23. Widimsky P, Budesinsky T, Vorac D, et al. Long distance transport for primary angio-plasty vs immediate thrombolysis in acute myocardial infarction. Final results of the randomized national multicentre trial–PRAGUE-2. Eur Heart J 2003; 24:94.
24. Grines CL, Westerhausen DR Jr, Grines LL, et al. A randomized trial of transfer for primary angioplasty versus on-site thrombolysis in patients with high-risk myocar-dial infarction: the Air Primary Angioplasty in Myocardial Infarction study. J Am Coll Cardiol 2002; 39:1713.
25. Dalby M, Bouzamondo A, Lechat P, et al. Transfer for primary angioplasty versus immediate thrombolysis in acute myocardial infarction: a meta-analysis. Circulation 2003; 108:1809–1814.
26. Gibson CM, Pride YB, Frederick PD, et al. Trends in reperfusion strategies, door-to-needle and door-to-balloon times, and in-hospital mortality among patients with ST-segment elevation myocardial infarction enrolled in the National Registry of Myocardial Infarction from 1990 to 2006. Am Heart J 2008; 156:1035–1044.
27. Krumholz HM, Bradley EH, Nallamothu BK, et al. A campaign to improve the timeli-ness of primary percutaneous coronary intervention: door-to-balloon: an alliance for quality. JACC Cardiovasc Interv 2008; 1:97–104.
28. Ting HH, Krumholz HM, Bradley EH, et al. Implementation and integration of pre-hospital ECGs into systems of care for acute coronary syndrome: a scientific state-ment from the American Heart Association Interdisciplinary Council on Quality of Care and Outcomes Research, Emergency Cardiovascular Care Committee, Coun-cil on Cardiovascular Nursing, and Council on Clinical Cardiology. Circulation 2008; 118:1066–1179.
29. Moyer P, Feldman J, Levine J, et al. Implications of the mechanical (PCI) vs throm-bolytic controversy for ST segment elevation myocardial infarction on the organiza-tion of emergency medical services: the Boston EMS experience. Crit Path Cardiol 2004; 3:53–61.
30. Ting HH, Rihal CS, Gersh BJ, et al. Regional systems of care to optimize timeliness of reperfusion therapy for ST-elevation myocardial infarction: the Mayo Clinic STEMI Protocol. Circulation 2007; 116:729–736.
31. Henry TD, Sharkey SW, Burke MN. A regional system to provide timely access to percutaneous coronary intervention for ST-elevation myocardial infarction. Circula-tion 2007; 16:721–728.
32. Le May MR, So DY. Dionne R, et al. A citywide protocol for primary PCI in ST-segment elevation myocardial infarction. N Engl J Med 2008; 358:231–240.
33. Manari A, Ortolani P, Guastaroba P, et al. Clinical impact of an inter-hospital trans-fer strategy in patients with ST-elevation myocardial infarction undergoing primary angioplasty: the Emilia-Romagna ST-segment elevation acute myocardial infarction network. Eur Heart J 2008; 29:1834–1842.

34. Kalla K, Christ G, Karnik R, et al; for the Vienna STEMI Registry Group. Implementation of guidelines improves the standard of care: the Viennese registry on reperfusion strategies in ST-elevation myocardial infarction (Vienna STEMI registry). Circulation 2006; 113:2398–2405.
35. Bradley EH, Curry LA, Webster TR, et al. Achieving rapid door-to-balloon times: how top hospitals improve complex clinical systems. Circulation 2006; 113:1079–1085.
36. Bradley EH, Herrin J, Wang Y, et al. Strategies for reducing the door-to-balloon time in acute myocardial infarction. N Engl J Med 2006; 355:2308–2320.
37. Larson DM, Menssen KM, Sharkey SW, et al. "False-positive" cardiac catheterization laboratory activation among patients with suspected ST-segment elevation myocardial infarction. JAMA 2007; 298:2754–2760.
38. O'Donoghue M, Boden WE, Braunwald E, et al. Early invasive vs conservative treatment strategies in women and men with unstable angina and non-ST-segment elevation myocardial infarction: a meta-analysis. JAMA 2008; 300:71–80.
39. Prasad A, Mathew V, Holmes DR Jr, et al. Current management of non-ST-segment-elevation acute coronary syndrome: reconciling the results of randomized controlled trials. Eur Heart J 2003; 24:1544–1553.

14 Utilization of Facilitated and Rescue Angioplasty

Rajiv Gulati and Bernard J. Gersh

Division of Cardiovascular Diseases, Mayo Clinic, Rochester, Minnesota, U.S.A.

INTRODUCTION

The pivotal animal experiments of Reimer et al., which demonstrated the wave-front phenomenon of myocardial necrosis (1), led to the correct assumption that restoration of flow in an infarct artery would salvage myocardium and improve clinical outcomes. Indeed, reperfusion therapy has transformed the management of ST-segment elevation myocardial infarction over the last 30 years. Considerable endeavor has been undertaken in comparing the two principal reperfusion modalities: fibrinolysis and primary percutaneous coronary intervention (PPCI). Many randomized trials as well as a pooled meta-analyses have led to the consensus that, all things being equal, PPCI is the preferred therapy when performed by experienced operators in accredited institutions (2), leading to fewer deaths, reinfarctions, and strokes than fibrinolysis. The benefits of PPCI over fibrinolysis may relate to the achievement of infarct vessel TIMI 3 flow in the vast majority, stabilization of the ruptured, unstable plaque resulting in less reocclusions and the avoidance of hemorrhagic complications (particularly intracranial hemorrhage) associated with fibrinolysis.

Current data suggest that for the greatest clinical gain, achievements of first door-to-balloon time of 90 minutes or less should be the goal (3). However, the fact that only 40% of the U.S. population identifies a hospital with a PPCI program as the closest facility to their home and only 80% reside within 60 minutes of a PPCI-capable facility underscores the difficulties encountered in widespread attainment of such times. Indeed, only a minority of U.S. patients transferred from an index hospital to a PCI center currently achieve first door-to-balloon times of less than 120 minutes.

Difficulties in achieving rapid percutaneous reperfusion because of access to a PCI center or delays in interhospital transfer makes understandable the appeal of combining validated reperfusion therapies with fibrinolytic therapy administered immediately and percutaneous intervention performed subsequently. Despite disappointing initial evidence generated in the 1980s for the use of a combined fibrinolytic and invasive approach, improvements in adjunctive pharmacology (antithrombotic and antiplatelet regimens) and the widespread use of stents have justified re-evaluation of such an approach in the contemporary era. Currently, for patients treated with fibrinolysis as the initial reperfusion strategy, there are three options for subsequent care (Fig. 1):

1. Facilitated PCI (transfer for immediate angiography and PCI, if indicated).

Facilitated	Transfer for immediate angiography and PCI, if indicated, usually in less than 3 hr.
Pharmacoinvasive	Immediate transfer to PCI center. If failure to reperfuse, perform angiography and rescue PCI. If successful reperfusion, perform early routine angiography and PCI at between 3 and 24 hr.
Delayed guided	Transfer for angiography and PCI only if evidence of recurrent ischemia, for example, reinfarction, angina, positive stress test.

FIGURE 1 Approaches available for management after initial fibrinolytic therapy.

2. Pharmacoinvasive approach (immediate transfer and rescue PCI if there is evidence of failed reperfusion, or mandatory routine angiography and PCI within a 3–24-hour time window).
3. Ischemia-guided PCI (transfer for angiography and PCI only if evidence of recurrent ischemia, for example, re-occlusion, angina, positive stress test).

FACILITATED PCI

The term facilitated PCI refers to mandatory angiography and PCI after fibrinolytic therapy, usually within a three-hour window. It is important to distinguish this approach from a pharmacoinvasive approach in which, if there is evidence of reperfusion, the policy is to wait at least three hours for routine angiography and PCI to be performed. A pharmacoinvasive approach therefore combines rescue PCI with routine deferred PCI within 3 to 24 hours.

The combination of fibrinolytic administration with immediate transfer for angiography and PCI, in theory, might enable swift pharmacologic reperfusion (and reduction in ischemia) to be a bridge to mechanical stabilization, thereby

---

KEY POINTS

Rescue PCI is the preferred strategy for failure to reperfuse after fibrinolytics.

A pharmacoinvasive approach of rescue PCI, if indicated, or early routine PCI within 3 to 24 hours results in better outcomes than standard therapy after fibrinolytics and is a recommended strategy.

Facilitated PCI has been shown to result in worse outcomes than standard therapy after fibrinolytics and is in general not a recommended strategy.

Facilitated PCI may have a role in high-risk patients who present early and who have a long transfer time.

negating the effects of a time delay to PCI. Of course, any potential positive effect would have to be balanced with the known downsides of fibrinolytic therapy, namely, increased serious bleeding, the potential for intraplaque hematoma, and fibrinolytic-enhancement of platelet activation, which may hamper PCI. The term facilitated PCI has been used to refer to a number of pharmacotherapies prior to PCI, including full-dose or half-dose fibrinolytic agents, alone or with glycoprotein IIb/IIIa inhibitors. Unfortunately, and perhaps surprisingly, studies to date in total have not yielded this strategy to be successful and, in some cases, have revealed facilitated PCI to confer worse outcomes compared with PCI alone.

Rationale
The rationale for facilitated PCI is that early pharmacologic reperfusion would offset the negative effects of a delay in transfer to a PCI facility. Indeed, indirect evidence in support of this hypothesis came from trials of primary PCI. Several studies, including the early PAMI trials, indicated that patients who had TIMI 2 or 3 flow prior to PCI (i.e., spontaneous reperfusion) had greater myocardial salvage and lower rates of early and late mortality. This supports the intuitive suspicion that early pharmacologically assisted patency of the infarct artery might result in improved outcomes with subsequent PCI. It is important to point out that the outcome of any reperfusion strategy directly depends on the duration of ischemia prior to treatment. Within the first two to three hours of an evolving myocardial infarction, the time to treatment (regardless of treatment type) is the critical determinant of myocardial salvage and clinical outcome, with a 30-minute delay being associated with an 8% increase in relative mortality ant one year. After three hours, there remains a benefit from reperfusion therapy, but the time to treatment is less important. The main goal during this period is to open the infarct-related artery, which is better performed with PCI than fibrinolytic therapy.

Results of Randomized Trials and Meta-Analyses
Initial studies using balloon angioplasty alone and pharmacotherapies that are currently considered obsolete have limited relevance in the current era and will thus not be discussed in this chapter. The CAPITAL AMI trial of 170 patients with STEMI, randomized patients to treatment with full-dose tenecteplase alone or full-dose tenecteplase with subsequent immediate transfer for PCI (4). Although there were no differences in mortality between the groups, patients in the facilitated arm were better off in terms of the composite primary endpoint of death, recurrent MI, recurrent unstable ischemia or stroke, and the improvement in large part being driven by a reduction in recurrent ischemia. The principal limitation of this study was the very small number of patients and the subsequent inability to demonstrate differences in hard endpoints. In contrast, the ASSENT-4 trial was a much larger study of patients presenting with STEMI of <6 hours duration, who were scheduled to undergo PPCI with an anticipated one to three hours delay (5). Patients were randomized to full-dose tenecteplase facilitated PCI ($n = 829$) or PCI with placebo ($n = 838$). The primary endpoint was a composite of death, heart failure, or shock within 90 days. The Data Safety and Monitoring Board terminated the study prior to completion because of a statistically significant increase in in-hospital mortality in the facilitated PCI group

(6% vs. 3%). This was largely due to a higher rate of stroke, primarily hemorrhagic stroke in the facilitated arm. Moreover, the rate of primary composite endpoint was statistically worse in the facilitated arm (19% vs. 13%). Notably, most subgroups indicated a worse outcome with facilitated PCI, including early symptom onset (when fibrinolysis may be most beneficial), anterior MI and diabetes. Limitations of the trial include the lack of heparin infusion after bolus and the restriction if glycoprotein IIb/IIIa usage to bailout situations during PCI. Moreover, the open-label design may have induced operator bias. Patients treated with tenecteplase were less likely to undergo PCI at the time of catheterization, presumably directly because of higher rates of TIMI 3 flow. This may have led to this group being disadvantaged by not undergoing stent-based culprit vessel stabilization.

Keeley et al. published a pooled analysis of 17 randomized trials of facilitated PCI versus PPCI, which included the ASSENT-IV study (6). Facilitated PCI was, as expected, associated with significantly higher rates of TIMI 3 flow (37% vs. 15%) prior to PCI. However, as with ASSENT-IV, facilitated PCI was also associated with significantly higher mortality (5% vs. 3%). The higher mortality was driven by patients receiving full-dose fibrinolytic therapy, with no signal of mortality risk with half-dose fibrinolytic therapy. The most recent study involving a half-dose fibrinolytic facilitated strategy, the FINESSE trial, is another neutral trial at the 90-day endpoint (7). In this study, 2452 patients with STEMI were randomized in a 1:1:1 fashion to half-dose reteplase with early abciximab, half-dose reteplase with abciximab given in the cath lab and early abciximab alone. As seen with other studies described above, a greater proportion of patients treated with combination therapies achieved TIMI 3 flow and ST-segment resolution prior to PCI. However, there was no significant difference between the groups in the composite endpoint of all cause death, ventricular fibrillation more than 48 hours after randomization, cardiogenic shock, and heart failure. Moreover, combination therapy was associated with an increase in intracranial hemorrhage and increase in TIMI major and minor bleeding.

Why Has Facilitated PCI Not Been Shown to Improve Clinical Outcome?

In part, this may simply be due to the fact that the major benefit for any reperfusion strategy is confined to those presenting within 2 to 3 hours. In the ASSENT-IV study, the median symptom to fibrinolysis commencement time was $2^1/_2$ hours. If one then takes into consideration the time required for pharmacologic effect, the total ischemic time is beyond three hours. Likewise in the FINESSE trial, the median time from symptom onset to reperfusion was approximately 4.3 hours, which being outside the early period, in the fairly time-independent phase, may not be expected to significantly reduce mortality. In clinical practice, door-to-balloon times are often much longer than in randomized trials. This may in part be due to distances involved, weather conditions, and less-efficient strategies at the PCI center. Moreover, the time from symptom to presentation remains disappointingly long. In the United States, the median time to presentation is 114 minutes. Data from the GRACE registry have shown that the time to presentation has actually lengthened over time (120 minutes in 2000 and 133 minutes in 2006), despite the fact that door-to-balloon times have shortened (from 40 to 34 minutes for fibrinolysis and from 99 to 80 minutes for primary PCI).

Early studies of primary PCI consistently demonstrated spontaneous reperfusion to confer better clinical outcomes. Why has this not been the case with pharmacologically assisted reperfusion prior to PCI? This probably relates, in part, to the range of deleterious effects associated with fibrinolysis independent of its effect on epicardial coronary flow. Fibrinolysis-induced platelet activation and intramural coronary hemorrhage will promote recurrent ischemia. Myocardial hemorrhage (which occurs after PCI only in the setting of fibrinolytic therapy) will promote infarct extensions and propensity to ventricular rupture. Access-site bleeding and intracranial hemorrhage are much more likely in the setting of recent fibrinolytic therapy. All patients undergoing facilitated PCI are exposed to these risks, whereas only about 25% will potentially benefit by incremental early restoration of TIMI 3 flow (8).

PHARMACOINVASIVE APPROACH

The pharmacoinvasive strategy combines immediate transfer and rescue PCI for failed reperfusion with immediate transfer and routine early PCI within 3 to 24 hours. Rescue PCI will be discussed in the next section. A strategy of routine PCI between 3 and 24 hours after fibrinolytic therapy was evaluated in the GRACIA-1, SIAM-III, and CARESS-in-AMI studies among others (9–11). In all the three studies, routine early PCI resulted in better outcomes than conservative therapy. Furthermore, the WEST study suggested that a pharmacoinvasive approach (rescue and early invasive) resulted in similar outcomes to primary PCI (12). The two most recent studies of a pharmacoinvasive approach, TRANSFER-AMI and NORDISTEMI, add additional evidence that this strategy is superior to a conservative approach and highlights the importance of timing of PCI as a potential explanation for the relatively poorer outcomes with a facilitated approach (13,14). The TRANSFER-AMI study randomized 1059 STEMI patients who were receiving fibrinolysis at non-PCI hospitals to immediate transfer and PCI within six hours or standard therapy. PCI was performed in 98% and 89% of the early PCI and standard groups, respectively. The early PCI group suffered statistically fewer composite ischemic events without higher bleeding rates. The NORDISTEMI trial randomized 266 STEMI patients in rural Norway who lived more than 90 minutes from a PCI center to fibrinolytic therapy with or without transfer for early PCI. There was a statistically significant reduction in the composite ischemic endpoint at 12 months in the PCI transfer group.

PHARMACOINVASIVE VS. FACILITATED APPROACHES

The Importance of Timing of PCI

Median times of fibrinolysis to balloon inflation were 163 and 230 minutes in the TRANSFER-AMI and NORDISTEM pharmacoinvasive studies, respectively, contrasting with 90 and 104 minutes in the ASSENT-IV and FINESSE facilitated studies, respectively. Thus one could argue that the times to PCI were too short in the facilitated PCI studies, with persisting excessive fibrinolytic activity leading to increased complications. Another important difference between the facilitated and phamacoinvasive approaches was that thienopyridines were administered with fibrinolytics in the latter. The lack of dual antiplatelet administration in the facilitated studies could quite conceivably have led to more thrombotic complications.

Is There a Role for Facilitated PCI?

The latest AHA and ESC guidelines argue against a strategy of transfer for immediate PCI after fibrinolysis given the data outlined above, suggesting a tendency toward harm with this approach. However, two recent retrospective analyses from the largest trials of facilitated PCI, FINESSE and ASSENT-4, suggest this may not be the end of the story (15,16).

In the FINESSE retrospective analysis, patients were stratified by presentation to a non-PCI vs. PCI center, symptom to randomization time, and TIMI risk score. Not surprisingly, mortality was directly related to TIMI risk score. Interestingly, patients with a TIMI score ≥ 3, those presenting to a non-PCI center and those randomized <4 hours after symptom onset exhibited a significant improvement in the 90-day combined endpoint of death, early ventricular fibrillation, cardiogenic shock, and heart failure with a facilitated approach. More so, these groups exhibited a statistically significant improvement in one-year survival with a facilitated versus conservative approach. This is all the more noteworthy in that patients with high risk, presenting early to a non-PCI center is exactly the group that might be expected to benefit from a facilitated approach. In this regard, a retrospective analysis of the ASSENT-4 trial concluded that few patients in this study fit the target population, namely, those with long delays to PCI, for whom facilitated PCI was designed. In fact, patients randomized to a facilitated approach in the prehospital setting had the lowest 90-day mortality of all groups. The authors suggested caution in extrapolating the initial results of ASSENT-4 to the clinical setting where patients may present early but face a long transfer time to a PCI center.

SUMMARY

The success of any reperfusion strategy depends on the time to administration. However, in the United States, less than 5% of patients undergoing PPCI achieve a door-to-balloon time of <90 minutes, often because of initial presentation to a non-PCI center and delays incurred by transfer. The concept of a combined approach, namely, initial fibrinolysis at presentation with subsequent transfer for angiography and PCI is therefore appealing. Options after fibrinolytic therapy include a facilitated approach (immediate transfer for angiography and PCI) or a pharmacoinvasive approach comprising immediate transfer and rescue PCI for failed reperfusion or early routine PCI within 3 to 24 hours. Studies have consistently shown the early routine PCI (performed in this time window after successful fibrinolysis) to be superior to conservative therapy. On the other hand, studies of a facilitated strategy, defined as transfer for immediate angiography and PCI, usually in less than three hours have in general a worse outcome. It seems likely that the marked difference in findings between studies of facilitated versus a pharmacoinvasive strategy is due to timing of PCI, which if performed too early after fibrinolysis (<3 hours) may suffer from the downside of residual fibrinolytic activity. In general, facilitated PCI with immediate PCI after fibrinolytic therapy has not been recommended because of data demonstrating significant increases in mortality, reinfarction, and stroke. However, recent retrospective evaluation of two large contemporary trials suggests that there may be a role for facilitated PCI in patients who present early and with a long projected transfer time. Whether alternative pharmacologic regimens, with efficacy in restoring infarct artery patency but without attendant deleterious effects, may offer additional hope for a facilitated strategy remains to be determined.

RESCUE PCI

Rationale for Pursuing a Rescue Approach
Fibrinolytic therapy remains the principal index treatment for the majority of patients presenting with STEMI worldwide. Even with newer fibrin-specific agents, fibrinolysis achieves normal epicardial blood flow in only 50% to 60%. Moreover, anything less than TIMI 3 flow after reperfusion therapy confers an increased risk of mortality. A recent meta-analysis suggests that about 125,000 patients per year in the United States will not achieve successful reperfusion with fibrinolytic therapy administered as primary therapy, leaving considerable scope for pursuing additional approaches to ensure normalization of flow in the infarct artery (17).

Diagnosis of Failed Reperfusion
Rescue PCI as defined by the AHA/ACC constitutes PCI within 12 hours after failed fibrinolysis for patients with continuing or recurrent myocardial ischemia. Although the gold standard for diagnosing failed reperfusion is diagnostic angiography, it is generally not a clinical practice to pursue angiography in all cases purely for the purposes of making this diagnosis. The accuracy of diagnosing failed reperfusion by noninvasive means remains a clinical challenge. It is generally accepted that successful reperfusion can be diagnosed clinically by resolution of pain, complete ST-segment resolution, and development of reperfusion arrhythmias. However, given the nonspecific nature of pain as a symptom of ongoing ischemia and rarity of complete ST-segment resolution even with successful reperfusion, it is generally felt best to maintain a high index of suspicion of failure to reperfuse and to consider earlier angiography if uncertainty remains. The ACC/AHA guidelines consider a $\leq$50% reduction of ST-segment elevation on a follow-up ECG 60 to 90 minutes after fibrinolysis to be suggestive of reperfusion and $\geq$70% reduction being considered complete resolution.

Studies of Rescue PCI in the Stent Era
Two contemporary randomized trials and one recent meta-analysis have provided important information that has helped defining the optimal treatment strategy for failed reperfusion after fibrinolysis. The MERLIN randomized study recruited 307 patients with fibrinolytic-treated STEMI (90% streptokinase) and less than 50% improvement in ST segment elevation at 60 minutes (18). Patients were randomized to PCI (50% stent rate, 85% TIMI 3 flow at completion) or conservative therapy. Anterior MIs comprised 40% and 48% of groups, respectively. Glycoprotein IIb/IIIa inhibitors were used in only 3.3% of cases. The primary endpoint of the study was 30 days mortality, and there was no significant difference between the groups. The PCI group experienced fewer revascularizations but more strokes and more bleeding requiring transfusions. This study may have less relevance to current practice given the lower usage of antiplatelet therapy and low stent rates. Perhaps the major limitation of this trial was the choice of mortality as the primary endpoint, which, given the sample size, was unlikely to have been shown to be statistically different.

The most relevant randomized data for current practice comes from the REACT study, a multicenter trial of 427 patients who failed to achieve 50% resolution of ST-segment elevation at 90 minutes postfibrinolysis (19). Patients with cardiogenic shock were excluded. The study did suffer from slow recruitment and eventually was prematurely terminated due to low enrollment. Patients were randomized in a 1:1:1 fashion to intravenous heparin, repeat fibrinolysis with a fibrin-specific agent or rescue PCI (69% stent rate), which was performed within 12 hours of pain onset if angiography indicated less than TIMI 3 flow and a stenosis of >50% in the infarct artery. The mean additional delay to PCI over repeat fibrinolysis was 84 minutes. Glycoprotein IIb/IIIa usage was 43%. The primary endpoint of the study was a composite of death, nonfatal reinfarction, stroke, or severe heart failure at six months. This composite endpoint was significantly reduced in the rescue group at six months. In addition, freedom from repeat revascularization was improved in the rescue PCI group at 86.7% compared with 76.5% with repeat fibrinolytic therapy and 79.3% in the conservative arm. There was a trend toward lower all-cause mortality in the rescue arm (6.2% vs. 12.7% with repeat fibrinolysis and 12.8% with intravenous heparin). Most recently, the REACT group has published long-term data (20). Importantly, there was a significant reduction in long-term mortality in the rescue arm (median follow up 4.4 years). Mortality was 11.2% in the rescue group, 22.3% with repeat fibrinolysis and 22.4% with intravenous heparin, suggesting rescue PCI to be the treatment of choice in the setting of failure to reperfuse with fibrinolytic therapy.

A meta-analysis of 908 pooled patients from six randomized studies suggested a nonsignificant 25% risk reduction in one to four year mortality, with a rescue PCI approach over conservative therapy. Rescue PCI was also associated with a significant reduction in reinfarction and risk of developing heart failure, although also with a significantly greater risk of stroke.

The AHA/ACC guidelines currently indicate a class I recommendation for rescue PCI in the setting of cardiogenic shock in patients <75 years, with severe heart failure and hemodynamically significant ventricular arrhythmias. Class IIa recommendations are indicated for suitable older patients in cardiogenic shock, patients with hemodynamic or electrical instability or with persistent ischemic symptoms. Similarly, on the basis of data outlined above, a class IIa recommendation (level of evidence B) is given for a rescue PCI strategy in patients with ECG evidence of failed fibrinolysis and at least a moderate area of myocardium at risk as defined either by anterior MI, inferior MI with RV involvement or precordial ST segment depression. A stronger recommendation was not given in part because of the lack of consensus with all randomized studies. One scenario occasionally encountered in this setting for which there is little evidence to guide is the finding of TIMI 3 flow at angiography with significant stenosis and/or thrombus. There may now also be evidence of reperfusion clinically. Should PCI be performed immediately in the setting of angiographic thrombus and fibrinolytic activity or should it be deferred for a period? Most would move forward with PCI in this setting, but it is worth noting that there is no strong evidence to support this.

In general, it is felt best to maintain a low threshold for angiography and rescue PCI when there is doubt about reperfusion, given the poor outcomes when reperfusion has not occurred. Whether additional studies using newer pharmacotherapies (including antiplatelet therapies) will influence future recommendations remains to be seen. Regardless of future developments, it appears unlikely that a strategy of repeat fibrinolysis or conservative therapy alone will prove to be better than a mechanical approach.

REFERENCES

1. Reimer KA, Lowe JE, Rasmussen MM, et al. The wavefront phenomenon of ischemic cell death. 1. Myocardial infarct size vs duration of coronary occlusion in dogs. Circulation 1977; 56(5):786–794.
2. Keeley EC, Boura JA, Grines CL. Primary angioplasty versus intravenous thrombolytic therapy for acute myocardial infarction: a quantitative review of 23 randomised trials. Lancet 2003; 361(9351):13–20.
3. McNamara RL, Wang Y, Herrin J, et al. Effect of door-to-balloon time on mortality in patients with ST-segment elevation myocardial infarction. J Am Coll Cardiol 2006; 47(11):2180–2186.
4. Le May MR, Wells GA, Labinaz M, et al. Combined angioplasty and pharmacological intervention versus thrombolysis alone in acute myocardial infarction (CAPITAL AMI study). J Am Coll Cardiol 2005; 46(3):417–424.
5. Primary versus tenecteplase-facilitated percutaneous coronary intervention in patients with ST-segment elevation acute myocardial infarction (ASSENT-4 PCI): randomised trial. Lancet 2006; 367(9510):569–578.
6. Keeley EC, Boura JA, Grines CL. Comparison of primary and facilitated percutaneous coronary interventions for ST-elevation myocardial infarction: quantitative review of randomised trials. Lancet 2006; 367(9510):579–588.
7. Ellis SG, Tendera M, de Belder MA, et al. Facilitated PCI in patients with ST-elevation myocardial infarction. N Engl J Med 2008; 358(21):2205–2217.
8. Stone GW, Gersh BJ. Facilitated angioplasty: paradise lost. Lancet 2006; 367(9510):543–546.
9. Fernandez-Aviles F, Alonso JJ, Castro-Beiras A, et al. Routine invasive strategy within 24 hours of thrombolysis versus ischaemia-guided conservative approach for acute myocardial infarction with ST-segment elevation (GRACIA-1): a randomised controlled trial. Lancet 2004; 364(9439):1045–1053.
10. Scheller B, Hennen B, Hammer B, et al. Beneficial effects of immediate stenting after thrombolysis in acute myocardial infarction. J Am Coll Cardiol 2003; 42(4):634–641.
11. Di Mario C, Dudek D, Piscione F, et al. Immediate angioplasty versus standard therapy with rescue angioplasty after thrombolysis in the Combined Abciximab REteplase Stent Study in Acute Myocardial Infarction (CARESS-in-AMI): an open, prospective, randomised, multicentre trial. Lancet 2008; 371(9612):559–568.
12. Armstrong PW. A comparison of pharmacologic therapy with/without timely coronary intervention vs. primary percutaneous intervention early after ST-elevation myocardial infarction: the WEST (Which Early ST-elevation myocardial infarction Therapy) study. Eur Heart J 2006; 27(13):1530–1538.
13. Cantor WJ, Fitchett D, Borgundvaag B, et al. Routine early angioplasty after fibrinolysis for acute myocardial infarction. N Engl J Med 2009; 360(26):2705–2718.
14. Bohmer E, Hoffmann P, Abdelnoor M, et al. Efficacy and safety of immediate angioplasty versus ischemia-guided management after thrombolysis in acute myocardial infarction in areas with very long transfer distances results of the NORDISTEMI (NORwegian study on DIstrict treatment of ST-Elevation Myocardial Infarction). J Am Coll Cardiol 2010; 55(2):111–113.
15. Herrmann HC, Lu J, Brodie BR, et al. Benefit of facilitated percutaneous coronary intervention in high-risk ST-segment elevation myocardial infarction patients presenting to nonpercutaneous coronary intervention hospitals. JACC Cardiovasc Interv 2009; 2(10):917–924.
16. Ross AM, Huber K, Zeymer U, et al. The impact of place of enrollment and delay to reperfusion on 90-day post-infarction mortality in the ASSENT-4 PCI trial: assessment

of the safety and efficacy of a new treatment strategy with percutaneous coronary intervention. JACC Cardiovasc Interv 2009; 2(10):925–930.

17. Wijeysundera HC, Vijayaraghavan R, Nallamothu BK, et al. Rescue angioplasty or repeat fibrinolysis after failed fibrinolytic therapy for ST-segment myocardial infarction: a meta-analysis of randomized trials. J Am Coll Cardiol 2007; 49(4):422–430.

18. Sutton AG, Campbell PG, Graham R, et al. A randomized trial of rescue angioplasty versus a conservative approach for failed fibrinolysis in ST-segment elevation myocardial infarction: the Middlesbrough Early Revascularization to Limit INfarction (MERLIN) trial. J Am Coll Cardiol 2004; 44(2):287–296.

19. Gershlick AH, Stephens-Lloyd A, Hughes S, et al. Rescue angioplasty after failed thrombolytic therapy for acute myocardial infarction. N Engl J Med 2005; 353(26):2758–2768.

20. Carver A, Rafelt S, Gershlick AH, et al. Longer-term follow-up of patients recruited to the REACT (Rescue Angioplasty Versus Conservative Treatment or Repeat Thrombolysis) trial. J Am Coll Cardiol 2009; 54(2):118–126.

15 Opportunities and Challenges of Stem Cell Therapy: Is there a Role in AMI?

Barry H. Trachtenberg

Department of Medicine, Cardiovascular Division, University of Miami Miller School of Medicine, Miami, Florida, U.S.A.

Joshua M. Hare

Department of Medicine, Cardiovascular Division, University of Miami Miller School of Medicine, and Interdisciplinary Stem Cell Institute, Miami, Florida, U.S.A.

INTRODUCTION

Traditional management of myocardial infarction (MI) focuses on limiting the extent of ischemia by combining medical therapies with strategies such as percutaneous coronary interventions (PCI), coronary artery bypass surgery, or thrombolytic therapy to restore blood flow to the ischemic myocardium. Medications such as 3-hydroxy-3-methylglutaryl coenzyme A (HMG-CoA) reductase inhibitors, angiotensin converting-enzyme inhibitors (ACEI), beta-blockers, antiplatelet and anticoagulant therapies, coupled with early intervention to stop the progression of myocyte damage have clearly had an impact on the morbidity and mortality of coronary artery disease. These medications and revascularization have helped bring about a dramatic improvement in life expectancy throughout the Western world.

Despite these therapeutic advances, even patients who have early revascularization are left with significant myocyte damage and some degree of scar tissue due to the healed infarction. As a result, not only is coronary artery disease the number one cause of mortality in the world, but the morbidity and economic burden associated with ischemic heart disease is also tremendous.

While some therapies such as ACEI or aldosterone antagonists are effective at ameliorating remodeling of the failing heart, there is currently no established therapy that actually leads to tissue regeneration. As such, the promise of stem cell therapy as a strategy to regenerate or repair myocardial tissue fulfills a true unmet need. Therefore, there is considerable interest and anticipation of the potential of stem cell therapies in the treatment of acute and chronic myocardial ischemia.

STEM CELL BACKGROUND

Stem cells are defined by two properties—the ability to self-replicate and the capacity to differentiate into a variety of lineages (1) and can be broadly categorized into embryonic stem cells and adult stem cells. Embryonic stem cells, which have the advantage of pluripotency (capacity to differentiate into all cell lineages), have not been studied extensively in humans with myocardial ischemia

153

due largely to ethical concerns and potential teratoma formation (1). Adult stem cells under active investigation are bone marrow-derived stem cells, circulating stem cells, cells from a variety of nonhematopoietic sources, and tissue-resident stem cells (cardiac stem cells). Bone marrow stem cells comprise mesenchymal stem cells, hematopoietic stem cells, and "side population" cells. As far as clinical development is concerned, the majority of human trials in heart disease utilize autologous whole bone marrow.

The exact mechanism(s) explaining the beneficial effects of cell-based therapeutic responses remain controversial. Acute and subacute ischemia leads to a rise in serum levels of vascular endothelial growth factor (VEGF) and stromal cell-derived factor (SDF)-1 as well as in the number of endogenous circulating CD34+ mononuclear cells. Thus, ischemia enhances mobilization and homing of endogenous endothelial or hematopoietic stem cells. Many animal and human trials have demonstrated improved myocardial functioning after delivery or mobilization of stem cells despite the fact that the underlying mechanism is not entirely clear. Contemplated mechanisms include cell engraftment and differentiation, release of paracrine growth factors, cell fusion, and the stimulation and regeneration of resident cardiac stem cells niches (2).

Another important concept in stem cell therapies involves the donor source. As opposed to autologous cells, stem cells can also be cultured from healthy donors and expanded for storage and allogeneic use in a multitude of patients without the need for individual bone marrow biopsies in every patient. Data have shown that allogeneic MSCs do not stimulate a T cell response and thus are not rejected by recipients (3). A key disadvantage of autologous cells is that patients who have ischemic cardiomyopathy have a decline in number and regenerative capacity of BM and circulating stem cells; (4) thus, patients who suffer from cardiomyopathy may not only have damaged myocardium but also a lessened capacity for repair (3,4).

STRATEGIES TO MOBILIZE ENDOGENOUS CELLS

Given the notion that there are reservoirs of precursor cells at remote sites from the injured organ, various methods to enhance mobilization and engraftment of circulating stem cells have been sought. Since granulocyte colony-stimulating factor (G-CSF) is widely available and endogenous levels positively correlate with CD34+ levels (5), G-CSF administration has been tested in multiple preclinical and clinical trials. Animal studies and several pilot studies in humans have demonstrated evidence of reverse remodeling with the administration of G-CSF in the periinfarct period. However, larger randomized, placebo-controlled studies showed no significant improvement in infarct size or ejection fraction in patients who had a recent ST segment elevation MI treated with percutaneous intervention (6,7). Studies have shown that the intracoronary injection of G-CSF mobilized stem cells may improve ejection fraction in patients with acute MI (Fig. 1) though data is conflicting in regards to chronic MI (8,9). In terms of safety, while small studies suggested the possibility of increased restenosis rates in patients treated with G-CSF, this was not demonstrated in larger, better designed trials (6,7). Other mobilization strategies that have shown potential for benefits include erythropoietin, SDF-1, tumor necrosis factor-alpha, and placental growth factor.

(A) Acute myocardial infarction

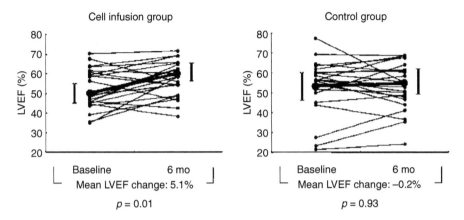

(B) Old myocardial infarction

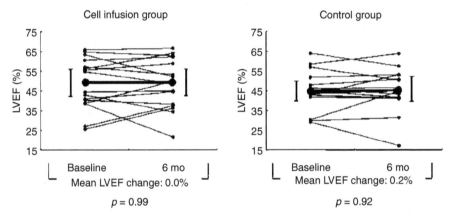

FIGURE 1 The effect of intracoronary infusion of granulocyte colony-stimulating factor (G-CSF) mobilized peripheral blood stem cells at baseline and after six months in (**A**) patients with AMI and (**B**) patients with chronic ischemia. There was a significant improvement in EF ($P = 0.01$) in the AMI group but not in the chronic ischemia group. Small dots represent individual patients, large dots represent the mean, and vertical bars show standard deviation. *Source*: From Ref. 9.

DELIVERY TECHNIQUES

Several different routes of SC delivery have been used in clinical trials: (*i*) intravenous (IV), (*ii*) intracoronary (IC), (*iii*) transendocardial (TE) via intraventricular catheter systems, (*iv*) direct epicardial injection during open-heart surgery or via thoracotomy, and (*v*) retrograde via the coronary venous system.

The IC route, used with or without a balloon occlusion catheter to prevent backflow, has the theoretical advantages of being able to directly target ischemic or infarcted myocardial tissue by injecting cells into the infarct-related artery (Fig. 2). In addition, this route is less invasive then surgery and easy

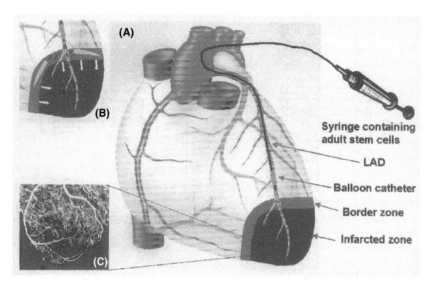

FIGURE 2 Intracoronary delivery of stem cells. (**A**) The balloon catheter is placed in the infarct-related artery proximal to the border zone of the infarction. The balloon is inflated to prevent backflow and cells are infused. (**B**) Cartoon depicting cells migrating (arrows) to the area of infarct via the infarct-related vasculature (*dots*). (**C**) Depicts supply of blood flow within infracted area. *Source*: From Ref. 16.

to perform for interventional cardiologists. Potential disadvantages include washout and microvascular obstruction, particularly with MSCs (3) or skeletal myoblasts (10).

The IV route, due to its simplicity and low cost, has the potential to delivery cells to the largest population of patients. Potential disadvantages of IV application of stem cells include early distribution to the lungs with possible pulmonary toxicity, damage to other organs, and poor myocardial retention. However, we have shown no evidence of toxicity to the lungs or other organs in a double-blinded randomized trial of IV MSCs (11).

Several TE injection catheter-based systems are available (Fig. 3). Some, such as the Noga Myostar injection catheter (12) and Biocardia helical catheter (13), have shown safety and efficacy in human trials. Advantages include the ability to directly target damaged myocardium without the need for surgery and avoidance of potential microvascular obstruction. Disadvantages include the potential for perforation and a steep learning curve for a more technically complex delivery compared to the IC or IV route.

Epicardial delivery during surgery was the first method of stem cell delivery to be tested. A key advantage is that it can be injected (with direct visualization of the myocardium by the surgeon) at the time of open-heart surgery, although the fact that it must coincide with a major operation also severely reduces the pool of potential recipients. Retrograde coronary venous delivery is promising but its use has been limited to small number of animal studies.

There are very few studies comparing methods of delivery. A study by Perin et al. compared the IC versus TE route in a canine model with acute

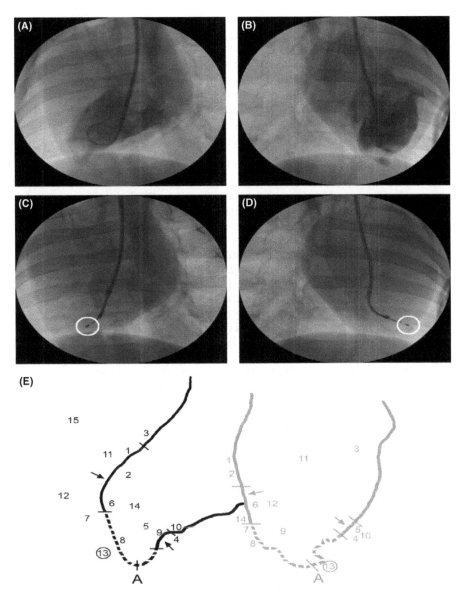

FIGURE 3 Transendocardial technique in male swine. A left ventricular (LV) gram was obtained in lateral (**A**) and anterior–posterior (**B**) fluoroscopic projections. End-diastolic LV endocardial borders were traced manually, and areas of hypokinesia (*arrows*) and akinesia (*dashed lines*) were defined (**E**). Delivery of mesenchymal stem cells using the Stiletto Endocardial Direct Injection Catheter System (Boston Scientific) into the akinetic infarct area in orthogonal projections (**C** and **D**) and its correlation on the tracing map (injection site 13) (**E**) is shown. *Source*: From Ref. 38.

MI. Compared to the IC route, dogs injected via the TE route had evidence of greater cell retention and a significant improvement in LVEF (14). In a small study directly comparing TE, IC, and IV delivery of MSC in ischemia-induced swine, the IC method had the highest amount of cellular engraftment within the infarct zone. Engraftment with the TE route was greater than IV delivery. However, TE delivery had less engraftment to other organs other than the heart, and IC injections were more likely to be associated with microvascular obstruction (15). More robust studies are needed to determine the optimal mode of delivery to enhance retention while limiting toxicity.

ACUTE ISCHEMIA

The studies of stem cells in the setting of acute MI have shown that delivery of stem cells is generally safe, and the majority of studies have shown a modest improvement in ejection fraction or infarct size. However, the heterogeneity of the trials complicates the interpretation of the data. For example, the published trials use different delivery techniques, cell types, cell processing and culturing methods, methods of assessing myocardial function, and variable timing of cell delivery in relation to the sentinel event. Most studies have been limited by relatively small sample sizes and the lack of long-term follow-up.

The IC route has been used in the majority of human trials. A study by Strauer et al. (16). was the first study to use IC transplantation of autologous BMCs in humans. Ten patients received the cells five to nine days post transmural MI and subsequent revascularization. Although the sample size was small and was compared to a nonrandomized control, a three-month follow-up showed a significant decrease in infarct size and left ventricular end-systolic volume. Larger studies followed, such as the Reinfusion of Enriched Progenitor cells and Infract Remodeling in Acute Myocardial Infraction study (REPAIR-AMI) (17), which showed that IC BMCs three to seven days post AMI and revascularization led to improved ejection fraction (measured by left ventricular angiography) at four months and a decrease in the combined endpoint of death, recurrent MI, and need for revascularization at one year (18).

While many additional studies showed improvements in ejection fraction and/or cardiac geometry, two studies showed less promising results. One study randomized 100 patients who received PCI for an acute ST elevation MI followed by IC stem cell injections or standard medical care and found no significant improvement in ejection fraction, LV end-diastolic volume (LVEDV), or infarct size (19). Another study demonstrated decreased infarct size and enhanced regional systolic function but no improvement in LVEF (20). This study injected cells into the infarct-related coronary artery 24 hours after PCI, which was performed at a median of 4 hours from symptom onset. It is possible that the early administration of stem cells after AMI in this study may have mitigated the effects.

Because of the discrepancy in data and the limited number of subjects in each study, two different meta-analyses have been performed. A meta-analysis by Abdel-Latif et al. (21) included 18 studies (12 randomized and 6 cohort studies) with a total sample size of 999 patients (Table 1). The majority (>92%) used IC delivery, and most studies involved unfractionated BM mononuclear cells. Eight of the 18 trials included patients with chronic myocardial ischemia. The pooled data revealed a statistically significant 3.7% improvement in LVEF versus

TABLE 1 Forest Plot of Unadjusted Difference in Mean (with 95% Confidence Intervals) Improvement in Left Ventricular Ejection Fraction in Patients Treated with Bone Marrow-Derived Cells Compared with Controls

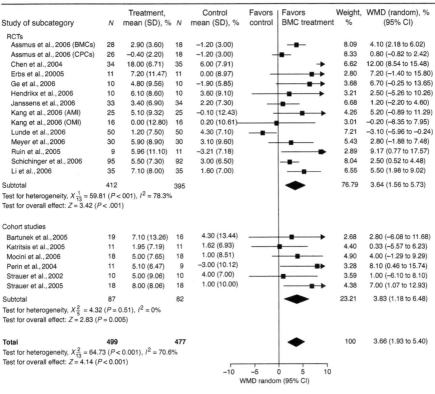

Study of subcategory	N	Treatment, mean (SD), %	N	Control mean (SD), %	Weight, %	WMD (random), % (95% CI)
RCTs						
Assmus et al., 2006 (BMCs)	28	2.90 (3.60)	18	−1.20 (3.00)	8.09	4.10 (2.18 to 6.02)
Assmus et al., 2006 (CPCs)	26	−0.40 (2.20)	18	−1.20 (3.00)	8.33	0.80 (−0.82 to 2.42)
Chen et al., 2004	34	18.00 (6.71)	35	6.00 (7.91)	6.62	12.00 (8.54 to 15.48)
Erbs et al., 20005	11	7.20 (11.47)	11	0.00 (8.97)	2.80	7.20 (−1.40 to 15.80)
Ge et al., 2006	10	4.80 (9.56)	10	−1.90 (5.85)	3.68	6.70 (−0.25 to 13.65)
Hendrikx et al., 2006	10	6.10 (8.60)	10	3.60 (9.10)	3.21	2.50 (−5.26 to 10.26)
Janssens et al., 2006	33	3.40 (6.90)	34	2.20 (7.30)	6.68	1.20 (−2.20 to 4.60)
Kang et al., 2006 (AMI)	25	5.10 (9.32)	25	−0.10 (12.43)	4.26	5.20 (−0.89 to 11.29)
Kang et al., 2006 (OMI)	16	0.00 (12.80)	16	0.20 (10.61)	3.01	−0.20 (−8.35 to 7.95)
Lunde et al., 2006	50	1.20 (7.50)	50	4.30 (7.10)	7.21	−3.10 (−5.96 to −0.24)
Meyer et al., 2006	30	5.90 (8.90)	30	3.10 (9.60)	5.43	2.80 (−1.88 to 7.48)
Ruin et al., 2005	9	5.96 (11.10)	11	−3.21 (7.18)	2.89	9.17 (0.77 to 17.57)
Schichinger et al., 2006	95	5.50 (7.30)	92	3.00 (6.50)	8.04	2.50 (0.52 to 4.48)
Li et al., 2006	35	7.10 (8.00)	35	1.60 (7.00)	6.55	5.50 (1.98 to 9.02)
Subtotal	412		395		76.79	3.64 (1.56 to 5.73)

Test for heterogeneity, $X^2_{13} = 59.81$ ($P < 001$), $I^2 = 78.3\%$
Test for overall effect: $Z = 3.42$ ($P < .001$)

Cohort studies						
Bartunek et al., 2005	19	7.10 (13.26)	16	4.30 (13.44)	2.68	2.80 (−6.08 to 11.68)
Katritsis et al., 2005	11	1.95 (7.19)	11	1.62 (6.93)	4.40	0.33 (−5.57 to 6.23)
Mocini et al., 2006	18	5.00 (7.65)	18	1.00 (8.51)	4.90	4.00 (−1.29 to 9.29)
Perin et al., 2004	11	5.10 (6.47)	9	−3.00 (10.12)	3.28	8.10 (0.46 to 15.74)
Strauer et al., 2002	10	5.00 (9.06)	10	4.00 (7.00)	3.59	1.00 (−6.10 to 8.10)
Strauer et al., 2005	18	8.00 (8.06)	18	1.00 (10.00)	4.38	7.00 (1.07 to 12.93)
Subtotal	87		82		23.21	3.83 (1.18 to 6.48)

Test for heterogeneity, $X^2_5 = 4.32$ ($P = 0.51$), $I^2 = 0\%$
Test for overall effect: $Z = 2.83$ ($P = 0.005$)

| **Total** | 499 | | 477 | | 100 | 3.66 (1.93 to 5.40) |

Test for heterogeneity, $X^2_{13} = 64.73$ ($P < 0.001$), $I^2 = 70.6\%$
Test for overall effect: $Z = 4.14$ ($P < 0.001$)

WMD random (95% CI): −10, −5, 0, 5, 10

Source: From Ref. 21: Please refer to source for additional details on references.

controls, as well as decreased infarct size and LV end-systolic volume. Another systematic review, which differed in that it included only acute MI patients and randomized controlled trials (13 trials, total $n = 818$), yielded similar conclusions. In this review, autologous BM cells post-AMI led to significant improvement in LVEF (mean increase 2.99%), decreased left ventricular end-systolic volume (LVESV), and myocardial lesion area (22). An assessment of clinical outcomes yielded trends favoring BMC treatment but none of these outcomes reached statistical significance (Table 2). Both studies concluded that the injection of cells was safe without any statistically significant increase in adverse events such as malignancies, restenosis, reinfarction, or arrhythmias. It is important to note that the long-term follow-up was limited in the majority of the studies; the longest follow-up included in these meta-analyses was 18 months in the former review and 6 months in the latter.

A critical question is whether the increase in LVEF is sustained long-term or not; the data in this regard are conflicting. For example, the BOne marrOw transfer to enhance ST elevation infarct regeneration (BOOST) trial (23) showed a significant improvement in LVEF 6 months after stem cell injection versus

TABLE 2 Summary of Clinical Outcomes in a Meta-Analysis of Randomized Controlled Trials of Autologous BMCs in AMI

Outcome	No. of trials	Time point measure[a]	Relative risk (95% CI)	*P*-value
Mortality	5	1–12 months	0.62 (0.22, 1.76)	0.37
Morbidity				
Reinfarction	7[b]	<30 days (1)	0.33 (0.01, 7.81)	0.49
		1–4 months (4)	0.61 (0.12, 2.96)	0.54
		12 months (1)	0.08 (0.00, 1.37)	0.08
Arrhythmias	1	Not known	0.57 (0.21, 1.53)	NA
Restenosis	7[b]	6 months (5)	1.10 (0.68, 1.80)	0.69
		12 months (1)	0.34 (0.01, 813)	0.51
Readmission	4[b]	1–6 months (2)	0.61 (0.25, 1.52)	0.29
		12 months (1)	0.15 (0.01, 278)	0.2
Revascularization	6[b]	1–6 months (2)	0.55 (0.19, 1.62)	0.28
		12 months (1)	0.71 (0.42, 1.20)	0.2
Adverse events	5[c]	Not reported in all studies	NA	NA
Quality of life	2	21 day to 6 months	Not measured	NA
Reoperation	1	12 months	0.61 (0.39, 0.95)	NA

NA, not applicable.
[a]Number of trials that measured the outcome at each time point is in brackets.
[b]One study did not report the time point at which the outcome was measured.
[c]Adverse events not always reported in full details to allow statistical analysis.
Source: From Ref. 22.

controls, but after 18 months the control group had also improved considerably so that the difference was no longer statistically significant (24). In contrast, data from the Transplantation of Progenitor Cells and Regeneration Enhancement in Acute Myocardial Infarction (TOPCARE-AMI) trial showed lasting improvement in LVEF compared to controls at 12 months (25).

Analysis of data from the REPAIR-AMI trial showed that patients treated with stem cells who had a lower baseline LVEF (stratified by the median LVEF 48.9%) gained the most benefit, with an absolute increase in EF that was three times that of the control group (17). The meta-analyses did not have enough information to stratify patients according to baseline LVEF.

Another key factor that may affect the outcome is the timing of the delivery of cells. Some data suggest that the acute inflammatory response in the first four to five days post-MI inhibits cell engraftment (16) and that delaying the infusion of cells after AMI is more effective than early administration. In the REPAIR-AMI study, there was a significant effect of treatment in patients at least five days post-AMI but none if <5 days. The meta-analysis by Martin-Rendon et al. also indicated that improvement in LVEF was greater if infused later (>7 days).

OTHER CELL TYPES

Increasingly, mesenchymal stem cells have been studied in cardiac repair. MSCs, while representing only ~1/10,000 nucleated BM cells, are easily isolated and expanded. Additional advantages of MSCs include increased ability to home to areas of injured myocardium compared to BMCs and the capacity to differentiate into a variety of tissue types (11). The first human trial with MSCs injected autologous cells via the IC method approximately 18 days post-STEMI and percutaneous intervention, showing a significant improvement in LVEF and infarct size versus controls at 6 months (26). However, due to their relatively large size, IC infusion of MSCs may cause microvascular obstruction and infarction. TE catheter-based delivery of allogeneic MSCs in pigs with anterior wall MIs resulted in decreased infarct size, attenuation of wall thinning, and dramatic improvements in cardiac function (27).

Recent data have shown that the IV delivery of allogeneic MSCs to human patients in the postinfarction setting is safe. There was no evidence of pulmonary toxicity or ectopic tissue formation after six months. In addition, patients with anterior wall MIs who were treated with IV MSCs had significant improvement in LVEF versus controls (11). A subset of patients who had serial cardiac MRIs also showed an increase in LVEF and decrease in LVEDV and LVESV versus the placebo group. While larger and more long-term studies are clearly warranted to further demonstrate safety and efficacy, this relatively simple technique may obviate the need for more invasive procedures.

Skeletal myoblasts are myofiber precursor cells that have the capacity for renewal and differentiation and are vital to repair injured skeletal muscle. They can be harvested in an autologous manner from skeletal muscle biopsies and amplified easily in culture. Other advantages include high resistance to ischemia and low risk of tumorigenicity. Disadvantages include the fact that they do not differentiate into cardiomyocytes and they have an arrhythmogenic propensity when injected into the myocardium, presumably due to their lack of electrical coupling with cardiomyocytes. Early studies showed an increase in ventricular arrhythmias (28), necessitating prophylactic cardioverter/defibrillator implantation in subsequent trials. Due to the relatively large size of the cells and thus increased risk of microvascular obstruction with the IC route of delivery, the epicardial approach has been used in most trials. Several small studies have shown an improvement in regional and global LVEF, although a recent, larger randomized placebo-controlled trial of epicardial myoblast transplantation in patients with ischemic cardiomyopathy undergoing coronary surgery failed to show a significant difference by echocardiography at six months (29).

The recent discovery of cardiac stem cells (CSCs) has generated a great deal of enthusiasm. These multipotent cells are capable of self-renewal and regeneration of damaged myocardium in vivo. Examination of hearts of patients who died from acute ischemic insults demonstrates a substantially increased population of CSCs. In the chronic setting, there was a sizeable drop in the number of CSCs, suggesting a model of ischemic cardiomyopathy associated with a dysfunction or decline in CSCs (30). Animal studies have suggested that the mobilization and injection of CSCs is associated with regeneration of myocardial tissue, decreased mortality (31), and formation of new coronary arteries (32). While these studies show great promise for the potential therapeutic benefit of CSCs, there have been no published trials of CSC transplantation in humans thus far.

CHRONIC ISCHEMIA

There is considerably less data on stem cell transplantation in patients with chronic ischemia, and much of the literature that exists involves small sample sizes. Many of the initial pilot trials involved delivery of cells at the time of

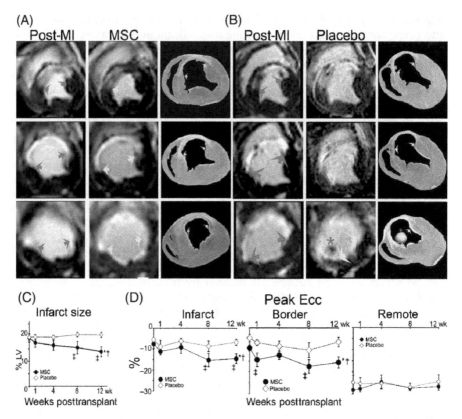

FIGURE 4 Twelve weeks post-MI, swine received transendocardial delivery of allogeneic MSC ($n = 6$) or placebo ($n = 4$). Infarct size and regional myocardial function were assessed by delayed gadolinium enhancement MRI. (**A** and **B**) Sequential short axis heart sections from base (*top*) to apex (*bottom*) of MRI images depicting the infarct extension (*white*) before treatment and 12 weeks following MSC therapy. Also shown are comparable gross pathology sections. Arrows delineate the infarct extension and the asterisk illustrates the presence of a thrombus in a placebo animal. (**C**) Reduction in infarct size following 8 and 12 weeks post-MSC transplantation versus placebo (*$P < 0.001$ within MSC group ANOVA, †$P < 0.05$ between groups ANOVA, ‡$P < 0.001$ vs. preinjection status by Student Newman–Keuls test). (**D**) Myocardial strain analysis represented by peak Eulerian circumferential shortening (Ecc) decreased in response to MSC treatment in infarct (*Left*) and border (*Center*) areas but remained constant in the remote uninfarcted zone (*Right*) (*$P < 0.05$ for ANOVA within MSC group, †$P < 0.05$ ANOVA between groups, ‡$P < 0.05$ vs. preinjection status by Student Newman–Keuls test). *Source*: From Ref. 36.

coronary artery bypass surgery, thus making it difficult to separate the effects of the transplantation from those of revascularization. However, a recent study of 40 patients with chronic ischemia randomized to CABG alone *or* CABG plus intramyocardial BMC injection showed a statistically significant improvement of LVEF and LVESV at six months in the BMC group (33).

In addition to the epicardial route, other studies have explored the IC and TE routes of stem cell delivery in chronic ischemia. One of the early trials of IC BMC delivery demonstrated a powerful effect on LVEF (increasing 15% increase at three months) (34) while larger, randomized studies showed a smaller but significant effect on LVEF (increasing 2.9% at three months) versus placebo or versus patients injected with circulating progenitor cells (35). One of the first studies to use the TE route was an open-labeled study using electromechanical mapping and injection with a NOGA catheter in patients with chronic CAD and evidence of hibernating myocardium. This procedure was found to be safe and showed a significant improvement in LVEF, cardiac geometry, and decreased perfusion defects by single photon emission computed tomography at four months (12).

A recent study of allogeneic MSCs injected transendocardially in swine with chronic ischemia not only showed improvement in cardiac function versus controls but also showed evidence of differentiation into cardiomyocytes, vascular smooth muscle cells, and endothelial cells (36) (Fig. 4). There are several ongoing trials of stem cell delivery in humans with chronic ischemia whose results will be highly anticipated.

Many studies of stem cells in chronic ischemia have utilized crude measures of systolic function and cardiac geometry obtained from two-dimensional echocardiography and angiography as outcomes. The increasing availability and usage of cardiac magnetic resonance imaging and computed tomography allow much more sophisticated and perhaps more relevant outcomes, such as infarct size, myocardial first-pass perfusion, and regional wall motion, to be assessed (i.e., Fig. 4). These tools should be used routinely in future studies. Ultimately, however, stem cells will be judged on whether they favorably affect clinical outcomes.

CONCLUSIONS

In the past few years, there has been an abundance of literature, debate, publicity, and controversy surrounding stem cells and their potential to repair a damaged heart. Current limitations in the widespread therapeutic application of stem cells include a mechanism of action that is not entirely known, poor cell retention, and perhaps most importantly, a lack of robust studies showing a significant difference in clinical outcomes. On the other hand, most studies have shown that transplantation of stem cells is safe and modestly effective. While clearly not yet reaching the highly anticipated therapeutic effects, two large meta-analyses have demonstrated that stem cells at the current state leads to an average improvement in ejection fraction of about 3% to 4% and evidence of reverse remodeling. It has been noted that comparable improvements in ejection fraction have occurred in other landmark AMI trials (37).

There is a multitude of ongoing research attempting to find the optimal cell type, dose, delivery method, mobilization strategy, and patient population. As these factors are adjusted and optimized, larger, multicentered placebo-controlled trials are clearly needed to advance the field.

REFERENCES

1. Burt RK, Loh Y, Pearce W, et al. Clinical applications of blood-derived and marrow-derived stem cells for nonmalignant diseases. JAMA 2008; 299(8):925–936.
2. Boyle AJ, Schulman SP, Hare JM, et al. Is stem cell therapy ready for patients? Stem Cell Therapy for Cardiac Repair. Ready for the Next Step. Circulation 2006; 114(4):339–352.

3. Zimmet JM, Hare JM. Emerging role for bone marrow derived mesenchymal stem cells in myocardial regenerative therapy. Basic Res Cardiol 2005; 100(6):471–481.
4. Kissel CK, Lehmann R, Assmus B, et al. Selective functional exhaustion of hematopoietic progenitor cells in the bone marrow of patients with postinfarction heart failure. J Am Coll Cardiol 2007; 49(24):2341–2349.
5. Leone AM, Rutella S, Bonanno G, et al. Endogenous G-CSF and CD34+ cell mobilization after acute myocardial infarction. Int J Cardiol 2006; 111(2):202–208.
6. Ripa RS, Jorgensen E, Wang Y, et al. Stem cell mobilization induced by subcutaneous granulocyte-colony stimulating factor to improve cardiac regeneration after acute ST-elevation myocardial infarction: result of the double-blind, randomized, placebo-controlled stem cells in myocardial infarction (STEMMI) trial. Circulation 2006; 113(16):1983–1992.
7. Zohlnhofer D, Ott I, Mehilli J, et al. Stem cell mobilization by granulocyte colony-stimulating factor in patients with acute myocardial infarction: a randomized controlled trial. JAMA 2006; 295(9):1003–1010.
8. Erbs S, Linke A, Schuler G, et al. Intracoronary administration of circulating blood-derived progenitor cells after recanalization of chronic coronary artery occlusion improves endothelial function. Circ Res 2006; 98(5):e48.
9. Kang HJ, Lee HY, Na SH, et al. Differential effect of intracoronary infusion of mobilized peripheral blood stem cells by granulocyte colony-stimulating factor on left ventricular function and remodeling in patients with acute myocardial infarction versus old myocardial infarction: the MAGIC Cell-3-DES randomized, controlled trial. Circulation 2006; 114(suppl 1):I145–I151.
10. Angelini P, Markwald RR. Stem cell treatment of the heart: a review of its current status on the brink of clinical experimentation. Tex Heart Inst J 2005; 32(4):479–488.
11. Hare JM, Traverse J, Henry T, et al. A randomized, double-blind placebo controlled dose escalation study of intravenous adult human mesencyhal stem cells after acute myocardial infarction. J Am Coll Cardio 2009; 54(24):2287–2289.
12. Perin EC, Dohmann HF, Borojevic R, et al. Transendocardial, autologous bone marrow cell transplantation for severe, chronic ischemic heart failure. Circulation 2003; 107(18):2294–2302.
13. de la Fuente LM, Stertzer SH, Argentieri J, et al. Transendocardial autologous bone marrow in chronic myocardial infarction using a helical needle catheter: 1-year follow-up in an open-label, nonrandomized, single-center pilot study (the TABMMI study). Am Heart J 2007; 154(1):77–79.
14. Perin EC, Silva GV, Assad JA, et al. Comparison of intracoronary and transendocardial delivery of allogeneic mesenchymal cells in a canine model of acute myocardial infarction. J Mol Cell Cardiol 2008; 44(3):486–495.
15. Freyman T, Polin G, Osman H, et al. A quantitative, randomized study evaluating three methods of mesenchymal stem cell delivery following myocardial infarction. Eur Heart J 2006; 27(9):1114–1122.
16. Strauer BE, Brehm M, Zeus T, et al. Repair of infarcted myocardium by autologous intracoronary mononuclear bone marrow cell transplantation in humans. Circulation 2002; 106(15):1913–1918.
17. Schachinger V, Erbs S, Elsasser A, et al. Intracoronary bone marrow-derived progenitor cells in acute myocardial infarction. N Engl J Med 2006; 355(12):1210–1221.
18. Schachinger V, Erbs S, Elsasser A, et al. Improved clinical outcome after intracoronary administration of bone-marrow-derived progenitor cells in acute myocardial infarction: final 1-year results of the REPAIR-AMI trial. Eur Heart J 2006; 27(23):2775–2783.
19. Lunde K, Solheim S, Aakhus S, et al. Intracoronary injection of mononuclear bone marrow cells in acute myocardial infarction. N Engl J Med 2006; 355(12):1199–1209.
20. Janssens S, Dubois C, Bogaert J, et al. Autologous bone marrow-derived stem-cell transfer in patients with ST-segment elevation myocardial infarction: double-blind, randomised controlled trial. Lancet 2006; 367(9505):113–121.
21. Abdel-Latif A, Bolli R, Tleyjeh IM, et al. Adult bone marrow-derived cells for cardiac repair: a systematic review and meta-analysis. Arch Intern Med 2007; 167(10):989–997.

22. Martin-Rendon E, Brunskill SJ, Hyde CJ, et al. Autologous bone marrow stem cells to treat acute myocardial infarction: a systematic review. Eur Heart J 2008; 29(15):1807–1818.
23. Wollert KC, Meyer GP, Lotz J, et al. Intracoronary autologous bone-marrow cell transfer after myocardial infarction: the BOOST randomised controlled clinical trial. Lancet 2004; 364(9429):141–148.
24. Meyer GP, Wollert KC, Lotz J, et al. Intracoronary bone marrow cell transfer after myocardial infarction: eighteen months' follow-up data from the randomized, controlled BOOST (BOne marrOw transfer to enhance ST-elevation infarct regeneration) trial. Circulation 2006; 113(10):1287–1294.
25. Assmus B, Schachinger V, Teupe C, et al. Transplantation of Progenitor Cells and Regeneration Enhancement in Acute Myocardial Infarction (TOPCARE-AMI). Circulation 2002; 106(24):3009–3017.
26. Chen SL, Fang WW, Ye F, et al. Effect on left ventricular function of intracoronary transplantation of autologous bone marrow mesenchymal stem cell in patients with acute myocardial infarction. Am J Cardiol 2004; 94(1):92–95.
27. Amado LC, Saliaris AP, Schuleri KH, et al. Cardiac repair with intramyocardial injection of allogeneic mesenchymal stem cells after myocardial infarction. Proc Natl Acad Sci U S A 2005; 102(32):11474–11479.
28. Menasche P, Hagege AA, Vilquin JT, et al. Autologous skeletal myoblast transplantation for severe postinfarction left ventricular dysfunction. J Am Coll Cardiol 2003; 41(7):1078–1083.
29. Menasche P, Alfieri O, Janssens S, et al. The Myoblast Autologous Grafting in Ischemic Cardiomyopathy (MAGIC) trial: first randomized placebo-controlled study of myoblast transplantation. Circulation 2008; 117(9):1189–1200.
30. Urbanek K, Torella D, Sheikh F, et al. Myocardial regeneration by activation of multipotent cardiac stem cells in ischemic heart failure. Proc Natl Acad Sci U S A 2005; 102(24):8692–8697.
31. Urbanek K, Rota M, Cascapera S, et al. Cardiac stem cells possess growth factor-receptor systems that after activation regenerate the infarcted myocardium, improving ventricular function and long-term survival. Circ Res 2005; 97(7):663–673.
32. Tillmanns J, Rota M, Hosoda T, et al. Formation of large coronary arteries by cardiac progenitor cells. Proc Natl Acad Sci U S A 2008; 105(5):1668–1673.
33. Stamm C, Kleine HD, Choi YH, et al. Intramyocardial delivery of CD133+ bone marrow cells and coronary artery bypass grafting for chronic ischemic heart disease: safety and efficacy studies. J Thorac Cardiovasc Surg 2007; 133(3):717–725.
34. Strauer BE, Brehm M, Zeus T, et al. Regeneration of human infarcted heart muscle by intracoronary autologous bone marrow cell transplantation in chronic coronary artery disease: the IACT Study. J Am Coll Cardiol 2005; 46(9):1651–1658.
35. Assmus B, Honold J, Schachinger V, et al. Transcoronary transplantation of progenitor cells after myocardial infarction. N Engl J Med 2006; 355(12):1222–1232.
36. Quevedo HC, Hatzistergos KE, Oskouei BN, et al. Allogeneic mesenchymal stem cells restore cardiac function in chronic ischemic cardiomyopathy via trilineage differentiating capacity. Proc Natl Acad Sci U S A 2009; 106(33):14022–14027.
37. Reffelmann T, Konemann S, Kloner RA. Promise of blood- and bone marrow-derived stem cell transplantation for functional cardiac repair: putting it in perspective with existing therapy. J Am Coll Cardiol 2009; 53(4):305–308.
38. Schuleri KH, Amado LC, Boyle AJ, et al. Early improvement in cardiac tissue perfusion due to mesenchymal stem cells. Am J Physiol Heart Circ Physiol 2008; 294(5):H2002–H2011.

Primary Angioplasty in Health Care Delivery: The European Model

Jacob Thorsted Sorensen, Christian Juhl Terkelsen, and Steen Dalby Kristensen

Department of Cardiology B, Aarhus University Hospital, Skejby, Denmark

BACKGROUND

In Europe, in the 1990s, primary percutaneous coronary intervention (PPCI) evolved as a viable and feasible reperfusion strategy for STEMI patients. Pioneering efforts on both sides of the Atlantic demonstrated the superiority of primary angioplasty over fibrinolysis (1,2) and efforts in the Netherlands and the Czech Republic helped establish PPCI as an option to a wider population. Trials such as the Maastricht trial (3), the AirPAMI study (4), and the Prague trials (5,6) made it clear that a better outcome could be achieved with PPCI, even though patients had to be transported a considerable distance to tertiary PCI centers. The trials also suggested that transport of these critically ill patients is safe. The European setup, using a "hub and spoke" system, relies heavily on impeccable logistics and an excellent infrastructure.

In 2003, the DANAMI-2 trial (7), comparing fibrinolysis to PPCI, revolutionized the treatment of STEMI patients in Denmark almost overnight. Later on meta-analyses also documented a mortality benefit achieved from PPCI compared to fibrinolysis (8,9). The fact that PPCI proved to be superior made it necessary to develop a system in which patients were diagnosed rapidly and transferred immediately from noninvasive hospitals in rural regions to PPCI centers operating on a 24/7 basis. Furthermore, observational data indicated that the benefit of reducing treatment delay before initiation of PPCI was of the same magnitude as that achieved when reducing treatment delay before fibrinolysis, that is, a 2% reduction in mortality for each hour of reduction in treatment delay (10). Thus, the benefit of reducing treatment delay by one hour is comparable with the benefit of PPCI over fibrinolysis or that obtained by the introduction of aspirin therapy or fibrinolysis in the 1980s. This highlights the importance of reducing treatment delay irrespective of reperfusion strategy.

In an effort to shorten the time from symptom onset to treatment it became imperative to establish the diagnosis of myocardial infarction as soon as possible and furthermore to try and bypass admission at the local hospitals by diagnosing patients before hospital arrival. In Denmark, this lead to the introduction of prehospital ECG recording, transmission, and interpretation, initially in a single region (11), but from 2006 covering the entire country.

Even though PPCI has proven superior to fibrinolysis it is not a universally available reperfusion modality. Furthermore, PPCI is associated with an extra logistic delay, and there must be a point beyond which the benefit of PPCI over

TABLE 1 Danish Core Strategies to Reduce System Delay in All Patients with ST Elevation Myocardial Infarction (STEMI) Treated with Primary Percutaneous Coronary Intervention (PPCI)

1. Establish large-volume emergency medical services
2. Ensure short response time of 5–7 min for the EMS system
3. EMS personnel should be able to record ECGs
4. If EMS personnel is not capable of establishing the diagnosis of STEMI then the ECGs should be transmitted wirelessly to a hospital-based physician
5. Prehospital activation of the catheterization laboratory
6. Prehospital rerouting to a PPCI center bypassing the local hospital
7. Admit patients directly to the catheterization laboratory, bypassing the intensive care unit, the coronary care unit, and the emergency department at the interventional hospital
8. Establish large-volume PPCI centers running 24-7-365 with a sufficient number of procedures and operators to ensure a door-to-balloon time <30 min
9. Enable return transfer to local hospital within 12–24 hr after PCI to ensure continuity in the cardiac rehabilitation program

Source: From Ref. 15.

fibrinolysis is outweighed by this delay. In the following we will address core strategies aimed at increasing the number of patients eligible for PPCI.

PRIMARY PCI FOR ALL PATIENTS—THE DANISH CORE STRATEGIES

The European and American STEMI guidelines recommend PPCI as the preferred reperfusion therapy if performed by an experienced team, in a timely manner (i.e., within 90–120 minutes of first medical contact) (12,13). However, the extra delay acceptable for performing PPCI instead of administering fibrinolysis is debatable, and may explain some of the differences in use of PPCI at each side of the Atlantic. When looking at fibrinolysis, first, it cannot be initiated instantaneously; second, its effects are not immediate; and third, it is only available in the prehospital phase in very few regions/countries. Furthermore, recent data indicate that the benefit achieved from PPCI is comparable to the benefit achieved from fibrinolysis even if 120 minutes extra is spent to perform PPCI (14,15). It could be argued that the guideline recommendations only take a few of the possible, logistic STEMI scenarios into account. Another option would be to balance the choice of reperfusion strategy according to the alternative reperfusion strategies available in the region of interest.

As proponents for a widespread PPCI strategy, we will in the following address various core strategies aimed at reducing treatment delay and increasing the number of patients eligible for PPCI. It is of paramount importance to focus on every step that may influence treatment delay from symptom onset to initiation of reperfusion therapy (Table 1).

PREHOSPITAL PHASE

The prehospital phase of acute coronary syndromes (ACS) comprises the time from symptom onset until admission to the hospital. This phase is important because one-third of AMI patients dies in the prehospital phase without receiving treatment (16), and also because optimal prehospital logistics is the key to the implementation of a successful regional PPCI strategy.

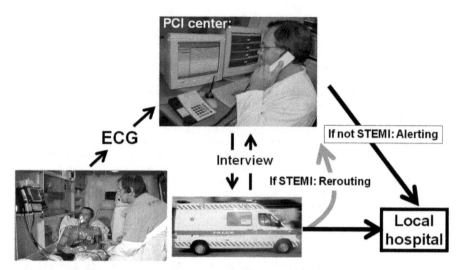

FIGURE 1 The Danish prehospital organization. The ECG is recorded by paramedics and transmitted to a telemedicine center. The ECG is interpreted and the patient interviewed over the phone by an experienced cardiologist. The patient is referred to a local hospital or rerouted directly to an interventional center depending on the findings.

Patients should be encouraged to contact the health care system when experiencing chest pain or discomfort. Immediate telephone contact to the emergency medical services (EMS) is preferable, whereas self-presenting should be avoided. The EMS systems should have short response times of maximum five to seven minutes. After initial clinical assessment and stabilization of the patient, an ECG should be recorded. If the EMS personnel are not trained to diagnose STEMI, the ECG should be transmitted wirelessly to a hospital-based physician for interpretation. Some regions rely on a computer algorithm to diagnose STEMI; with the current advances in this technology, this method could be feasible in some regions.

After having established the diagnosis of STEMI, reperfusion therapy should be initiated as soon as possible. To increase the number of patients eligible for PPCI a strategy of rerouting the patients directly to the interventional hospital is preferable (Fig. 1). Prehospital diagnosis combined with rerouting to interventional centers can reduce treatment delay by more than one hour (Fig. 2) (11).

The catheterization laboratory should be alerted as soon as a diagnosis of STEMI is established.

LOCAL HOSPITAL PHASE

Preferably the local hospitals should be bypassed. Self-presenters at local hospitals should be transferred as soon as possible to an interventional hospital. In this setting, chest pain patients should have an ECG recorded immediately after arrival at the local hospital and if symptoms and ECG findings are consistent with STEMI the EMS should be contacted for immediate transfer of the patient to an interventional hospital.

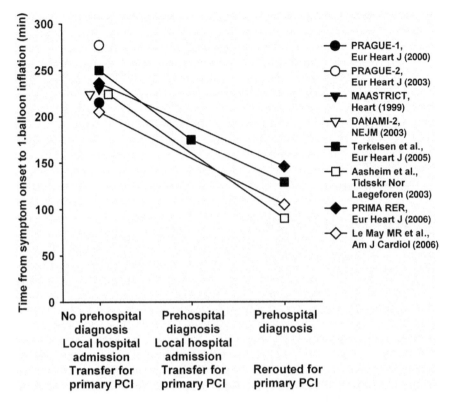

FIGURE 2 Time from symptom onset until first balloon inflation in patients with ST elevation myocardial infarction treated with primary percutaneous coronary intervention. Stratified according to prehospital diagnostic and referral strategy. *Source*: Adapted from Ref. 21.

INTERVENTIONAL CENTER

When approaching the interventional center, the EMS personnel should alert the attending cardiologist of the imminent arrival. This ensures that the patient can be taken directly to the catheterization laboratory bypassing the emergency department (ED), the coronary care unit (CCU), and the intensive care unit (ICU). If the patient has unstable hemodynamics or is in respiratory distress, intensive care physicians should be notified before arrival to monitor and stabilize the patient during the invasive procedures.

To ensure optimal door-to-balloon times of 30 minutes or less, large-volume interventional centers should be established. This will guarantee a sufficient number of physicians to ensure a 24/7 on call system in which the catheterization laboratory can be ready within 15 to 20 minutes. A large number of acute admissions will also enable invasive cardiologists to have enough interventions to ensure a high success and low complication rate (17).

The Danish strategy involves return transfer to the local hospitals 12 to 24 hours after PCI for initiation of optimal, adjuvant medical therapy and rehabilitation.

TABLE 2 Frequency and Distribution of Reperfusion Therapy (%) in Selected Countries in Europe

Country	Type of reperfusion			
	Primary angioplasty (%)	Fibrinolysis (%)	No reperfusion (%)	Total number of reperfusion (%)
Denmark	75	5	20	80
Italy	45	15	40	60
Finland	45	40	15	85
Austria	35	35	30	70
Belgium	59	31	10	90
UK	24	55	21	79

Source: Adapted from Ref. 20.

OTHER EUROPEAN EXPERIENCES

Other countries in Europe have alternative approaches to delivering high-standard STEMI care. In Sweden, despite the low population density in some areas combined with the long distances and rugged terrain, an admirable effort has been made to introduce PPCI to most patients, thanks to a very effective transport network. In this "real-world" scenario, Stenestrand et al. (18) have shown that PPCI is feasible also in rural areas, and that PPCI is superior to even prehospital fibrinolysis also when the extra delay associated with performing PPCI instead of administering prehospital fibrinolysis is more than two hours.

Also in urban areas with heavy traffic, impressive efforts are made to deliver PPCI to the large majority of patients. In Vienna, this process of introducing a city-wide protocol for optimal STEMI care has been documented in the trial by Kalla et al. (19).

Recently, a review of treatment strategies in selected European countries has been published (20). The paper not only illustrates the differences between the countries, but also shows an impressive effort to introduce PPCI in order to provide optimal care in Europe (Table 2).

SUMMARY

Although wide variations in prehospital and in-hospital organization exist, along with varying infrastructural and geographical challenges, the main focus for treating STEMI patients today should be on reducing the time from symptom onset to treatment. Several options are available for achieving this goal, but all imply the need for an optimal prehospital setup combined with initiatives to improve communication and collaboration between the EMS providers and interventional cardiologists.

REFERENCES

1. Zijlstra F, de Boer MJ, Hoorntje JC, et al. A comparison of immediate coronary angioplasty with intravenous streptokinase in acute myocardial infarction. N Engl J Med 1993; 328(10):680–684.
2. Grines CL, Browne KF, Marco J, et al. A comparison of immediate angioplasty with thrombolytic therapy for acute myocardial infarction. The Primary Angioplasty in Myocardial Infarction Study Group. N Engl J Med 1993; 328(10):673–679.

3. Vermeer F, Oude Ophuis AJ, vd Berg EJ, et al. Prospective randomised comparison between thrombolysis, rescue PTCA, and primary PTCA in patients with extensive myocardial infarction admitted to a hospital without PTCA facilities: a safety and feasibility study. Heart 1999; 82(4):426–431.
4. Grines CL, Westerhausen DR Jr, Grines LL, et al. A randomized trial of transfer for primary angioplasty versus on-site thrombolysis in patients with high-risk myocardial infarction: the Air Primary Angioplasty in Myocardial Infarction study. J Am Coll Cardiol 2002; 39(11):1713–1719.
5. Widimsky P, Groch L, Zelizko M, et al. Multicentre randomized trial comparing transport to primary angioplasty vs immediate thrombolysis vs. combined strategy for patients with acute myocardial infarction presenting to a community hospital without a catheterization laboratory. The PRAGUE study. Eur Heart J 2000; 21(10):823–831.
6. Widimsky P, Budesinsky T, Vorac D, et al. Long distance transport for primary angioplasty vs. immediate thrombolysis in acute myocardial infarction. Final results of the randomized national multicentre trial—PRAGUE-2. Eur Heart J 2003; 24(1):94–104.
7. Andersen HR, Nielsen TT, Rasmussen K, et al. A comparison of coronary angioplasty with fibrinolytic therapy in acute myocardial infarction. N Engl J Med 2003; 349(8):733–742.
8. Boersma E. Does time matter? A pooled analysis of randomized clinical trials comparing primary percutaneous coronary intervention and in-hospital fibrinolysis in acute myocardial infarction patients. Eur Heart J 2006; 27(7):779–788.
9. Keeley EC, Boura JA, Grines CL. Primary angioplasty versus intravenous thrombolytic therapy for acute myocardial infarction: a quantitative review of 23 randomised trials. Lancet 2003; 361(9351):13–20.
10. De Luca G, Suryapranata H, Ottervanger JP, et al. Time delay to treatment and mortality in primary angioplasty for acute myocardial infarction: every minute of delay counts. Circulation 2004; 109(10):1223–1225.
11. Terkelsen CJ, Lassen JF, Norgaard BL, et al. Reduction of treatment delay in patients with ST-elevation myocardial infarction: impact of pre-hospital diagnosis and direct referral to primary percutanous coronary intervention. Eur Heart J 2005; 26(8):770–777.
12. Antman EM, Hand M, Armstrong PW, et al. 2007 focused update of the ACC/AHA 2004 guidelines for the management of patients with ST-elevation myocardial infarction: a report of the American College of Cardiology/American Heart Association Task Force on Practice Guidelines. J Am Coll Cardiol 2008; 51(2):210–247.
13. Van de WF, Bax J, Betriu A, et al. Management of acute myocardial infarction in patients presenting with persistent ST-segment elevation: the Task Force on the Management of ST-Segment Elevation Acute Myocardial Infarction of the European Society of Cardiology. Eur Heart J 2008; 29(23):2909–2945.
14. Terkelsen CJ, Sorensen JT, Nielsen TT. Is there any time left for primary percutaneous coronary intervention according to the 2007 updated American College of Cardiology/American Heart Association ST-segment elevation myocardial infarction guidelines and the D2B alliance? J Am Coll Cardiol 2008; 52(15):1211–1215.
15. Terkelsen CJ, Christiansen EH, Sorensen JT, et al. Primary PCI as the preferred reperfusion therapy in STEMI: it is a matter of time. Heart 2009; 95(5):362–369.
16. Lowel H, Lewis M, Hormann A. Prognostic significance of prehospital phase in acute myocardial infarct. Results of the Augsburg Myocardial Infarct Registry, 1985–1988. Dtsch Med Wochenschr 1991; 116(19):729–733.
17. Canto JG, Every NR, Magid DJ, et al. The volume of primary angioplasty procedures and survival after acute myocardial infarction. N Engl J Med 2000; 342(21):1573–1580.
18. Stenestrand U, Lindback J, Wallentin L. Long-term outcome of primary percutaneous coronary intervention vs. prehospital and in-hospital thrombolysis for patients with ST-elevation myocardial infarction. JAMA 2006; 296(14):1749–1756.
19. Kalla K, Christ G, Karnik R, et al. Implementation of guidelines improves the standard of care: the Viennese registry on reperfusion strategies in ST-elevation myocardial infarction (Vienna STEMI registry). Circulation 2006; 113(20):2398–2405.

20. Knot J, Widimsky P, Wijns W, et al. How to set up an effective national primary angio-plasty network: lessons learned from five European countries. EuroIntervention 2009; 5(3):299–309.
21. Andersen HR, Sørensen JT, Terkelsen CJ. Fast-track Primary Percutaneous Coronary Intervention in Patients with ST-elevation Myocardial Infarction. Interv Cardiol 2006; Sept.; 10–11.

16b Primary Angioplasty in Health Care Delivery: The North American Model

Faisal Latif, Kintur Sanghvi, and Cindy L. Grines

Cardiovascular Section, William Beaumont Hospital, Royal Oak, Michigan, U.S.A.

Coronary artery disease is the number one cause of death in North America. Over 1.1 million Americans suffer an acute MI (AMI) every year including 650,000 new cases and 450,000 recurrences (1). Approximately 460,000 of these are fatal (1). About half of those deaths occur within the first hour of onset of symptoms and before the patient reaches the hospital. If the patient receives medical attention, numerous therapies have proven to be beneficial. Primary percutaneous coronary intervention (PPCI) is associated with higher rates of reperfusion and lower rates of death, stroke, and reinfarction, when compared to fibrinolytics (2). Although PPCI is the dominant reperfusion strategy in patients with AMI, fewer than 40% of them achieve a door-to-balloon time of 90 minutes. Furthermore, in the United States, approximately one-third of patients with STEMI do not receive any reperfusion therapy despite availability and absence of any contraindication (3).

Currently, US health care system faces many serious challenges, including 16% uninsured population and a skyrocketing health care expenditure ($2.2 trillion in 2007). We shall briefly discuss the issues related to existing systems and discuss various initiatives by governing agencies to resolve those problems.

EMERGENCY MEDICAL SERVICES (EMS)

The United States boasts a well equipped and trained EMS available to >90% of the population (4). American Heart Association (AHA) and National Heart, Lung, and Blood Institute (NHLBI) have carried out public awareness campaigns aimed at reducing time delay between symptom onset and hospital presentation as well as timely activation of EMS. The EMS system is operated by governmental as well as private or volunteer providers, and thus the standards and protocols can differ, as opposed to the centralized emergency systems in place in European countries (5).

A minority (10%) of EMS systems have electronic ECG transmission capabilities, a system that holds enough promise to significantly decrease reperfusion times, should be implemented universally. A mandate exists to deliver the patient to the nearest facility even when fibrinolysis may be contraindicated and the facility does not provide primary PCI. If a patient is brought to a non–PCI capable facility and primary PCI is deemed necessary, it is not unusual for the unacceptable delay in patient transportation. Furthermore, critically ill patients often require stabilization before transport. Some regional EMS systems have successfully established the protocol of en route 12 lead-EKG, prehospital thrombolytics or activation of primary PCI team.

PRIMARY PERCUTANEOUS CORONARY INTERVENTION CENTERS

The traditional program established for EMS is to transport the patient with AMI to the nearest hospital. Many hospitals in close proximity have designated chest pain centers and therefore possess PPCI capabilities. This has required "the physician to go to the patient" instead of the "patient coming to the physician." Currently, in many areas, the interventional cardiologist covers three or four PPCI hospitals located within a 5- to 10-mile radius. This leads to a reduction in volume of PPCI for any given hospital, which can ultimately affect quality of care. The outcomes of low-volume hospitals are not as robust as those of high-volume centers. In the National Registry of AMI, U.S. centers that performed >48 PPCI yearly had the greatest benefit of PPCI over fibrinolytic therapy, when compared to centers performing lesser number of PPCI (6). Reportedly, there are many hospitals with PPCI facilities that are staffed by interventional cardiologists who do not meet the minimum requirements of 75 PCIs per year, or the hospital does not perform at least 200 coronary interventions per year of which at least 36 are PPCI for ST elevation myocardial infarction, as mandated by the ACC/AHA guidelines for management of ST elevation myocardial infarction (4). This is in contrast to ESC guidelines that do not provide for a minimum number of procedures as a prerequisite for performing PPCI (7). The ACC/AHA guidelines have also indicated that not all the catheterization laboratories equipped for PPCI can provide high quality care to patients with AMI. This could be related to lack of 24-hour staffing or the volume of cases may be insufficient for the team to acquire and maintain skills required for rapid PPCI reperfusion strategies. This calls for development of centers of excellence, rather than many low-volume centers. However, one must take into consideration the transport constraints involved in meeting the 90-minute door-to-balloon time. Some observers have recommended that the current default program of transporting patients with suspect myocardial infarction to the nearest hospital should be obsolete (8). In an editorial comment on this observation, it was mentioned that "PPCI should not be performed in low-volume hospitals unless there are substantial overriding concerns about geographic or socio-economic status" (9). Therefore, there possibly exists a need for development of the state-of-the-art tertiary care regional centers, instead of multiple small centers within a small radius. Interestingly, door-to-balloon times are inversely related to hospital volume for PPCI procedures (8,10).

GEOGRAPHIC CONSIDERATIONS

The United States and Canada have vast areas of uninhabited or scantly inhabited land, which makes it challenging to provide PPCI services to the whole population. In 2003, the Society of Chest Pain Centers launched the first accreditation program for hospitals in the United States (11). There are more than 1500 hospitals in the United States that have either a certified or self-designated chest pain center. An analysis of NCDR data from 2005 to 2006 revealed that in the United States, for >50% of patients transferred for PPCI (i.e., PPCI not available at the hospital where the patient initially presented), the door-to-balloon time was between 2 to 4 hours and in about 20% of the transferred patients it was >4 hours (12). This is despite the fact that almost 80% of adult U.S. population lived within 60 minutes of driving time of a PPCI hospital in the year 2000 (13). The proportion of patients eligible for primary PCI has likely increased now with more and more hospitals providing angioplasty. The median driving time varies from 8 minutes on the west coast to 36 minutes in the rural population in the Midwest (13), and >40% population lived in areas where a PPCI facility was the closest hospital. Moreover, an increasing number of hospitals are performing PPCI without surgical backup, a class IIb indication, per ACC/AHA guidelines (4,14).

Transportation time occupies a key importance in the care of AMI in North America. In the trial Air PAMI, average transportation time was 43 minutes as opposed to 10 minutes in the Danish trial (DANAMI-2) and 30 minutes in the Czech trial (PRAGUE-2) (8). In the United States, majority of the "transfer time" is spent waiting for the ambulance to pick up the patient from the initial hospital. In other countries, the patient is never taken off the stretcher and the EMS staff and vehicle do not leave the patient, which results in major reduction in time delays. There is now a nationwide initiative to perform prehospital ECGs and for the EMS to activate the cardiac catheterization laboratory. Prehospital ECGs allow early diagnosis and bypassing hospitals that do not provide PPCI. As arbitrary as a 90-minute door-to-balloon time is, it may be that a longer window for reperfusion may still lead to better outcomes compared to fibrinolytics (15).

FINANCIAL BURDEN

The United States spends a larger share of its GDP on health care than does any other major industrialized nation (16). The total direct and indirect cost of cardiovascular diseases in the United States is estimated at $448.5 billion in 2008, of which $140 billion is hospital expenditure (17). A variety of payers foot the bill. Approximately 14% of U.S. population (40 million) were covered by Medicare, 12% (36 million) by Medicaid, 69% (200 million) insured by private insurance, and 16% (45 million) were uninsured in 2003 (18). However, in contrast to many other developed countries, as a law in the United States, any person presenting to the emergency room with an AMI, or for that matter, any emergency, is rendered full standard care regardless of insurance, race, religion or ethnicity. The hospital is partially reimbursed for taking care of uninsured patient from the Centers for Medicare and Medicaid Services (CMS) or the state budget for emergency Medicaid. Physician performing the procedure may or may not be reimbursed; however, he or she cannot refuse to care for the patient and is legally liable in the event of failure to provide appropriate standard care.

A common misperception exists that PPCI costs more than fibrinolytics. However, the Canadian STAT study and others demonstrated a lower cost of hospitalization for PPCI compared to thrombolytics for patients with AMI (19).

An important difference between North American and European financial model is the substitution of hospital charges for actual costs incurred by the health service. Breakdown of the hospital charges indicate that professional fees form a significant component, which is not a feature of most national health care systems in Europe (20). However, in the United States, reimbursement to the interventional cardiologists is the same for primary PCI as it is for elective percutaneous coronary intervention, and for a single vessel procedure in our region averages $800 to $900.

Clopidogrel discontinuation after PPCI, often due to lack of insurance, remains a critical issue. The practice of the use of bare metal stents for PPCI may help curtail stent thrombosis in these patients. This is in contrast to some

European centers, which use DES in the majority of PPCI, but clopidogrel discontinuation related to insurance issues is less prevalent due to the presence of a public health system.

90-MINUTE DOOR-TO-BALLOON TIME

The ACC/AHA guidelines established a 90-minute door-to-balloon time as a goal for ST elevation myocardial infarction. The U.S. model for PPCI continues to evolve as more modern devices come into practice. The "door-to-balloon time" is now considered "door-to-device time" and if instead of balloon, a thrombectomy device or a stent is initially used, it is considered as the reperfusion time (21). Although the data are scant, an increasing number of hospitals are adapting a prehospital digital transmission of ECG to activate the PPCI team before the patient reaches the hospital to minimize reperfusion time. Some hospitals have adapted an on-site interventional cardiologist and catheterization laboratory staff that remain in the hospital 24/7 to meet the 90-minute door-to-balloon time.

Additionally, continuing education of paramedical personnel and emergency room physicians for recognition of ECG criteria for ST elevation MI and contraindications to fibrinolytic therapy are the cornerstones of performance measures being scrutinized (12).

QUALITY OF CARE

Multiple initiatives have been taken by government agencies and organizations to improve the door-to-balloon time and overall care of STEMI patients (Fig. 1).

American College of Cardiology (ACC) has embarked on a national initiative to achieve a door-to-balloon time of $</= 90$ minutes for at least 75% of non-transfer primary PCI across the nation (www.d2balliance.org). D2B: An Alliance for Quality™ advocates the adoption of six key, evidenced-based strategies for reducing door-to-balloon times, which include the following:

1. Emergency Department physician activates the cath lab;
2. One call activates the cath lab;
3. Cath lab team ready in 20 to 30 minutes;
4. Prompt data feedback;
5. Senior management commitment;
6. Team-based approach.

Use of real-time performance feedback on door-to-balloon times to drive the quality improvement effort is one of the core measures. Each participating hospital reports their current system or mechanism to monitor their door-to-balloon times. Some of these systems might include the NCDR-ACTION Registry™, AHA's Get With the Guidelines or various proprietary software packages. A prehospital ECG to activate the cath lab and having a cardiologist in the hospital 24/7 are some of the other initiatives adopted by hospitals locally.

CMS has formulated a "pay-for performance" program intended to align financial incentives with desired improvements in patient care. As a result of this, door-to-balloon time of less than 90 minutes is being achieved more than 70% of the time in hospitals reporting their outcome data. Other measures of quality include primary and secondary prevention care measures based on evidence. For example, in the hospitals reporting data, patients with AMI received

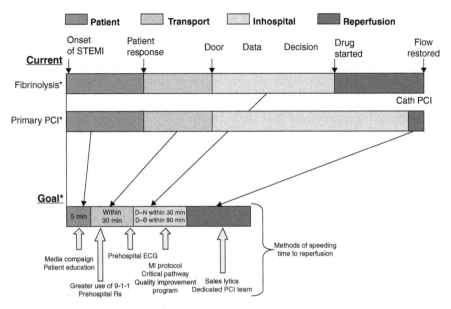

FIGURE 1 Major components of time delay between onset of symptoms in ST elevation MI and restoration of flow in the infarct-related artery. Time to initiate fibrinolytic therapy is the "door-to-needle" time and the time to achieve flow in the infarct-related artery is the D–B (door-to-balloon) time. *These bar graphs are meant to be semi-quantitative and not to scale. *Abbreviations*: Cath, catheterization; PCI, percutaneous coronary intervention; min, minutes. *Source*: From Ref. 4.

Aspirin (ASA) on arrival 94% of the time, ASA at discharge 91%, and door-to-thrombolysis time of <30 minutes was achieved in 41% of the patients. Public reporting of data allows hospitals to compare themselves and strive to become a top performer (www.hospitalcompare.hhs.gov).

CONCLUSION
Despite challenges and flaws, the overall state of care for patients with AMI in the United States continues to improve. Implementation of quality measures is producing results and is a model for different health care systems, which face similar challenges.

REFERENCES
1. www.nhlbi.nih.gov/health/dci/Diseases/HeartAttack/HeartAttack_WhatIs.html. Accessed March 16, 2009.
2. Keeley, EC, Boura JA, Grines CL. Primary angioplasty versus intravenous thrombolytic therapy for acute myocardial infarction: a quantitative review of 23 randomized trials. Lancet 2003; 361:13–20.
3. Fox KA. An international perspective on acute coronary syndromes care: insights from the Global registry of Acute Coronary Events. Am Heart J 2004; 148:S40–S45.
4. Antman EM, Anbe DT, Armstrong PW, et al. ACC/AHA guidelines for the management of patients with ST-elevation myocardial infarction. J Am Coll Cardiol 2004; 44:671–719.
5. McGinn AP, Rosamond WD, Goff DC Jr, et al. Trends in prehospital delay time and use of emergency medical services for acute myocardial infarction: experience in 4 US communities from 1987–2000. Am Heart J 2005; 150:392–400.

6. Magid DJ, Calonge BN, Rumsfeld JS, et al. Relation between hospital primary angioplasty volume and mortality of patients with acute MI treated with primary angioplasty vs thrombolytic therapy. JAMA 2000; 284(24):3131–3138.
7. De Werf FV, Ardissino D, Betriu A, et al. Management of acute myocardial infarction in patients presenting with ST-segment elevation. Eur Heart J 2003; 24:28–66.
8. Topol EJ, Kereiakes DJ. Regionalization of care for acute ischemic heart disease. Circulation 2003; 107:1463–1466.
9. Jollis JG, Romano PS. Volume-outcome relationship in acute myocardial infarction: the balloon and the needle. JAMA 2000; 284:3169–3170.
10. Cannon CP, Gibson CM, Lambrew CT, et al. Relationship of symptom onset to balloon time and door-to-balloon time with mortality in patients undergoing primary angioplasty for acute myocardial infarction. JAMA 2000; 283:2941–2947.
11. http://www.scpcp.org/dnn/AboutUs/tabid/83/Default.aspx. Accessed February 21, 2010.
12. Chakrabarti A, Krumholz HM, Wang Y, et al. Time-to-perfusion in patients undergoing interhospital transfer for primary percutaneous intervention in the U.S.: an analysis of 2005 and 2006 data from the National Cardiovascular Data Registry. J Am Coll Cardiol 2008; 51:2442–2443.
13. Nallamothu BK, Bates ER, Krumholz HK, et al. Driving times and distances to hospitals with percutaneous coronary intervention in the United States. Circulation 2006; 113:1189–1195.
14. Wharton TP, Grines LL, Grines CL, et al. Primary angioplasty in acute myocardial infarction at hospitals with no surgery on-site (the PAMI-No SOS Study) versus transfer to surgical centers for primary angioplasty. J Am Col Cardiol 2004; 43:1943–1950.
15. Stenestrand U, Lindback J, Wallentin L. Long-term outcome of primary percutaneous coronary intervention vs prehospital and inhospital thrombolysis for patients with ST-elevation myocardial infarction. JAMA 2006; 296(14):1749–1756.
16. www.cdc.gov/nchs/data/hus/hus07.pdf#executivesummary. Accessed March 20, 2009.
17. Rosamond W, Flegal K, Furie K, et al. Heart disease and stroke statistics—2008 update: a report from the American Heart Association Statistics Committee and Stroke Statistics Committee. Circulation 2008; 117;e25–e146.
18. DeNavas-Walt C, Proctor BD, Mills RJ. Income, poverty, and health insurance coverage in the United States: 2003. Current population reports P60–226. Washington, DC:U.S. Census Bureau; August 2004. http://www.census.gov/prod/2004pubs/p60-226.pdf. Accessed February 21, 2010.
19. Le May MR, Davies RF, Labinaz M, et al. Hospitalization costs of primary stenting versus thrombolysis in acute myocardial infarction. Circulation 2003; 108:2624–2630.
20. Melikian N, Morgan K, Beatt KJ. Can the published cost analysis data for delivery of an efficient primary angioplasty service be applied to the modern National Health Service? Heart 2005; 91(10):1262–1264.
21. Masoudi FA, Bonow RO, Brindis RG, et al. ACC/AHA 2008 statement on performance measurement and reperfusion therapy: A report of the ACC/AHA task force on performance measures (Work Group to address the challenges of performance measurement and reperfusion therapy). Circulation 2008; 118:2649–2661.

Primary Angioplasty in Health Care Delivery: The Economics

Allan J. Wailoo

Health Economics and Decision Science, School of Health and Related Research, University of Sheffield, Sheffield, U.K.

INTRODUCTION

It is now generally recognized and accepted that decision makers in health care systems the world over include as part of their considerations the economic aspects of alternative approaches to managing patients. Even in the United States, where there is strong and vocal resistance to such moves, there is already a widespread use of economic evaluation in the private health care sector and increasing pressure for publicly funded elements to make use of such analyses (1). Internationally, institutions like the National Institute for Health and Clinical Excellence (NICE) in the U.K. National Health Service (NHS) have helped to drive the adoption and development of methods for economic evaluation.

Commonly cited pressures driving these decisions are aging populations, technological advances, and the costs of those technologies (particularly in pharmaceuticals); other calls on government budgets and a general need for more rational and transparent decision making.

The rationale is straightforward: All health care systems are resource constrained relative to all the potentially beneficial treatments that could be provided. Such scarcity means that decisions entail opportunity costs: If resources are used in one way, providing a particular treatment such as primary angioplasty, those same resources cannot then be used to generate benefits for other patients. Thus, the concept of cost in economic evaluation is very different from a simple financial one. Although the terminology refers to "cost-effectiveness" and "cost benefit" analyses, at the very heart of economic evaluation is the need to compare health benefits between those patients who gain (the benefits or effects) and those who lose (the costs). Economic evaluation provides a systematic framework in which these competing benefits can be considered.

Economic evaluation is not motivated by a desire to cut costs but to ensure that high-cost treatments generate correspondingly high benefits, that at least offset the health benefits displaced elsewhere in the health care system. In order to ensure that population health is maximized, it is important to accurately identify and value the costs and benefits associated with treatments such as primary angioplasty and relevant comparators. In the following sections, I outline some of the key issues in assessing cost-effectiveness of primary angioplasty, previous studies, and ongoing challenges.

ECONOMIC EVALUATION AND PRIMARY ANGIOPLASTY

It is generally accepted that primary angioplasty is a more effective reperfusion strategy than pharmacological treatment using thrombolytics at least in certain circumstances. In those same circumstances it has been suggested that primary angioplasty is no more expensive than thrombolysis overall (2,3).

However, the assessment of cost-effectiveness of primary angioplasty compared to thrombolysis in real practice may not be so straightforward.

Measuring Costs

Primary angioplasty requires access to specialist staffing and technologically advanced facilities and equipment. It is therefore likely that the initial cost of primary angioplasty is greater than that of thrombolysis, particularly where high-cost drug-eluting stents are used.

Cardiac catheterization laboratories, while high-cost facilities to set up and run, are not used exclusively for primary angioplasty patients. The proportion of costs attributable to primary angioplasty is dependant, in part, on the degree to which the labs are used for other treatments. Lieu et al. (4) reported relative cost-ineffectiveness for primary angioplasty where catheterization laboratories operate at low volumes, raising the issue of how primary angioplasty may need to be delivered via regional centers to be cost-effective.

These costs will also vary according to whether the system provides primary angioplasty 24 hours a day or only during standard working hours, and how any out-of-hours cover is staffed.

Studies consistently show that the initial higher treatment costs of primary angioplasty are offset to some extent by reduced length of hospital stay, although the magnitude of this difference varies by study and is sometimes reported as median differences rather than means, which should be the focus for economic evaluation (2,3,5,6).

A more general issue to consider is how primary angioplasty may be delivered in clinical practice rather than in the context of clinical trials. Some studies have analyzed cost data from clinical trials (2,3) and found no significant differences within the trial period or subsequent follow-up.

However, many differences in costs between thrombolysis and primary angioplasty occur in the medium to long term, well beyond the scope of clinical trials. The proportion of patients undergoing subsequent coronary interventions is a significant driver of cost-effectiveness (5), and it is possible that thrombolysis followed by mandated subsequent angiography is a further strategy worthy of future consideration. In the long term, differences in the rates of reinfarction and stroke lead to potential cost differences between treatments over a patient's entire lifetime.

Measuring Outcomes

The health benefits of primary angioplasty are established from clinical trials in terms of mortality, nonfatal reinfarction, and nonfatal stroke as a function of the additional treatment time delay (7).

While it is important that decision making is based on the entirety of this evidence and associated uncertainty, it is also clear that the evaluation framework should reflect all benefits. Economic evaluations that focus on life years gained will underestimate important elements of patients' health benefit and make comparisons across diverse treatments and patient groups more difficult. Primary angioplasty must compete for limited resources with interventions affecting patients across health services.

For these reasons, the outcome measure of choice in economic evaluation is the Quality Adjusted Life Year (QALY), which combines concerns for mortality and morbidity into a single measure. With each year in full health given a weight of one, death assigned a value of zero, and a year in any intermediate health state assessed relative to these two anchor points, the concept of the QALY allows the health benefits from both improved mortality and morbidity to be reflected in the economic evaluation.

As with costs, QALYs will continue to differ between primary angioplasty and thrombolysis long beyond the duration of any clinical trial. It is obvious that a saved life generates QALYs into the future but the same is also true for reinfarction and stroke. These benefits can be reflected in any economic evaluation by extrapolating beyond the duration of a clinical trial. Several modeling studies have been conducted (5,4,8), with each concluding that primary angioplasty is cost-effective in most circumstances.

The time-dependent nature of the benefits from primary angioplasty is well recognized (7,9). Estimates of cost-effectiveness should be based on realistic times achievable in practice, which may differ from those observed in clinical trials, and adjust the trial-based estimates of effectiveness accordingly.

Delivery of Services

Since economic evaluation is comparative, it is essential that the nature of both the intervention and the comparator is clear and appropriate. Most studies to date have focused on primary angioplasty as a treatment compared to thrombolysis (4,8,10) since this is the focus of key clinical trials in the area (7) and thrombolysis is typically used in practice.

Wailoo et al. (5) provide an assessment of angioplasty-based services in the U.K. NHS, in which most patients receive primary angioplasty (67%) but some continue to receive thrombolysis (16%) or no reperfusion (17%) versus thrombolysis-based services, which make opportunistic use of primary angioplasty (4%) and lead to a greater percentage of patients receiving no reperfusion (23%).

The provision of primary angioplasty varies in many other ways that will influence cost-effectiveness.

It has been described above how there is likely to be a need for regional, primary angioplasty centers to achieve a degree of utilization of cardiac catheterization laboratories that reduces costs and maintains operator experience (11) but this must be balanced with the need to minimize treatment delay times. For example, Wailoo et al. suggest that transferring patients from one hospital to another primary angioplasty center may not be cost-effective. Identifying the optimal balance in terms of cost-effectiveness requires consideration of local circumstances, ambulance services, and geography. Whether the use of air ambulances to provide access to primary angioplasty for more rural populations can achieve such a balance requires investigation, alongside the role of prehospital thrombolysis (12).

CONCLUSIONS

Economic evaluation provides a framework for the systematic consideration of the costs and benefits of primary angioplasty. Studies to date have been conducted in several settings and are consistent in supporting primary angioplasty as a cost-effective intervention. However, the nature of delivering such an intervention in practice, in particular the time-dependent nature of both costs and benefits, means that these findings cannot be generalized uncritically.

Ultimately, the requirement for primary angioplasty to demonstrate cost-effectiveness may need to be made at a local level where alternative geographies, costs, and service delivery models for both angioplasty and thrombolysis can form part of the assessment.

REFERENCES

1. Neumann PJ, Rosen AB, Weinstein M. Medicare and cost-effectiveness analysis. New Engl J Med 2005; 353:1516–1521.
2. Stone GW, Grines CL, Rothbaum D, et al. Analysis of the relative costs and effectiveness of primary angioplasty versus tissue-type plasminogen activator: the Primary Angioplasty in Myocardial Infarction (PAMI) trial. The PAMI Trial Investigators. J Am Coll Cardiol 1997; 29:901–907.
3. de Boer MJ, van Hout BA, Liem AL, et al. A cost-effective analysis of primary coronary angioplasty versus thrombolysis for acute myocardial infarction. Am J Cardiol 1995; 76:830–833.
4. Lieu TA, Gurley RJ, Lundstrom RJ, et al. Projected cost-effectiveness of primary angioplasty for acute myocardial infarction. J Am Coll Cardiol 1997; 30:1741–1750.
5. Wailoo AJ, Hernandez M, Goodacre S, et al. Primary angioplasty versus thrombolysis for acute ST-elevation myocardial infarction in the UK NHS: an economic analysis of the National Infarct Angioplasty Project Pilots. Heart 2009. doi:10.1136/hrt.2009.167130. Accessed June 8, 2009.
6. Morgan KP, Leahy M, Sheehy C, et al. UK primary angioplasty cost effectiveness study (UK-paces) 30 day outcome data. Heart 2005; 91(suppl I):A27.
7. Asseburg C, Bravo Vergel Y, et al. Assessing the effectiveness of primary angioplasty compared with thrombolysis and its relationship to time delay: a Bayesian evidence synthesis. Heart 2007; 93:1244–1250.
8. Bravo Vergel Y, Palmer S, Asseburg C, et al. Is primary angioplasty cost effective in the UK? Results of a comprehensive decision analysis. Heart 2007; 93:1238–1243.
9. Rathore SS, Curtis JP, Chen J, et al. Association of door-to-balloon time and mortality in patients admitted to hospital with ST elevation myocardial infarction: national cohort study. BMJ 2009; 338:b1807.
10. Hartwell D, Colquitt J, Loveman, et al. Clinical effectiveness and cost-effectiveness of immediate angioplasty for acute myocardial infarction: systematic review and economic evaluation. Health Technol Assess 2005; 9:17.
11. BA Vakili, Kaplan R, Brown DL. Volume-outcome relation for physicians and hospitals performing angioplasty for acute myocardial infarction in New York state. Circulation 2001; 104:2155–2157.
12. Machecourt J, Bonnefoy E, Vanzetto G, et al. The Comparison of Angioplasty and Pre-Hospital Thrombolysis in Acute Myocardial Infarction (CAPTIM) Cost-Efficacy Sub-Study. J Am Coll Cardiol 2005; 45:4.

17 Special Management of Diabetic Patients with STEMI

Salvatore Brugaletta and Manel Sabaté

Interventional Cardiology Unit, University Hospital of Sant Pau, Barcelona, Spain

Diabetes mellitus (DM) currently affects more than 150 million people worldwide. It is usually associated with a number of metabolic and cardiovascular risk factors that contribute to a high rate of vascular events. Specifically, 80% of patients with DM will develop and possibly die from macrovascular disease and the risk of cardiovascular disease is two- to fourfold higher in DM patients than in non-DM patients. Indeed, a patient with DM has a high risk of experiencing a first myocardial infarction (MI) as someone without DM who has already had a MI. Up to 20% of all patients with an infarction have diabetes, and this figure is expected to increase. Moreover, up to 23% of DM patients with coronary heart disease were found to have silent ischemia and experienced poor outcomes following acute events (1,2). Diabetic patients who sustain a STEMI still have double mortality compared with nondiabetic patients. Diabetes was associated with impaired postprocedural TIMI 3 flow, myocardial blush grade, complete ST segment resolution, and more distal embolization (3).

PHARMACOLOGICAL THERAPY

DM patients have an increased atherothrombotic risk, to which contribute not only hyperglycemia and insulin resistance, but more importantly proinflammatory and prothrombotic status (4,5). In particular, the prothrombotic status is related to endothelial dysfunction, impaired fibrinolysis, increased coagulation factors, and increased platelet reactivity (Fig. 1). Since platelets play a role in the development of atherothrombotic events, the dysfunctional status of platelets in DM patients may contribute to the enhanced atherothrombotic risk of these patients. And this highlights the pivotal role of antiplatelet agents not only in a chronic therapy but also more importantly in the acute setting, such as the acute coronary syndromes.

Aspirin (ASA)

It is the first antiplatelet agent of choice for secondary prevention of ischemic events in patients with atherothrombotic disease, including in patients with DM. The American Diabetes Association (ADA) recommends the use of aspirin as a secondary prevention measure in diabetic patients with atherosclerotic disease (6). This recommendation is supported by data from two large meta-analyses of major secondary prevention trials by the Antithrombotic Trialists' Collaboration (7,8).

In a large population ($n = 22,701$) of healthy men that included 533 diabetic patients, the U.S. Physicians' Health Study found that among DM subjects on

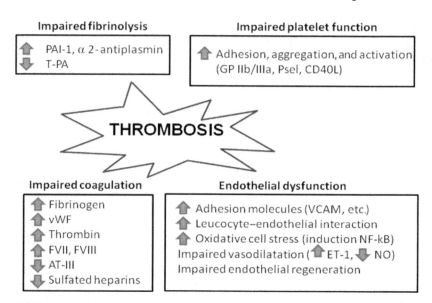

FIGURE 1 Mechanisms leading to the prothrombotic state in individuals with diabetes mellitus. *Source*: Adapted from Ref. 12.

ASA therapy there was a significantly lower incidence of MI rate than those on placebo therapy (9). These results are also supported by the Early Treatment Diabetic Retinopathy Study (ETDRS), which enrolled type 1 and type 2 diabetic men and women, about 48% of whom with a history of cardiovascular disease. This study, a primary and secondary prevention trial, showed that the relative risk for MI in the first five years in those patients randomized to ASA therapy was significantly lower than those randomized to placebo (10). Finally, in the Hypertension Optimal Treatment (HOT) study, addressing antihypertensive treatment in 18,790 individuals, 1501 of whom had DM, showed that ASA therapy resulted in an additional 15% reduction in the risk of cardiovascular events over that seen with antihypertensive therapy (11).

Interestingly, DM patients have been considered clinically unresponsive to the cardioprotective effects of ASA (12). The Heart Outcomes Prevention Evaluation trial, for example, demonstrated a 50% higher cardiovascular events rate in those with compared to those without diabetes despite aspirin therapy (13). And in the Primary Prevention Project, aspirin use was not associated with cardiovascular protection in those with, but a 40% decrease in cardiovascular death in those without diabetes (14). In a cohort study of 2499 patients with acute coronary syndromes, patients with diabetes experience less effective mortality reduction from aspirin use (15).

Despite all these controversial data, it is unclear how to optimize ASA therapy in diabetic patients. There is no good evidence to date that increasing ASA dose would be useful, especially without increasing the risk of bleeding (16). Probably the best option is to associate ASA with other antiplatelet agents with different mechanism of action.

Thienopyridines

The retrospective analysis of the CAPRIE study in the diabetic subgroup showed a superiority of clopidogrel compared to aspirin, attributable to its more potent antiplatelet effect with more efficient inhibition of hyper-reactive diabetic platelet: only 15.6% of diabetic patients on clopidogrel therapy developed the composite vascular primary endpoint versus 17.7% of those on ASA alone therapy (17,18).

Also in the CURE trial, the rate of primary outcome (composite vascular death, MI or stroke) was much higher in the diabetic cohort of patients. The use of clopidogrel in this subgroup reduced the rate of this endpoint, but had borderline statistical significance (14.2% rate of primary endpoint in diabetic cohort on clopidogrel vs. 16.7% in diabetic cohort on placebo) (19). The high event rates may be in part attributed to the persistence of increased platelet reactivity in DM patients even when on dual antiplatelet therapy compared to non-DM.

As for ASA, the phenomenon of the hyporesponsiveness to clopidogrel has emerged in diabetic patients (20), which is potentially related to the need of insulin therapy (21). The huge individual variability demonstrated in response to clopidogrel has provoked a controversy, regarding the optimal clopidogrel loading and maintenance dose regimens. Some studies have demonstrated that a 600 mg load dose of clopidogrel produces superior inhibition as compared to 300 mg (22,23). Use of high loading doses, in fact, may provide higher concentration of substrate for the metabolic activation of the drug by CYP3A4 isoenzyme, increasing the amount of the active metabolite and the inhibition of platelets activation, an effect very important in the acute scenario. Recently, it has also been shown that in high risk type 2 DM patient a 150 mg daily maintenance dose of clopidogrel is associated with enhanced antiplatelet effects compared with 75 mg (24). Moreover, another study enrolling 749 DM patients, of which 81 admitted at the hospital with ST-segment acute MI, showed that a longer duration of clopidogrel use may be associated with a lower incidence of death or MI in both the bare metal stent (BMS) and drug-eluting stent (DES) groups (25).

The treatment for failed antiplatelet therapy in diabetic patients is as yet undefined. Initially, physicians should ensure patient compliance, also minimizing drug–drug interactions. Moreover, in diabetic patients they must reach an optimal control of glucose levels, minimizing platelet reactivity. However, the optimal dose to use remains controversial. The addition of clopidogrel to ASA is logical given its distinct mechanism of action: ASA resistance patients have platelets that are more sensitive to ADP (26). This concept is supported by the CURE and CREDO trials, which demonstrated an additive clinical benefit of clopidogrel to aspirin in high-risk patients (19,27,28). Increasing maintenance doses or loading doses of clopidogrel may be an alternative. The antiplatelet therapy for Reduction of Myocardial Damage during Angioplasty (ARMYDA-2) study showed the benefit of 600 mg of clopidogrel compared with 300 mg as pretreatment in reducing periprocedural MI in patients undergoing PCI (23). The usefulness of increasing doses of clopidogrel has been further recently supported by the Intracoronary Stenting and Antithrombotic Regimen: Choose Between 3 High Oral Doses for Immediate Clopidogrel Effect trial (ISAR-CHOICE) (29). Regarding diabetic patients, the Optimizing Antiplatelet Therapy in Diabetes Mellitus (OPTIMUS) study showed that a 150-mg maintenance dose of clopidogrel is associated with enhanced antiplatelet effects compared with 75 mg (22).

However, although high dose resulted in a marked platelet inhibition, a considerable number of patients still remained below the therapeutic threshold of posttreatment platelet reactivity used in this study, suggesting the need for more potent P2Y12 inhibitors or alternative antithrombotic regimens in these high-risk patients. Current guidelines state class IIb indication with a level of evidence C only in patients in whom stent thrombosis may be catastrophic or lethal (such as unprotected left main, bifurcating left main, and last patent coronary vessel) may the dose of clopidogrel be increased to 150 mg per day if <50% inhibition of platelet aggregation is demonstrated (30).

However, although the use of a 150 mg maintenance dose of clopidogrel in patients with type 2 DM and with <50% platelet inhibition has been shown associated with enhanced antiplatelet effects, these effects are nonuniform and a considerable number of patients persist with inadequate platelet inhibition (24).

Probably the use of more potent P2Y12 inhibitors, with their more uniform effect, could help us to resolve this problem. Prasugrel, a third generation P2Y12 inhibitor, fulfils these criteria as it shows more potent and less variable antiplatelet effects compared with clopidogrel (31). Recently, the TRITON-TIMI 38 trial showed significantly reduced rates of ischemic events, including stent thrombosis, in patients presenting with acute coronary syndromes undergoing PCI treated with prasugrel compared with clopidogrel (31). The net clinical benefit achieved with prasugrel in the general study population was obtained despite the occurrence of an increased risk of bleeding. Importantly, in this trial the greatest risk reduction was observed in the diabetic population ($n = 3146$) (rate of primary endpoint, defined as death from cardiovascular causes, nonfatal MI or nonfatal stroke, in diabetic patients on prasugrel 12.2% vs. diabetic patients on clopidogrel 17.0% with 30% relative risk reduction) (32). In these patients prasugrel was not associated with an increased risk of major bleedings compared with clopidogrel. The functional impact of prasugrel versus clopidogrel among selected diabetic patients is currently being evaluated in the OPTIMUS-3 study.

Interestingly, a recent randomized trial evaluated role of cilostazol in a possible triple antiplatelet therapy in diabetic patients, receiving a DES. It enrolled 400 patients (almost 22% admitted at hospital with STEMI), randomized to receive a standard double antiplatelet therapy or triple therapy, and showed that after nine months major adverse cardiac events, including death, MI, and TLR tended to be lower in the triple than in the standard group (3.0% vs. 7.0%, $P = 0.066$) (33).

Glycoprotein IIb/IIIa Receptor Antagonists

In a meta-analysis of six trials of intravenous glycoprotein IIb/IIIa inhibitors in ACS patients, in which 22% had DM ($n = 6458$), these drugs significantly reduced mortality at 30 days in DM patients (34). The effect of these inhibitors in diabetic individuals was even greater in the patients who underwent PCI during the index hospitalization. Among the more than 22,000 patients in all these trials who did not have DM, glycoprotein IIb/IIIa blockers did not improve survival. Of note, these trials were performed in an era of limited use of clopidogrel, which has challenged the need for glycoprotein IIb/IIIa receptor antagonists in diabetes patients. In fact, the ISAR-SWEET (Intracoronary Stenting and Antithrombotic Regimen: is Abciximab a superior way to Eliminate Elevated Thrombotic Risk in Diabetics) trial did not show any impact of abciximab on the one-year risk of death and MI in stable DM patients, undergoing PCI after pretreatment with a 600 mg loading dose of clopidogrel at least two hours before procedure (35). BRAVE-3 (Bavarian Reperfusion Alternatives Evaluation-3) trial showed that in acute ST-segment elevation MI patients within 24 hours from symptom, upstream administration of abciximab on top of clopidogrel (600 mg loading dose) is not associated with a reduction in infarct size: this result was not different in the DM cohort (36). The ISAR-REACT 2 (Intracoronary Stenting and Antithrombotic: Regimen Rapid Early Action for Coronary Treatment 2) trial, however, showed that abciximab significantly reduces the risk of adverse clinical events (death, MI, urgent target vessel revascularization occurring within 30 days) in patients with non-STEMI ACS undergoing PCI after pretreatment with high loading dose of clopidogrel: the benefit was observed across all subgroups, including DM patients (37).

However, although standard dosing of GP IIb/IIIa receptor antagonists achieve $\geq$80% platelet inhibition in most patients, interindividual variations in receptor blockade may even occur leading to a suboptimal platelet inhibition (38). Inadequate platelet inhibition using GP IIb/IIIa inhibitors has been associated with a higher risk of adverse events (39). Variations in platelet count, density of GP IIb/IIIa receptors, plasma levels of platelet cofactors, and genetic factors may affect the functional response to given plasma levels of a GP IIb/IIIa antagonist, and thus lead to interindividual variation in responsiveness (40). In the recent double-blind, prospective, randomized trial 3T/2R an intensified platelet inhibition with high dose of tirofiban was evaluated in patients who were poor responders to aspirin, clopidogrel or both. It enrolled 263 low-risk patients, of which almost 26% were diabetic patients, and demonstrated that an intensified platelet inhibition with tirofiban lowers the incidence of MI after elective coronary intervention (41).

Overall, current guidelines support the use of glycoprotein IIb/IIIa receptor antagonists in DM patients with ACS undergoing PCI (42,43).

Adjunctive Pharmacological Therapy in Diabetics

At the time of admission for an acute coronary syndrome, DM patients usually show a deterioration of the glucometabolic state, reflecting an acute stress response to sudden impairment of left ventricle function, which appears to have an effect on outcome. Higher glucose levels on admission are indeed associated with increased mortality rates in diabetic patients presenting with STEMI (44). Strict attention to the glycemic control by use of insulin infusion followed by multiple-dose insulin treatment has been shown to reduce long-term mortality as compared with routine oral antidiabetic therapy (45,46). In the recent DIGAMI-2 study (1253 patients), however, mortality did not differ significantly between diabetic patients randomized to either acute insulin infusion followed by insulin-based long-term glucose control, insulin infusion followed by standard glucose control, or standard glucometabolic management, probably reflecting a lack of difference in glucose control among the three groups (47). As hyperglycemia remained one of the most important predictors of outcome in this study, it appears to be reasonable to keep glucose levels within normal ranges in diabetic patients. In this regard, target glucose levels between 90 and 140 mg/dL (5 and 7.8 mmol/L) have been advocated (48). However, special care needs to be taken to avoid blood glucose levels below 80 to 90 mg/dL (4.4 to

5 mmol/L), as hypoglycemia-induced ischemia might also affect outcome in diabetic patients with acute coronary syndromes (49). The NICE-SUGAR trial, for example, showed in a cohort of 6104 patients admitted to an intensive care unit that a conventional glucose control (blood glucose target of 180 mg or less per deciliter) resulted in lower mortality than did a intensive treatment (blood glucose target of 81 to 108 mg per deciliter) (50).

Relatively new hypoglycemic agents, such as rosiglitazone, were pointed out as a strategy for the prevention of restenosis in diabetic patients. Rosiglitazone is a member of the class of drugs known as thiazolidinediones: these drugs are peroxisome proliferators-activated receptor (PPAR)-γ agonists, potentially able to increase insulin sensitivity, decrease inflammation, endogenous fibrinolysis, and glycemic control, as well as reduce neointimal proliferation after PCI in DM patients (51). However, a recent report of a meta-analysis of treatment trials of rosiglitazone, as compared either with other therapies for type 2 diabetes or with placebo, showed that rosiglitazone was associated with a significant increase in the risk of MI and a borderline risk of death from cardiovascular causes (52). So the role of these agents as adjunctive therapy for diabetics undergoing PCI has to be revised.

In any event, reducing coronary risk from diabetes requires a multifactorial approach to manage all atherogenic influences (53). Long-term, targeted, intensive use of proven therapies for the traditional coronary risk factors must be widely promoted for patients with diabetes, particularly following ACS. As with lipid levels, more stringent targets for patients with diabetes may be better all around.

REVASCULARIZATION IN DIABETICS PRESENTING WITH ACUTE CORONARY SYNDROMES

Primary PCI is the treatment of choice in diabetics presenting with acute MI. Cardiac surgery in the setting of ST elevation MI is only indicated when coronary anatomy is not suitable for a percutaneous intervention.

Diabetics with unstable angina/non-STEMI or STEMI faces a much higher risk of mortality within one year of their acute coronary syndromes than non-diabetics (54,55). Risk of dying the first year after an acute cardiac syndrome (ACS) event for a diabetic patient with UA/NSTEMI is almost the same as that of a nondiabetic patient with STEMI. These data have been demonstrated in the analysis comparing diabetics and nondiabetics enrolled in the primary angioplasty in myocardial infarction (PAMI) study (54). This analysis was set out to determine whether DM independently conferred poor prognosis in MI patients undergoing primary PCI. In hospital and six-month mortality rates and six-month MACE rate of the 626 patients with and the 3116 patients without diabetes were compared. Diabetics had worse baseline clinical characteristics, such as older age and later presentation, and had higher atherosclerotic burden (Fig. 2) (higher incidence of peripheral vascular disease, prior cerebrovascular accident, MI, PCI or CABG, and multivessel coronary artery disease). During the index hospitalization, diabetics had higher incidence of death (4.6% vs. 2.6%, $P = 0.005$), probably explained by the difference in baseline characteristics. However, diabetes was found to be an independent predictor of mortality at six-month follow-up (HR 1.53; 95% IC, 1.03–2.26, $P = 0.03$), also after adjustment for baseline clinical and angiographic differences.

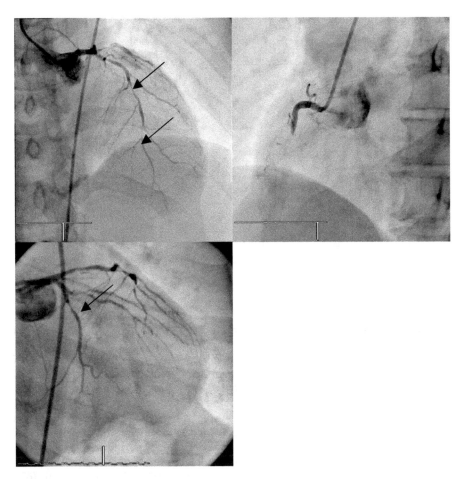

FIGURE 2 Atherosclerotic burden in DM patient previously asymptomatic admitted at the hospital with inferior STEMI. Note the diffuseness of the disease remote from the target site (*arrows*).

In another analysis, evaluating 11 thrombolysis in myocardial infarction (TIMI) clinical trials conducted between 1997 and 2006, performed to evaluate the influence of diabetes on mortality following ACS, a robust sample size of diabetics were included (10,613 out of the 62,036 total patients) (55). The authors found that mortality at 30 days was significantly higher among patients with DM than nondiabetics presenting with UA/NSTEMI (2.1% vs. 1.1%; $P < 0.001$) and STEMI (8.5% vs. 5.4%; $P < 0.001$). After adjustment for baseline characteristics and features and management of the ACS event, diabetes was independently associated with higher 30-day mortality after UA/NSTEMI (OR 1.78; 95% CI, 1.24–2.56) or STEMI (OR 1.40; 95% CI, 1.24–1.57). At the same time, mortality at one year was significantly higher among patients with diabetes than in patients without diabetes presenting with UA/NSTEMI (7.2% vs. 3.1%, $P < 0.001$) or STEMI (13.2% vs. 8.1%, $P < 0.001$) (Fig. 3). By one year following ACS, patients with diabetes and presenting UA/NSTEMI had a

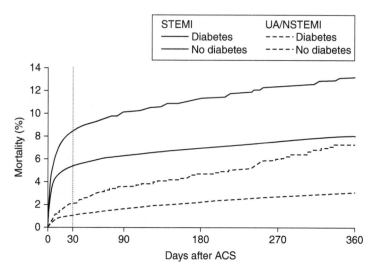

FIGURE 3 Cumulative incidence of all-cause mortality through one year after ACS, stratified by diabetes. *Source*: Adapted from Ref. 55.

mortality that approached patients without diabetes and presenting with STEMI (7.2% vs. 8.1%).

In other trials, such as GUSTO-1, OASIS registry, the GRACE multinational registry, DM was also identified as a significant contributor to in-hospital and six-month out of hospital mortality (56–58). In this regard, diabetes status was included in the TIMI risk score for both UA/NSTEMI and STEMI (59,60).

This worse outcome of diabetics compared to nondiabetics is present even after a successful PCI: DM has been identified as an independent predictor or restenosis (61). In a meta-analysis of 16 studies after stent implantation, angiographic restenosis (defined as $\geq$ 50% diameter stenosis at follow-up) occurred in 20.6% of non-DM patients as compared to 31.1% of DM patients ($P < 0.001$) (62). The pattern of restenosis is more severe as these patients typically show more proliferative and occlusive types of restenosis. The latter has been associated with increased long-term mortality and impaired left ventricular ejection fraction (63). The introduction of stents with the ability to elute medication with antiproliferative properties to directly tackle this mechanism of restenosis appeared as a revolution in treatment of DM patients.

Subgroup analysis of the SIRIUS trial including 279 DM patients, 131 receiving sirolimus-eluting stent (SES) and 148 BMS demonstrated favorable results toward SES with significant reduction in restenosis rates (50% for BMS vs. 17% for SES) and in major adverse cardiac events (25% for BMS vs. 9.2% for SES) (64). Similar results come from the TAXUS IV trial regarding use of paclitaxel-eluting stent (PES) in DM patients: use of PES compared to BMS reduced the risk of binary restenosis (70% reduction of in-segment restenosis) (65). Superiority of DES on the BMS in treatment of DM patients was confirmed by Massachusetts data analysis center registry: in a cohort of more than 5000 DM patients, of which 30% had ACS, DES was associated with reduced mortality, MI, and revascularization rates at three years follow-up compared to BMS (66).

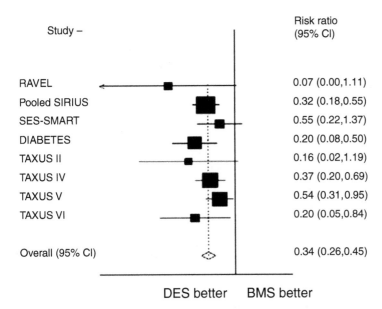

Study –		Risk ratio (95% CI)
RAVEL		0.07 (0.00,1.11)
Pooled SIRIUS		0.32 (0.18,0.55)
SES-SMART		0.55 (0.22,1.37)
DIABETES		0.20 (0.08,0.50)
TAXUS II		0.16 (0.02,1.19)
TAXUS IV		0.37 (0.20,0.69)
TAXUS V		0.54 (0.31,0.95)
TAXUS VI		0.20 (0.05,0.84)
Overall (95% CI)		0.34 (0.26,0.45)

DES better   BMS better

FIGURE 4 Meta-analysis of target lesion revascularization of DESs versus BMSs in patients with diabetes as reported by randomized controlled trials. *Source*: Adapted from Ref. 68.

The DIABETES trial was the only randomized multicenter controlled trial specifically designed in diabetics to assess the efficacy of SES versus BMS. It enrolled 160 patients, of which 50% with NSTEMI, randomized to SES or BMS, and showed after nine-month follow-up a significant lower target-lesion revascularization and major adverse cardiac event rates in the SES group (31.35 vs. 7.3% and 36.3 vs. 11.3%, respectively; both $P < 0.001$) (67).

These data were confirmed by a meta-analysis of all available data in DM patients that demonstrated the benefit of DES in terms of restenosis and target lesion revascularization (Fig. 4)(68).

However, despite these evidences, to date none of the trials was addressed to evaluate role of DES versus BMS in diabetic population in the setting of ST segment elevation acute MI.

CONCLUSION

DM patients represent a difficult category of patients to treat not only in an acute setting, but also in a chronic stable angina/silent ischemia pattern.

They are hyporesponders to the most common antiplatelet agents and probably only the new and recently commercialized antiplatelet drugs may help us to reach a good level of platelet inhibition. In an acute setting, it is very important the use of IIb/IIIa inhibitors in DM patient. As of today, the association of IIb/IIIa inhibitors on top of 600 mg loading dose of clopidogrel remains controversial.

Moreover, although there is a lack of direct data about the efficacy of DES in DM during MI, we could extrapolate from the trials in stable patients that use of DES could be associated with a better outcome in this population.

Diabetes should not therefore be considered a focal disease of coronary arteries, but rather a systemic and diffuse alteration involving myocardium, blood, platelet, etc. Thus, the best treatment of these patients is not only the use of more aggressive antiplatelet drugs and DES, but also to optimize the control of glycemia and of the other cardiovascular risk factors.

REFERENCES

1. Buse J, Ginsberg H, Bakris G, et al. Primary prevention of cardiovascular diseases in people with diabetes mellitus: a scientific statement from the American heart association and the American diabetes association. Diabetes Care 2007; 30:162–172.
2. Haffner SM, Lehto S, Ronnemaa T. Mortality from coronary heart disease in subjects with type 2 diabetes and in nondiabetics subjects with and without prior myocardial infarction. N Engl J Med 1998; 339:229–234.
3. De Luca G, Gibson CM, Bellandi F, et al. Diabetes mellitus is associated with distal embolization, impaired myocardial perfusion, and higher mortality in patients with ST-segment elevation myocardial infarction treated with primary angioplasty and glycoprotein IIb/IIIa inhibitors [published online ahead of print 2009]. Atherosclerosis.
4. Vinik AI, Erbas T, Park TS, et al. Platelet dysfunction in type 2 diabetes. Diabetes Care 2001; 24:1476–1485.
5. Ferroni P, Basili S, Falco A, et al. Platelet activation in type 2 diabetes. J Thromb Haemost 2004; 2:1282–1291.
6. Colwell J. American Diabetes Association. Aspirin therapy in diabetes (Position Statement). Diabetes Care 2003; 26:S87–S88.
7. Antithrombotic Trialists Collaboration. Collaborative meta-analyses of randomized trials of antiplatelet therapy for prevention of death, myocardial infarction, and stroke in high risk patients. BMJ 2002; 324:71–86.
8. Antiplatelet Trialists Collaboration. Collaborative overview of randomized trials of antiplatelets therapy. Prevention of death, myocardial infarction, and stroke by prolonged antiplatelet therapy in various categories of patients. BMJ 1994; 308:81–106.
9. Physicians'Health Study Research Group. Final report on the aspirin component of the ongoing Physicians'Health Study. N Engl J Med 1989; 321:129–135.
10. ETDRS Investigators. Aspirin effects on mortality and morbidity in patients with diabetes mellitus: Early Treatment Diabetic Retinopathy Study Report. JAMA 1992; 268:1292–1300.
11. Hansson L, Zanchetti A, Carruthers SG. Effects of intensive blood-pressure lowering and low-dose aspirin in patients with hypertension: principal results of the hypertensive optimal treatment randomized trial. Lancet 1998; 351:1755–1762.
12. Angiolillo DJ. Antiplatelet therapy in type 2 diabetes mellitus. Curr Opin Endocrinol Diabetes Obes 2007; 14:124–131.
13. Eikelboom JW, Hirsh J, Weitz JI, et al. Aspirin-resistant thromboxane biosynthesis and the risk of myocardial infarction, stroke, or cardiovascular death in patients at high risk for cardiovascular events. Circulation 2002; 105:1650–1655.
14. Sacco M, Pellegrini F, Roncaglioni MC, et al; on behalf of the PPP Collaborative Group. Primary prevention of cardiovascular events with low-dose aspirin and vitamin E in type 2 diabetic patients: results of the Primary Prevention Project (PPP) trial. Diabetes Care 2003; 26:3264–3272.
15. Cubbon RM, Gale CP, Rajwani A, et al. Aspirin and mortality in patients with diabetes sustaining acute coronary syndrome. Diabetes Care 2008; 31:363–365.
16. Patrono C, Garcia Rodriguez LA, et al. Low-dose aspirin for the prevention of atherothrombosis. N Engl J Med 2005; 353:2373–2383.
17. Bhatt D, Marso S, Hirsch A. Amplified benefit of clopidogrel versus aspirin in patients with diabetes mellitus. Am J Cardiol 2002; 90:625–628.

18. CAPRIE Steering Committee. A randomized, blinded, trial of clopidogrel versus aspirin in patients at risk of ischaemic events (CAPRIE). Lancet 1996; 348:1329–1339.
19. Yusuf S, Zhao F, Metha SR. Clopidogrel in Unstable Angina to Prevent Recurrent Events Trial Investigators. Effects of clopidogrel in addition to aspirin in patients with acute coronary syndromes without ST-segment elevation. N Engl J Med 2001; 345:494–502.
20. Angiolillo DJ, Fernandez-Ortiz A, Bernardo E, et al. Variability in individual responsiveness to clopidogrel: clinical implications, management and future perspectives. J Am Coll Cardiol 2007; 49:1505–1516.
21. Gurbel PA, Blinden KP, Hayes KM, et al. The relation of dosing to clopidogrel responsiveness and the incidence of high post-treatment platelet aggregation in patients undergoing coronary stenting. J Am Coll Cardiol 2005; 45:1392–1396.
22. Angiolillo DJ, Shoemaker SB, Desai B, et al. Randomized comparison of a high clopidogrel maintenance dose in patients with diabetes mellitus and coronary artery disease. Circulation 2007; 115:708–716.
23. Patti G, Colonna G, Pasceri V, et al. Randomized trial of high loading dose of clopidogrel for reduction of periprocedural myocardial infarction in patients undergoing coronary intervention. Circulation 2005; 111:2099–2106.
24. Angiolillo DJ, Costa MA, Shoemaker SB, et al. Functional effects of high clopidogrel maintenance dosing in patients with inadequate platelet inhibition on standard dose treatment. Am J Cardiol 2008; 101:440–445.
25. Brar SS, Kim J, Brar SK, et al. Long-term outcomes by clopidogrel duration and stent type in a diabetic population with de novo coronary artery lesions. J Am Coll Cardiol 2008; 51:2220–2227.
26. Zimmermann N, Wenk A, Kim U, et al. Functional and biochemical evaluation of platelet aspirin resistance after coronary artery bypass surgery. Circulation. 2003; 108:542–547.
27. Sabatine MS, Cannon CP, Gibson CM. Clopidogrel as Adjunctive Reperfusion Therapy (CLARITY)-Thrombolysis in Myocardial Infarction (TIMI) 28 Investigators. Addition of Clopidogrel to aspirin and fibrinolytis therapy for myocardial infarction with ST-segment elevation. CLARITY-TIMI 28 Investigators. N Engl J Med 2005; 352:1179–1189.
28. Steinhubl SR, Berger PB, Mann JT III, et al; CREDO Investigators. Clopidogrel for the Reduction of Events During Observation. Early and sustained dual oral antiplatelet therapy following percutaneous coronary intervention: a randomized controlled trial. JAMA 2002; 288:2411–2420.
29. von Beckerath N, Taubert D, Pogatsa-Murray G, et al. Absorption, metabolization, and antiplatelet effects of 300-, 600-, and 900-mg loading doses of clopidogrel: results of the ISAR-CHOICE (Intracoronary Stenting and Antithrombotic Regimen: Choose Between 3 High Oral Doses for Immediate Clopidogrel Effect) trial. Circulation 2005; 112:2946–2950.
30. Smith SC Jr, Feldman TE, Hischfeld JW Jr, et al. ACC/AHA/SCAI 2005 guideline update for percutaneous coronary intervention: a report of the American College of Cardiology/American Heart Association Task Force on Practice Guidelines (ACC/AHA/SCAI Writing Committee to Update the 2001 Guidelines for Percutaneous Coronary Intervention). J Am Coll Cardiol 2006; 47:e1–e121.
31. Wiviott SD, Braunwald E, McCabe CH, et al. Prasugrel versus clopidogrel in patients with acute coronary syndromes. N Engl J Med 2007; 357:2001–2015.
32. Wiviott, SD, Braunwald E, Angiolillo DJ, et al. Greater clinical benefit of more intensive oral antiplatelet therapy with prasugrel in patients with diabetes mellitus in the trial to assess improvement in therapeutic outcomes by optimizing platelet inhibition with prasugrel-thrombolysis in myocardial infarction 38. Circulation 2008; 118:1626–1636.
33. Lee SW, Park SW, Kim YH, et al. Drug-eluting stenting followed by cilostazol treatment reduces late restenosis in patients with diabetes mellitus. J Am Coll Cardiol 2008; 51:1181–1187.

34. Roffi M, Chew DP, Mukherjee D. Platelet glycoprotein IIb/IIIa inhibitors reduce mortality in diabetic patients with non-ST segment elevation acute coronary syndromes. Circulation 2001; 104:2767–277.
35. Mehilli J, Kastrati A, Schuhlen H. Intracoronary Stenting and Antithrombotic Regimen: Is Abciximab a Superior Way to Eliminate Elevated Thrombotic Risk in Diabetics (ISAR-SWEET) Study Investigators. Randomized clinical trial of abciximab in diabetic patients undergoing elective percutaneous coronary interventions after treatment with a high loading dose of clopidogrel. Circulation 2004; 110: 3627–3635.
36. Mehilli J, Kastrati A, Schulz S, et al. Abciximab in patients with acute ST-segment elevation myocardial infarction undergoing primary percutaneous coronary intervention after clopidogrel loading. A randomized double-blind trial. Circulation 2009; 119:1933–1940.
37. Kastrati A, Mehilli J, Neumann FJ. Intracoronary Stenting and Antithrombotic: Regimen Rapid Early Action for Coronary Treatment 2 (ISAR-REACT 2) Trial Investigators. Abciximab in patients with acute coronary syndromes undergoing percutaneous coronary intervention after clopidogrel pre-treatment: the ISAR-REACT 2 randomized trial. JAMA 2006; 295:1531–1538.
38. Mascelli MA, Lance ET, Damaraju L. Pharmacodynamic profile of short-term abciximab treatment demonstrates prolonged platelet inhibition with gradual recovery from GP IIb/IIIa receptor blockade. Circulation 1998; 97:1680–1688.
39. Steinhubl SR, Talley JD, Braden GA. Point-of-care measured platelet inhibition correlates with a reduced risk of an adverse cardiac event after percutaneous coronary intervention: results of the GOLD (AU-Assessing Ultegra) multicenter study. Circulation 2001; 103:2572–2578.
40. Rozalski M, Watala C. Antagonists of platelet fibrinogen receptor are less effective in carriers of Pl(A2) polymorphism of beta(3) integrin. Eur J Pharmacol 2002; 454:1–8.
41. Valgimigli M, Campo G, de Cesare N, et al. Intensifying platelet inhibition with tirofiban in poor responders to aspirin, clopidogrel or both agents undergoing elective coronary intervention. Results from the double-blind prospective, randomized tailoring treatment with tirofiban in patients showing resistance to aspirin and/or resistance to clopidogrel study. Circulation 2009; 119:3215–3222.
42. Braunwald E, Antman EM, Beasley JM; American College of Cardiology; American Heart Association. Committee on the management of Patients with Unstable Angina. ACC/AHA 2002 guideline update for the management of patients with unstable angina and non-ST-segment elevation myocardial infarction-summary article: a report of the American College of Cardiology/American Heart Association task force on practice guidelines (Committee on the Management of Patients with Unstable Angina). J Am Coll Cardiol 2002; 40:1366–1374.
43. Vorchheimer DA, Badimon JJ, Fuster V. Platelet glycoprotein IIb/IIIa receptors antagonists in cardiovascular disease. JAMA 1999; 281:1407–1414.
44. Capes SE, Hunt D, Malmberg K, et al. Stress hyperglycaemia and increased risk of death after myocardial infarction in patients with and without diabetes: a systematic overview. Lancet 2000; 355:773–778.
45. Malmberg K, Ryden L, Efendic S, et al. Randomized trial of insulin-glucose infusion followed by subcutaneous insulin treatment in diabetic patients with acute myocardial infarction (DIGAMI study): effects on mortality at 1 year. J Am Coll Cardiol 1995; 26:57–65.
46. Malmberg K, Norhammar A, Wedel H, et al. Glycometabolic state ad admission: important risk marker of mortality in conventionally treated patients with diabetes mellitus and acute myocardial infarction: long-term results from the Diabetes and Insulin-Glucose Infusion in Acute Myocardial Infarction (DIGAMI) study. Circulation 1999; 99:2626–2632.
47. Malmberg K, Ryden L, Wedel H, et al. Intensive metabolic control by means of insulin in patients with diabetes mellitus and acute myocardial infarction (DIGAMI 2): effects on mortality and morbidity. Eur Heart J 2005; 26:650–661.

48. Deedwania P, Kosiborod M, Barrett E, et al. A scientific statement from the American heart association diabetes committee of the council on nutrition, physical activity, and metabolism. Circulation 2008; 117:1610–1619.
49. Svensson AM, McGuire DK, Abrahamsson P, et al. Association between hyper- and hypoglycaemia and 2 year all-cause mortality risk in diabetic patients with acute coronary events. Eur Heart J 2005; 26:1245–1248.
50. The NICE-SUGAR Investigators. Intensive versus conventional glucose control in critically Ill patients. N Engl J Med 2009; 360:1283–1297.
51. Choi D, Kim SK, Choi SH, et al. Preventative effects of rosiglitazone on restenosis after coronary stent implantation in patients with type 2 diabetes. Diabetes Care 2004; 27:2654–2660.
52. Psaty BM, Furberg CD. Rosiglitazone and cardiovascular risk. N Engl J Med 2007; 356:2522–2524.
53. Gaede P, Vedel P, Larsen N, et al. Multifactorial intervention and cardiovascular disease in patients with type 2 diabetes. N Engl J Med 2003; 348:383–393.
54. Harjuai KJ, Stone GW, Boura J, et al. Comparison of outcomes of diabetic and non-diabetic patients undergoing primary angioplasty for acute myocardial infarction. Am J Cardiol 2003; 91:1041–1045.
55. Donahoe SM, Stewart GC, McCabe CH, et al. Diabetes and mortality following acute coronary syndromes. JAMA 2007; 298:765–775.
56. Mak KH, Moliterno DJ, Granger CB, et al. Influence of diabetes mellitus on clinical outcome in the thrombolytic era of acute myocardial infarction. GUSTO-I Investigators. Global Utilization of Streptokinase and Tissue Plasminogen Activator for Occluded Coronary Arteries. J Am Coll Cardiol 1997; 30:171–179.
57. Malmberg K, Yusuf S, Gerstein HC, et al. Impact of diabetes on long-term prognosis in patients with unstable angina and non-Q wave myocardial infarction: results of the OASIS (Organization to Assess Strategies for Ischemic Syndromes) Registry. Circulation 2000; 102:1014–1019.
58. Fox KA, Dabbous OH, Goldberg RJ. Prediction of risk of death and myocardial infarction in the six months after presentation with acute coronary syndrome: prospective observational study (GRACE). BMJ 2006; 333:1091.
59. Antman EM, Cohen M, Bernink PJ, et al. The TIMI risk score for unstable angina/non-ST elevation MI: a method for prognostication and therapeutic decision making. JAMA 2000; 284:835–842.
60. Morrow DA, Antman EM, Charlesworth A, et al. TIMI risk score for ST-elevation myocardial infarction: a convenient, bedside, clinical score for risk assessment at presentation: an intravenous nPA for treatment of infarcting myocardium early II trial substudy. Circulation 2000; 102:2031–2037.
61. Cutlip DE, Chauhan MS, Baim DS, et al. Clinical restenosis after coronary stenting: perspectives from multicenter clinical trials. J Am Coll Cardiol 2002; 40:2082–2089.
62. West NE, Ruygrok PN, Disco CM, et al. Clinical and angiographic predictors of restenosis after stent deployment in diabetic patients. Circulation 2004; 109:867–873.
63. Van Belle E, Ketelers R, Bauters C, et al. Patency of percutaneous transluminal coronary angioplasty sites at 6-month angiographic follow-up: a key determinant of survival in diabetics after coronary balloon angioplasty. Circulation 2001; 103:1218–1224.
64. Moussa I, Leon MB, Baim DS, et al. Impact of sirolimus eluting stents on outcome in diabetic patients. A SIRIUS substudy. Circulation 2004; 109:2273–2278.
65. Hermiller JB, Raizner A, Cannon L, et al. Outcomes with the polymer-based paclitaxel-eluting TAXUS stent in patients with diabetes mellitus: the TAXUS-IV trial. J Am Coll Cardiol 2005; 45:1172–1179.
66. Garg P, Normand SLT, Silbaugh TS, et al. Drug-eluting or bare-metal stenting in patients with diabetes mellitus. Results from the Massachusetts data analysis center registry. Circulation 2008; 118:2277–2285.

67. Sabate M, Jimenez-Quevedo P, Angiolillo DJ, et al. Randomized comparison of sirolimus-eluting stent versus standard stent for percutaneous coronary revascularization in diabetic patients: the diabetes and sirolimus-eluting stent (DIABETES) trial. Circulation 2005; 112:2175–2183.
68. Boyden TF, Nallamothu BK, Moscucci M, et al. Meta-analysis of randomized trials of drug-eluting stents versus bare metal stents in patients with diabetes mellitus. Am J Cardiol 2007; 99:1399–1402.

Yasir Abu-Omar
Department of Cardiothoracic Surgery, Papworth Hospital, Cambridge, U.K.

David P. Taggart
Department of Cardiothoracic Surgery, John Radcliffe Hospital and University of Oxford, Oxford, U.K.

INTRODUCTION

Myocardial infarction (MI) remains the leading cause of death in the developed world. Over the last 20 years, advances in medical and surgical management of ischemic heart disease, including thrombolysis, percutaneous coronary intervention, and coronary artery bypass surgery, have resulted in a significant reduction in mortality and morbidity associated with acute MI. In addition, development and evolution of mechanical support devices has widened the surgical armamentarium. However, complications including ventricular septal and free wall rupture, acute mitral regurgitation, and arrhythmias still occur and remain a challenge for the treating physician and surgeon. The most serious of those complications is the development of cardiogenic shock that is associated with 80% mortality.

Restoration of blood flow to the myocardium provides the best chance of survival following an acute MI. The timing of intervention remains highly debated mainly due to the temporal variation in the balance of risks and benefits following an acute coronary event.

REPERFUSION OF ISCHEMIC MYOCARDIUM

The role of surgical revascularization has changed significantly over the last three decades. Coronary artery bypass grafting (CABG) remains the most extensively studied surgical procedure ever undertaken with follow-up data extending to 20 to 30 years. It is highly effective in relieving the symptoms of IHD and improving life expectancy in certain anatomic patterns of disease particularly in those with severe disease and impaired left ventricular function (1). Furthermore, CABG is a remarkably safe therapy. Improvements in medical, anesthetic, and surgical management have ensured that its mortality has remained around 2% over the last decade despite the fact that it has been increasingly applied to an ageing and sicker patient population. Developments of thrombolytic and percutaneous techniques, however, offer other alternatives to surgery. The role of percutaneous coronary intervention is discussed in detail elsewhere in this book.

The increased and more widespread use of primary angioplasty has served to identify surgical candidates (e.g., those with failed angioplasty, unfavorable pattern of multivessel disease, and left main stem disease) early following acute

MI. However, surgical revascularization at this early stage is associated with increased mortality and morbidity. Earlier studies reported a mortality ranging from 5% to 30% (2,3). Consequently, revascularization in the acute setting was reserved to those with complications such as papillary muscle rupture, ventricular septal defect, or ventricular free wall rupture. Additional concern regarding the potential of early reperfusion resulting in hemorrhagic transformation and subsequent infarct extension along with the documented increased mortality from surgery in the acute setting has prompted many surgeons to delay revascularization for 4 to 6 weeks after the acute event. With emerging evidence from experience over the last decade, this practice has been challenged in favor of earlier revascularization.

TIMING OF SURGERY

There are no specific guidelines regarding the optimal timing for surgical intervention following acute MI. The ACC/AHA published guidelines state that "in patients who have had a ST-elevation MI (STEMI), CABG mortality is elevated for the first 3 to 7 days after infarction, and the benefit of revascularization must be balanced against this increased risk. Patients who have been stabilised (no ongoing ischemia, hemodynamic compromise, or life-threatening arrhythmia) after STEMI and who have incurred a significant fall in left ventricular function should have their surgery delayed to allow myocardial recovery to occur. If critical anatomy exists, revascularization should be undertaken during the index hospitalization (*Level of Evidence: B*). The Writing Committee believes that if stable STEMI patients with preserved LV function require surgical revascularization, then CABG can be undertaken within several days of the infarction without an increased risk" (4,5).

To date, there are no prospective randomized controlled trials comparing early versus late revascularization following acute MI. However, several retrospective studies have been published with varying recommendations on the timing of surgery following acute MI ranging from 48 hours to over 30 days after the acute event (3,6,7).

Almost 20 years ago, DeWood et al. (8) reported a significant reduction in mortality in matched patients undergoing early revascularization (within 6 hours of onset of infarction) compared to medical management (2% vs. 11.5%; $P < 0.05$). In addition, favorable outcomes of improved longevity extended over to 10 years follow-up. While this study was retrospective and limited by potential selection bias, it demonstrated the safety and superiority of surgical revascularization compared to medical therapy alone. In the current era, however, the cohort of patients referred for surgical intervention has dramatically changed with a significantly higher proportion of patients referred following failure of other treatment modalities.

More recently, Lee et al. (9) reported their experience on the appropriate timing of surgical intervention after transmural MI. A retrospective multicenter analysis of over 32,000 patients from the New York cardiac surgery registry over a six-year period was carried out. Overall mortality with surgery was 3.3%. The mortality rate decreased with increasing time interval between CABG and onset of AMI (14.2% within six hours to 2.7% >15 day) (Fig. 1). Mortality decreased to 3.8% after three days of onset of infarction. The authors concluded that CABG

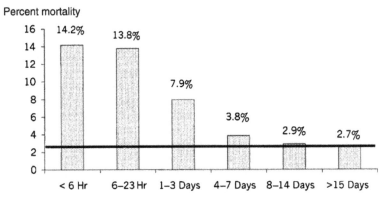

FIGURE 1 Hospital mortality versus timing of CABG. The *horizontal bar* represents the baseline mortality rate (2.7%) from the entire patient population. *Source*: From Ref. 9.

within three days of a transmural MI adds to the mortality risk and therefore a three-day wait is advocated in the absence of absolute indications for emergency surgery (9).

In a single-center study by Voisine et al., data from more than 7000 patients over a 15-year period undergoing CABG with a history of previous MI were analyzed. Patients were subdivided into five groups depending on the timing of surgery following acute MI. Mortality was highest up to one week following acute MI (but still displaying a reduction from 19% to 8%). Surgery performed one week after acute MI was associated with a mortality of 3.2% and thus the authors recommended delaying surgical intervention for that period of time (10).

In summary, CABG is indicated on an emergency basis following AMI in the presence of structural complications and persistent ischemia. Early surgery after transmural MI is associated with higher risk of mortality and stable patients may benefit from delay of surgery. The timing should be weighed through careful consideration of risks and benefits.

TRANSMURAL VERSUS NONTRANSMURAL MYOCARDIAL INFARCTION

Transmural MI is thought to be associated with differences in surgical outcome compared to nontransmural MI. Analysis from the New York State Cardiac Surgery Registry of over 44,000 patients reported a variation in the trend of mortality with CABG in transmural and nontransmural MI when the time delay is taken into consideration (11). In the transmural group, mortality was increased compared to the nontransmural group when CABG was performed within seven days of acute MI. Mortality peaked if CABG was performed within six hours in the nontransmural group and one day in the transmural group. Perioperative mortality was comparable in the two groups seven days after MI (11).

RISK FACTORS

Aside the timing of surgery, several risk factors are associated with increased mortality and morbidity following an acute infarction. Knowledge of these factors would aid in the perioperative assessment of risk and determining the optimal route for managing the individual patient. Curtis et al. identified several predictors of mortality through stepwise logistic regression analysis. Those factors include unstable angina, previous surgical revascularization, preoperative hypotension, nonelective surgery, preoperative cardiac arrest, and female sex (12).

In a study of 225 patients undergoing urgent CABG over a four-year period, Stuart et al. defined predictors of perioperative mortality using multivariate analysis. Significant independent predictors of mortality included the presence of a transmural anterior MI and the need for preoperative intra-aortic balloon pumping (13). In another study, Zaroff et al. attempted to generate a model to predict the risk of mortality for patients with acute MI undergoing CABG. Data from over 70,000 patients were used from the National Registry of Myocardial Infarction from selected U.S. hospitals. Logistic regression analysis identified the patients' age, previous CABG, heart failure on presentation, and the female gender as independent predictors of in-hospital death. A risk score was then generated that may aid in the decision-making for the timing of urgent CABG (14).

CARDIOGENIC SHOCK

Cardiogenic shock as a complication of acute MI affects 5% to 10% of patients and is the leading cause of in-hospital death in this group. Despite advances in the treatment strategies for patients with acute coronary syndromes, cardiogenic shock still carries a grave prognosis. It has a mortality rate of 80% (15) at one year and this figure has remained constant over the last two decades (16). In the "Global Use of Strategies to Open Occluded Coronary Arteries" (GUSTO-I), the incidence was 7.2% of approximately 41,000 patients with AMI (17). In GUSTO-I, 56% of all patients with cardiogenic shock died in hospital, regardless of the thrombolytic regimen used. Furthermore, patients treated with accelerated recombinant tissue plasminogen activator were significantly less likely to have shock; this finding suggests the possible benefit of early reperfusion associated with thrombolysis (17).

The diagnostic criteria for cardiogenic shock are (18):

- persistent hypotension (systolic blood pressure <90 mm Hg, or a fall of systolic blood pressure >30 mm Hg in hypertensive patients);
- poorly perfused extremities;
- decreased urine output;
- drowsiness or confusion;
- pulmonary capillary wedge pressure >18 mm Hg;
- cardiac index <1.8 L/min/m^2.

Development of cardiogenic shock is directly related to the extent of myocardial damage and is associated with loss of at least 40% of left ventricular muscle (19). In the setting of acute MI, STEMI is more frequently associated with cardiogenic shock compared with NSTEMI. In the prospective "Should We Revascularize Occluded Coronaries for Cardiogenic Shock?" (SHOCK) registry, 214 patients were found to have left ventricular failure and signs of shock; of these, only 14% did not have ST segment elevation (20). The GUSTO-IIb study also documents a significant difference in the incidence of cardiogenic shock, which was seen in 4.2% of patients with ST segment elevation but only 2.5% of those without ST segment elevation (21).

Cardiogenic shock is a syndrome of progressive deterioration due to a vicious cycle of infarction resulting in profound depression of cardiac output causing further coronary insufficiency and myocardial loss. The syndrome is not always associated with systemic vasoconstriction. Catastrophic loss of myocardium may not be the sole cause of cardiogenic shock. The SHOCK trial demonstrated the importance of the systemic inflammatory response syndrome in the development of cardiogenic shock even in individuals with modest depression in ejection fraction (22).

Several studies have reported the benefits of revascularization in the setting of cardiogenic shock following MI. The GUSTO-I trial reported a significant reduction in mortality rates in patients with cardiogenic shock undergoing revascularization with PCI or surgery. Mortality rates for PCI and CABG were 32% and 29%, respectively (17). This represents more than 50% reduction in mortality compared to medically treated cardiogenic shock. In the nonrandomized SHOCK trial registry of 884 with predominant left ventricular failure, the in-hospital mortality rates were 78.0% in patients treated medically, 46.4% in those treated with PCI, and 23.9% in those treated with CABG ($P < 0.001$). Patients with single vessel disease had similar in-hospital mortality rates regardless of whether they were treated with PCI or CABG (32.9% vs. 33.3%). Patients with two-vessel disease had higher in-hospital mortality with PCI than with CABG (42.2% vs. 17.7%; $P < 0.025$), as did patients with three-vessel disease (59.35% vs. 29.6%; $P < 0.0001$) (23).

In the international SHOCK trial, 302 patients who developed cardiogenic shock within 36 hours of the onset of acute MI were randomized to receive either emergency revascularization or initial medical stabilization. Eligible patients had either ST segment elevation, Q-wave infarction, new left bundle branch block, or a posterior infarct with anterior ST segment depression on the presenting ECG. Cardiogenic shock was due to predominant left ventricular failure. The trial demonstrated that patients undergoing revascularization within six hours of onset of cardiogenic shock have better survival compared to those undergoing no or delayed revascularization (46.7% vs. 33.6%) (15,24). Among patients randomized to emergency revascularization in the SHOCK trial, those selected for CABG were more likely to have diabetes and to have more severe coronary disease than those selected for PCI. Despite this disparity in risk factors between the two groups, the survival rates were 55.6% in the PCI group compared with 57.4% in the CABG group at 30 days ($P = 0.86$) and 51.9% compared with 46.8% ($P = 0.71$) respectively, at one year (25).

On the basis of the results presented above, it is no surprise that in the current European Society of Cardiology/American College of Cardiology guidelines, AMI with cardiogenic shock is listed as a class IA indication (i.e., a condition for which there is evidence for and/or general agreement that a given procedure/treatment is useful and effective) for PCI and a class IA indication for CABG if the patient has suitable coronary anatomy.

OFF-PUMP VERSUS ON-PUMP REVASCULARIZATION

While coronary revascularization using cardiopulmonary bypass remains the gold standard treatment for coronary artery disease, over the past decade, techniques of revascularization on the beating heart without the use of cardiopulmonary bypass (off-pump surgery) have evolved with an attempt to reduce the potential deleterious effects of extracorporeal circulation (26). Several trials have reported a significant reduction in morbidity with avoidance of cardiopulmonary bypass, while large observational studies have also reported a reduction in mortality (26). This mode of revascularization has been applied to patients with acute coronary syndromes.

In a small study by Mohr et al. (27), patients undergoing off-pump CABG within one week of AMI had a mortality of 1.7% demonstrating a significant improvement in comparison to studies undertaken using cardiopulmonary bypass. This difference was mainly attributed to the avoidance of cardiopulmonary bypass.

Rastan et al. reported their experience over a five-year period in a retrospective analysis of 638 patients, of whom 240 patients (38%) underwent CABG on the beating heart (28). Of the latter group, 116 (48%) underwent on-pump surgery and 124 (52%) had off-pump CABG. The remainder underwent conventional CABG using cardioplegic cardiac arrest. Using propensity score adjusted multiregression analysis, beating heart surgery was associated with reduced drainage loss, rate of transfusion, inotropic support, ventilation time, stroke rate, and intensive care stay (28). In the subset of patients with cardiogenic shock (17%), beating heart surgery was associated with a reduced incidence of stroke, inotropic support, renal failure, atrial fibrillation, and sternal wound complications. At five-year follow-up, the groups were comparable with respect to overall survival, major adverse cerebral and cardiovascular events, and repeat revascularization. This study is limited by the fact that it is nonrandomized and the presence of a selection bias to perform beating heart surgery on sicker patients. Notwithstanding these limitations, improved hospital outcomes were demonstrated with beating heart surgery. Others have also reported lower postoperative mortality and morbidity with the use of on-pump beating heart CABG (29).

In a series on 225 patients undergoing CABG following acute MI, Locker et al. (30) reported a significant reduction in mortality with avoidance of cardiopulmonary bypass (4.3% vs. 16.5%) in patients undergoing surgery within 48 hours of onset of symptoms. This difference was however less evident after 48 hours. An important finding of this study, however, was the reduced reintervention rate in the on-pump CABG group at late follow-up of up to nine years (30).

A recent randomized trial of 128 patients undergoing on-pump or off-pump CABG within 48 hours of ST segment elevation MI reported significant benefits associated with avoidance of cardiopulmonary bypass (31). In addition to reduction in mortality (1.6% vs. 7.7%), the authors reported reduced use of inotropes, duration of mechanical ventilation, reoperation for bleeding, duration in intensive care, and hospital stay. In addition, off-pump surgery was associated with reduced Troponin I release and improved cardiac function (assessed using transoesophageal echocardiography) (31).

In summary, off-pump CABG is a very safe and efficacious alternative to conventional revascularization, and in certain hands may have additional benefits of reduced mortality and morbidity. It should be increasingly utilized in the high-risk groups especially those with recent MI.

SUMMARY

In summary, surgical revascularization can be undertaken following acute MI with excellent results with appropriate timing and patient selection. Emergency surgery may be unavoidable in unstable patients and in those with mechanical complications. Perioperative mortality demonstrates a temporal decline following acute MI and the benefits of early revascularization have to be balanced against the increased risks associated with early operation. As no guidelines exist regarding the appropriate timing, judgment from experience tailored to the individual patient in the light of the evidence to date will continue to dictate the treatment strategy in this high-risk group.

REFERENCES

1. Yusuf S, Zucker D, Peduzzi P, et al. Effect of coronary artery bypass graft surgery on survival: overview of 10-year results from randomised trials by the Coronary Artery Bypass Graft Surgery Trialists Collaboration. Lancet 1994; 344:563–570.
2. Coleman WS, DeWood MA, Berg R Jr, et al. Surgical intervention in acute myocardial infarction: an historical perspective. Semin Thorac Cardiovasc Surg 1995; 7:176–183.
3. Dawson JT, Hall RJ, Hallman GL, et al. Mortality in patients undergoing coronary artery bypass surgery after myocardial infarction. Am J Cardiol 1974; 33:483–486.
4. Antman EM, Anbe DT, Armstrong PW, et al. ACC/AHA guidelines for the management of patients with ST-elevation myocardial infarction: a report of the American College of Cardiology/American Heart Association Task Force on Practice Guidelines (Committee to Revise the 1999 Guidelines for the Management of Patients with Acute Myocardial Infarction). Circulation 2004; 110:e82–e292.
5. Antman EM, Hand M, Armstrong PW, et al. 2007 Focused Update of the ACC/AHA 2004 Guidelines for the Management of Patients with ST-Elevation Myocardial Infarction: a report of the American College of Cardiology/American Heart Association Task Force on Practice Guidelines: developed in collaboration with the Canadian Cardiovascular Society endorsed by the American Academy of Family Physicians: 2007 Writing Group to Review New Evidence and Update the ACC/AHA 2004 Guidelines for the Management of Patients with ST-Elevation Myocardial Infarction, Writing on Behalf of the 2004 Writing Committee. Circulation 2008; 117:296–329.
6. Braxton JH, Hammond GL, Letsou GV, et al. Optimal timing of coronary artery bypass graft surgery after acute myocardial infarction. Circulation 1995; 92:II66–II68.
7. Deeik RK, Schmitt TM, Ihrig TG, et al. Appropriate timing of elective coronary artery bypass graft surgery following acute myocardial infarction. Am J Surg 1998; 176:581–585.
8. DeWood MA, Notske RN, Berg R Jr, et al. Medical and surgical management of early Q wave myocardial infarction. I. Effects of surgical reperfusion on survival, recurrent myocardial infarction, sudden death and functional class at 10 or more years of follow-up. J Am Coll Cardiol 1989; 14:65–77.
9. Lee DC, Oz MC, Weinberg AD, et al. Appropriate timing of surgical intervention after transmural acute myocardial infarction. J Thorac Cardiovasc Surg 2003; 125:115–119; discussion 119–120.
10. Voisine P, Mathieu P, Doyle D, et al. Influence of time elapsed between myocardial infarction and coronary artery bypass grafting surgery on operative mortality. Eur J Cardiothorac Surg 2006; 29:319–323.
11. Lee DC, Oz MC, Weinberg AD, et al. Optimal timing of revascularization: transmural versus nontransmural acute myocardial infarction. Ann Thorac Surg 2001; 71:1197–1202; discussion 1202–1194.
12. Curtis JJ, Walls JT, Salam NH, et al. Impact of unstable angina on operative mortality with coronary revascularization at varying time intervals after myocardial infarction. J Thorac Cardiovasc Surg 1991; 102:867–873.

13. Stuart RS, Baumgartner WA, Soule L, et al. Predictors of perioperative mortality in patients with unstable postinfarction angina. Circulation 1988; 78:I163–I165.
14. Zaroff JG, diTommaso DG, Barron HV. A risk model derived from the National Registry of Myocardial Infarction 2 database for predicting mortality after coronary artery bypass grafting during acute myocardial infarction. Am J Cardiol 2002; 90:1–4.
15. Hochman JS, Sleeper LA, White HD, et al. One-year survival following early revascularization for cardiogenic shock. JAMA 2001; 285:190–192.
16. Goldberg RJ, Samad NA, Yarzebski J, et al. Temporal trends in cardiogenic shock complicating acute myocardial infarction. N Engl J Med 1999; 340:1162–1168.
17. Holmes DR Jr, Bates ER, Kleiman NS, et al. Contemporary reperfusion therapy for cardiogenic shock: the GUSTO-I trial experience. The GUSTO-I Investigators. Global Utilization of Streptokinase and Tissue Plasminogen Activator for Occluded Coronary Arteries. J Am Coll Cardiol 1995; 26:668–674.
18. Holmes DR Jr. Cardiogenic shock: a lethal complication of acute myocardial infarction. Rev Cardiovasc Med 2003; 4:131–135.
19. Alonso DR, Scheidt S, Post M, et al. Pathophysiology of cardiogenic shock. Quantification of myocardial necrosis, clinical, pathologic and electrocardiographic correlations. Circulation 1973; 48:588–596.
20. Hochman JS, Boland J, Sleeper LA, et al. Current spectrum of cardiogenic shock and effect of early revascularization on mortality. Results of an International Registry. SHOCK Registry Investigators. Circulation 1995; 91:873–881.
21. Holmes DR Jr., Berger PB, Hochman JS, et al. Cardiogenic shock in patients with acute ischemic syndromes with and without ST-segment elevation. Circulation 1999; 100:2067–2073.
22. Hochman JS. Cardiogenic shock complicating acute myocardial infarction: expanding the paradigm. Circulation 2003; 107:2998–3002.
23. Webb JG, Sanborn TA, Sleeper LA, et al. Percutaneous coronary intervention for cardiogenic shock in the SHOCK Trial Registry. Am Heart J 2001; 141:964–970.
24. Hochman JS, Sleeper LA, Webb JG, et al. Early revascularization in acute myocardial infarction complicated by cardiogenic shock. SHOCK Investigators. Should We Emergently Revascularize Occluded Coronaries for Cardiogenic Shock. N Engl J Med 1999; 341:625–634.
25. White HD, Assmann SF, Sanborn TA, et al. Comparison of percutaneous coronary intervention and coronary artery bypass grafting after acute myocardial infarction complicated by cardiogenic shock: results from the Should We Emergently Revascularize Occluded Coronaries for Cardiogenic Shock (SHOCK) trial. Circulation 2005; 112:1992–2001.
26. Abu-Omar Y, Taggart DP. The present status of off-pump coronary artery bypass grafting. Eur J Cardiothorac Surg 2009; 36:312–321.
27. Mohr R, Moshkovitch Y, Shapira I, et al. Coronary artery bypass without cardiopulmonary bypass for patients with acute myocardial infarction. J Thorac Cardiovasc Surg 1999; 118:50–56.
28. Rastan AJ, Eckenstein JI, Hentschel B, et al. Emergency coronary artery bypass graft surgery for acute coronary syndrome: beating heart versus conventional cardioplegic cardiac arrest strategies. Circulation 2006; 114:I477–I485.
29. Miyahara K, Matsuura A, Takemura H, et al. On-pump beating-heart coronary artery bypass grafting after acute myocardial infarction has lower mortality and morbidity. J Thorac Cardiovasc Surg 2008; 135:521–526.
30. Locker C, Mohr R, Paz Y, et al. Myocardial revascularization for acute myocardial infarction: benefits and drawbacks of avoiding cardiopulmonary bypass. Ann Thorac Surg 2003; 76:771–776; discussion 776–777.
31. Fattouch K, Guccione F, Dioguardi P, et al. Off-pump versus on-pump myocardial revascularization in patients with ST-segment elevation myocardial infarction: a randomized trial. J Thorac Cardiovasc Surg 2009; 137:650–656; discussion 656–657.

Index

Milton Keynes UK
Ingram Content Group UK Ltd.
UKHW040101071024
449327UK00019B/723